DATE DUE

Allelopathy

PHYSIOLOGICAL ECOLOGY

A Series of Monographs, Texts, and Treatises

EDITED BY

T. T. KOZLOWSKI

University of Wisconsin
Madison, Wisconsin

T. T. KOZLOWSKI. Growth and Development of Trees, Volumes I and II — 1971

DANIEL HILLEL. Soil and Water: Physical Principles and Processes, 1971

J. LEVITT. Responses of Plants to Environmental Stresses, 1972

V. B. YOUNGNER AND C. M. McKELL (Eds.). The Biology and Utilization of Grasses, 1972

T. T. KOZLOWSKI (Ed.). Seed Biology, Volumes I, II, and III — 1972

YOAV WAISEL. Biology of Halophytes, 1972

G. C. MARKS AND T. T. KOZLOWSKI (Eds.). Ectomycorrhizae: Their Ecology and Physiology, 1973

T. T. KOZLOWSKI (Ed.). Shedding of Plant Parts, 1973

ELROY L. RICE. Allelopathy, 1974

In Preparation

T. T. KOZLOWSKI AND C. E. AHLGREN (Eds.). Fire and Ecosystems

Allelopathy

Elroy L. Rice

The University of Oklahoma
Department of Botany and Microbiology
Norman, Oklahoma

ACADEMIC PRESS   New York   San Francisco   London   1974

A Subsidiary of Harcourt Brace Jovanovich, Publishers

ACADEMIC PRESS, INC.
111 Fifth Avenue, New York, New York 10003

United Kingdom Edition published by
ACADEMIC PRESS, INC. (LONDON) LTD.
24/28 Oval Road, London NW1

Library of Congress Cataloging in Publication Data

Rice, Elroy Leon, Date
    Allelopathy.

    (Physiological ecology)
    Bibliography: p.
    1.   Allelopathy.   I.   Title.   [DNLM: 1.   Plants—
Physiology.   QK911 R495a 1974]
QK911.R5   581.5'24   73-18991
ISBN 0–12–587050–7

Contents

Preface   ix

1 Introduction

   I. Meaning and Origin of Term Allelopathy   1
  II. Suggested Terminology for Chemical Interactions
      between Plants of Different Levels of Complexity   2

2 Historical Account of Research on Allelopathy

   I. Higher Plants versus Higher Plants   3
  II. Higher Plants versus Microorganisms   11
 III. Microorganisms versus Higher Plants   15
 IV. Microorganisms versus Microorganisms   18

3 Roles of Allelopathy in Phytoplankton Succession

   I. Introduction   23
  II. Evidence for Importance of Allelopathy in
      Succession of Phytoplankton   24

4 Roles of Allelopathy in Old-Field Succession

   I. Introduction and Old-Field Succession in Central
      Oklahoma and Southeast Kansas   35

    II. Allelopathy and the Rapid Disappearance of the
        Pioneer Weed Stage   36
   III. Allelopathy and the Slowing of Succession
        Starting with Stage 2   52
   IV. General Conclusions   74

5   Inhibition of Nitrification by Vegetation; Increases during Succession and Pronounced Inhibition by Climax Ecosystems

    I. General Evidence for Chemical Inhibition of
      Nitrification by Vegetation   77
   II. Theoretical Basis for Selective Pressure against
       Nitrification   87
  III. Specific Evidence for Increases in Inhibition of
       Nitrification during Succession and in Climax
       Ecosystems   88
   IV. Conclusions   103

6   Roles of Allelopathy in Fire Cycle in California Annual Grasslands

    I. General Discussion of Fire Cycle   104
   II. Evidence for Role of Allelopathy   106
  III. Conclusions   124

7   Roles of Allelopathy in Patterning of Vegetation and Creation of Bare Areas

    I. Concepts of Patterning   126
   II. Patterning due to Allelopathic Effects of
       Herbaceous Species   128
  III. Patterning due to Allelopathic Effects of Woody
       Species   150

8   Allelopathy and the Prevention of Seed Decay before Germination

    I. Direct Production of Microbial Inhibitors by Seed
      Plants   174

II. Production of Microbial Inhibitors in Seed Coats by Soil Microorganisms 182
III. Conclusions 183

9   Impact of Allelopathy on Agriculture

I. Production by Crop Plants of Substances Inhibitory to Other Crop Plants 184
II. Allelopathic Effects of Crop Residues on Crop Plants 190
III. Allelopathic Effects of Weeds on Crop Plants and Vice Versa 205
IV. Allelopathy versus Nitrogen Fixation 210
V. Allelopathy and Seed Germination of Crop Plants 210
VI. The Roles of Allelopathy in Plant Infection 212
VII. Related Phenomena That Are Not Strictly Allelopathic 216

10   Impact of Allelopathy on Horticulture and Forestry

I. Roles in Horticulture 218
II. Roles of Allelopathy in Forestry 234

11   Plant Parts That Contain Inhibitors and Ways in Which Inhibitors Enter the Environment

I. Parts Known to Contain Inhibitors 237
II. Ways in Which Inhibitors Get Out of Plants 239

12   Chemical Nature of Inhibitors

I. Introduction 245
II. Types of Chemical Compounds Identified as Inhibitors 247
III. Unidentified Inhibitors 270

13   Mechanisms of Action of Inhibitors

I. Introduction 271
II. Mechanisms of Action 271

14   Factors Affecting Quantities of Inhibitors Produced by Plants

I. Introduction 295
II. Effects of Radiation 296
III. Mineral Deficiencies 300
IV. Water Stress 305
V. Temperature 307
VI. Allelopathic Agents 308
VII. Age of Plant Organs 310
VIII. Genetics 311

15   Interrelations of Allelopathy with Other Types of Chemical Interactions

I. Introduction 312
II. Chemical Interactions between Plants and Insects 313
III. Chemical Interaction between Plants and Animals Other than Insects 314

Bibliography 317

Index 345

Preface

No general monograph on the subject of allelopathy has been published previously in the English language, and none in any language since Grodzinsky's in 1965, in Russian. His book has not been translated and has had limited distribution outside the USSR. Moreover, much of the research that has established the field of allelopathy has been published since that time. The wide acceptance by ecologists of allelopathy as an important ecological phenomenon has occurred only within the past ten years. Thus, there appears to be a need for a general reference source in this field, both for researchers in the discipline and as an overview for those who desire to learn something about the subject.

Most significant contributions in the field, available at the time of writing, have been discussed; but no attempt has been made to include all publications that are in some way related to allelopathy. In fact, I have deliberately refrained from discussing the antibiotics involved primarily in medicine and most of the research concerned with biochemical interactions involved in plant diseases. My primary goal has been to discuss the broad ecological roles of allelopathy.

I have used the term allelopathy in the broad sense of Molisch (1937) to include biochemical interactions among plants of all levels of complexity, including microorganisms. Any restriction of this use does not make practical sense, as a perusal of this monograph will confirm. All levels of interaction are inextricably interwoven in ecological phenomena.

Most of my own research and that of my students reported here was supported by The National Science Foundation, for which I am grateful. I deeply appreciate the enthusiastic contributions of my graduate students, without whose help this monograph would not have been possible. I acknowledge with thanks the permissions granted by numerous authors and publishers to use previously published materials. The support and help of Dr. T. T. Kozlowski (editor of the Physiological Ecology Series) and of the staff of Academic Press are gratefully acknowledged.

Elroy L. Rice

Allelopathy

1

Introduction

I. MEANING AND ORIGIN OF TERM ALLELOPATHY

Several recent investigators have used the term allelopathy to refer to the deleterious effect that one higher plant has on another through the production of chemical retardants that escape into the environment (Martin and Rademacher, 1960a; Muller, 1966). Molisch (1937) coined the term to refer to biochemical interactions between all types of plants including microorganisms. His discussion indicated that he meant the term to cover both detrimental and beneficial reciprocal biochemical interactions. However, the term was derived from two Greek words meaning mutual harm.

I feel that the current use of the term, allelopathy, should include any direct or indirect harmful effect by one plant (including microorganisms) on another through the production of chemical compounds that escape into the environment. That is the way I will use the term throughout this book.

The salient point concerning allelopathy is that its effect depends upon a chemical compound being added to the environment by an allelopathic agent. Allelopathy is thus separated from competition involving the removal or reduction of some factor from the environment that is required by some other plant sharing the habitat. The factors that may be reduced by competition include water, minerals, food, and light.

Unfortunately, many biologists either consider allelopathy to be a part of competition or, worse, are completely unaware of the phenomenon of allelopathy. Virtually none of the papers I have read, which purported to demonstrate some aspect of competition, has in any way eliminated allelopathy as a possible cause of the observed results.

1

I agree with the suggestion of Muller (1969) that the term interference should be used to refer to the overall deleterious effects of one plant on another, thus encompassing both allelopathy and competition.

II. SUGGESTED TERMINOLOGY FOR CHEMICAL INTERACTIONS BETWEEN PLANTS OF DIFFERENT LEVELS OF COMPLEXITY

Grümmer (1955) suggested that special terms be adopted for the chemical inhibitors involved in allelopathy based on the type of plant producing the inhibitor and the type of plant affected. He recommended the commonly used term antibiotic for a chemical inhibitor produced by a microorganism and effective against a microorganism. He recommended Waksman's suggested term phytoncide for an inhibitor produced by a higher plant and effective against a microorganism. He suggested Gaumann's term marasmins for compounds produced by microorganisms and harmful to higher plants, and he coined the term kolines for chemical inhibitors produced by higher plants and effective against higher plants.

The antibiotics have been investigated chiefly in connection with the treatment of human ailments, and such investigations are not in the scope of the present ecological treatment of allelopathy. A small amount of work has been done on antibiotics, which is directly related to basic ecology, and this will be discussed elsewhere.

Marasmins are very important in the field of plant pathology and thus are obviously of great ecological significance. These compounds have been widely discussed in many papers and texts, so I will discuss them only rather briefly in future chapters. Most of the ecological work that has been done in the area of allelopathy has been concerned with phytoncides and kolines, and these will be considered in detail in the following chapters.

When a specific allelopathic substance is considered, it may have a sharply limited scope of action such that it is not effective against higher plants if it is an antibiotic. On the other hand, it may act like the antibiotic, patulin, which exhibits a marked toxicity for higher plants also (Grümmer, 1955). Additionally, there are many kolines that inhibit growth of microorganisms and many phytoncides that inhibit growth of higher plants (Floyd and Rice, 1967; W. H. Muller, 1965; Nagy et al., 1964; Rice, 1965a). There are no doubt marasmins that inhibit microorganisms also.

2

Historical Account of
Research on Allelopathy

I. HIGHER PLANTS VERSUS HIGHER PLANTS

DeCandolle (1832) was apparently one of the earliest scientists to suggest the possibility that some plants may excrete something from their roots which is injurious to other plants. He observed, for example, that thistles (*Cirsium*) in fields injure oats, euphorbe (*Euphorbia*) and *Scabiosa* injure flax, and rye plants (*Lolium*) injure wheat. He also described experiments of M. Macaire in which it was found that beans (*Phaseolus*) languish and die in water containing material previously exuded by roots of other individuals of the same species, whereas wheat flourishes in water charged with exudations from legumes. DeCandolle suggested that such excretions of roots could conceivably explain the exhaustion of soil by certain plants and thus the need for crop rotation.

DeCandolle's views were apparently given little credence by his contemporaries because it was almost 50 years before a similar suggestion appeared in the literature. Stickney and Hoy (1881) observed that vegetation under black walnut, *Juglans nigra*, is very sparse compared with that under most other commonly used shade trees. They pointed out also that no crop will grow under or very near it. Stickney stated that there is a question as to whether this is caused by water dripping from the tree, or by the tree being a gross feeder, thereby exhausting the soil. Hoy claimed, however, that the main reason vegetation does not thrive under these trees is the poisonous character of the drip. He said that the juice of the leaf is poisonous, and a solution made from it will keep off flies when applied to a horse.

Livingston (1905) presented convincing evidence that the failure of nonbog plaⁱts to grow in peat bogs is due to deleterious chemical substances, and that these substances account for the xerophytic habit of the plants that grow there.

Schreiner and his associates published a series of papers starting in 1907 in which they presented evidence that exhaustion of soil by single-cropping is due to addition of growth inhibitors to the soil by certain crop plants (Schreiner and Reed, 1907a,b, 1908; Schreiner and Shorey, 1909; Schreiner and Sullivan, 1909; Schreiner and Lathrop, 1911). Schreiner and Reed (1907b) demonstrated clearly that roots of seedlings of wheat (*Triticum*), oats (*Avena*), and certain other crop plants exude materials into the growing medium that elicit chemotropic responses by the roots of wheat and oat seedlings. Schreiner and Reed (1908) developed a technique that is still used for determining possible allelopathic effects of compounds obtained from the soil or from plants. They were able to show with this technique that many compounds previously identified from various plants were inhibitory to the growth and transpiration of wheat seedlings. Schreiner and Sullivan (1909) extracted an unidentified substance from soil fatigued by the growth of cowpeas, *Vigna catjang,* and found that the substance strongly inhibited the growth of cowpeas. Moreover, the soil from which the inhibitor was extracted was no longer inhibitory to the growth of cowpeas.

Cowles (1911) suggested that plant-produced toxins may be very important as causative agents in plant succession.

Pickering (1917, 1919) demonstrated that the leachate from trays containing certain species of grasses was inhibitory to the growth of apple seedlings. He designed his experiment such that mineral deficiencies, root interaction, shading, water deficiency, and oxygen exclusion were eliminated as possible causes of inhibition.

Magnus (1920) reported that the leaf sap of *Phacelia* and *Pelargonium* is inhibitory to the germination of some seeds, and Oppenheimer (1922) demonstrated that the tomato fruit (*Lycopersicum*) contains a strong inhibitor of seed germination.

Cook (1921) described the characteristic wilting of potato, *Solanum tuberosum,* and tomato, *Lycopersicum esculentum,* plants grown near *Juglans nigra,* black walnut. He also described the injurious effect of walnut on apple trees. These observations supported those of Stickney and Hoy (1881), and subsequently Massey (1925) did a careful study of the inhibitory effects of black walnut on alfalfa and tomato plants. In both cases, he found that the test plants wilted and died whenever their roots came in close contact with the walnut roots. This

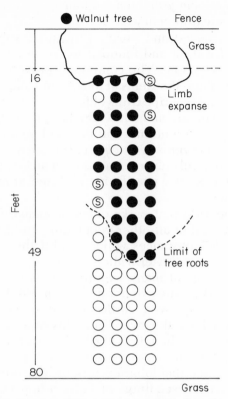

Fig. 1. Diagram showing conditions of tomato plants 8 weeks after setting plants in the immediate vicinity of a black walnut tree. Each circle indicates position in which a plant was set. Open circles indicate plants that remained healthy. Circles with S in them represent plants that died soon after transplanting. Closed circles indicate plants that wilted and died. (From Massey, 1925.)

effect was so definite that he could trace the extent of the walnut roots without removing soil just by observing the development of wilt in test plants (Fig. 1). There was no specific relationship between the region of greatest concentration of walnut roots and the wilting of tomatoes, which would be expected if the trouble were due to lowering of soil moisture. Apparently there is little or no poisoning of the soil, since the roots of the affected plants must be in close contact with those of the walnut. When several pieces of bark from walnut roots were placed in a water culture of tomato plants, the plants wilted and their roots browned within 48 hours. Addition of bark from walnut roots to soil in which tomato plants were growing caused the plants to grow poorly. Massey suggested that juglone or some similar substance may be the toxic constituent of walnut.

Davis (1928) extracted and purified the toxic substance from the hulls and roots of walnut and found it to be identical to juglone, 5-hydroxy-α-naphthaquinone. The compound proved to be a powerful toxin when injected into the stems of tomato and alfalfa plants.

Elmer (1932) found that ripe fruits of four varieties of apples—Winesap, Stayman, Jonathan, and Ben Davis—produced volatile substances that inhibited the normal sprout development of germinating potatoes. When nongerminated sections of potato tubers were exposed to the volatile substances, bud dominance was overcome. He found also that ripe Kieffer pear fruits inhibited growth of sprouts of germinating potatoes.

Waks (1936) reported that parks of black locust, *Robinia pseudoacacia*, are nearly void of all other vegetation, and bark and wood of black locust contain substances which inhibit the growth of barley.

Molisch (1937) coined the term allelopathy, as previously indicated, and he performed a great many experiments with ripe apple fruits which confirmed and greatly extended the results of Elmer (1932).

Loehwing (1937) reviewed earlier literature on plant-produced toxins and concluded that they were probably of no great significance. In my opinion, however, he failed to give any satisfactory reasons for arriving at this conclusion.

Bode (1940) reported that foliar excretions of *Artemisia absinthium* inhibited the growth of seedlings of *Foeniculum vulgare* and other species within approximately 1 m of the *Artemisia* plants. According to Bode, the leaves of this species have glandular hairs that excrete ethereal oils and the inhibitor absinthiin. This is formed especially during dry, hot weather and appears as numerous droplets on the surface of the hairs. When it rains, these droplets are washed away and spread on the neighboring plants. Funke (1943) confirmed and extended Bode's results with *Artemisia absinthium*. He measured the effects of a hedge of this species on a large number of test species planted near it and found that all were affected. No effect was noted in the same test species planted near a hedge of *Atriplex hortensis*. Funke found that fresh or pulverized leaves of *A. absinthium* dug into the soil retarded the germination of *Pisum sativum* seeds and permanently lowered the percent germination of *Phaseolus multiflorus* seed planted in the soil. Growth of *Phaseolus* was permanently retarded also by the *Artemisia* leaves. Subsequently, seed germination and seedling growth of numerous other species were found to be severely inhibited in soil in which *Artemisia* leaves were incorporated.

Benedict (1941) studied the reasons for the natural thinning of smooth brome, *Bromus inermis,* and he found that when oven-dried roots of smooth brome were placed in soil with seeds of that species, a significant reduction in the subsequent dry weight of the seedlings resulted. He obtained similar results by adding a leachate from an old culture of smooth brome to seedlings of the species. He thus established the production of a toxic substance by smooth brome roots.

Went (1942) investigated the relationship between certain shrubs and annual plants in a desert area in California. He reported that certain annuals were rarely associated with some shrubs unless the shrubs were dead; some annuals were chiefly associated with certain shrubs; and others showed no definite affiliations. He found that annuals were rarely associated with *Encelia farinosa* unless the shrub was dead. Went suggested that the observed relationships might be due to substances produced by living roots of the shrubs. Subsequently, Gray and Bonner (1948a,b) reported that the leaves of *Encelia farinosa* produce a substance that causes pronounced inhibition in growth of many other plants. They identified the compound as 3-acetyl-6-methoxybenzaldehyde and demonstrated that it is toxic to many plants, but not to *Encelia farinosa.* This inhibitor is produced primarily in the leaves and is released when the leaves fall to the ground and decompose. Evidence indicated that this inhibitor is relatively persistent in the soil.

Kuhn *et al.* (1943) reported that mountain ash, *Sorbus aucuparia,* produces parasorbic acid, an unsaturated lactone, which inhibits germination of *Lepidium* seeds in a dilution of 1:1000 and allows only 10–80% germination at 1:10,000.

Bonner and Galston (1944) observed that the edge rows in guayule, *Parthenium argentatum,* plantings at Salinas, California had much larger plants than the center rows and that the differences could not be eliminated by heavy watering and mineral application. Additionally, roots of adjacent plants did not intermingle but grew in entirely separate areas, and seedlings of guayule plants virtually never grew under larger guayule plants. On the other hand, such seedlings were commonly found growing under other kinds of shrubs. Experiments were designed to determine if guayule produces a growth inhibitor. Initial experiments indicated that leachates from pots of 1-year-old guayule plants were very inhibitory to guayule seedlings but not to tomato seedlings. In another type of experiment performed in sand culture, guayule seedlings were planted in sand adjacent to a 1-year-old guayule plant. In addition, other guayule seedlings were planted in fresh sand in a glass jar, and the jar was placed in an excavation in the sand under the older guayule plant so that the shading effect on all seedlings was the same. Thus, the seedlings in the glass jar were not subjected to any possible inhibiting material that might be present in the sand around the older plant. Seedlings growing under the guayule plant had a high mortality rate and grew slowly if not contained in glass jars, whereas those grown under the same conditions, but in a separate glass jar, had good growth and a lower mortality. Results of this experiment supported those of the initial one, indicating that roots of guayule plants excrete a toxin.

Subsequent experiments with nutrient solutions and distilled water leachates of roots of guayule plants enabled Bonner and Galston to identify the toxin as *trans*-cinnamic acid. This compound is highly toxic to guayule seedlings, with significant growth reduction resulting from as little as 1 mg/liter of culture solution. Guayule seedlings were found to be at least 100 times as sensitive to cinnamic acid as tomato seedlings, which explains why tomato seedlings were not affected by the leachates of the guayule plants in the initial experiments.

In later work, Bonner (1946) found that cinnamic acid is toxic to the growth of guayule plants in soil also. Incorporation of 10 mg of cinnamic acid in 1500 gm of soil, making a concentration of less than 1 part in 100,000, significantly depressed the growth of the plants over a period of 6 weeks. He found that this toxin is unstable in the soil, however, and decreases with time. It does not disappear in sterilized soil, so obviously it is decomposed by microorganisms. Apparently it has to be added to the soil continuously to be effective as a koline, as has since been demonstrated in numerous instances with other kolines.

McCalla and Duley (1948) reported that soaking corn grains for 24 hours in an extract of sweet clover markedly inhibited subsequent germination and growth. An extract made with 1 gm sweet clover tops (cut when 18–24 inches high) in 5 ml of distilled water reduced the percentage germination of corn from 95% in the control to 33% after soaking 24 hours in the extract. The subsequent top growth of the corn seedlings after 3 days was reduced from 2.8 cm in the control to 0.3 cm in the test, and the root growth was reduced from 6.4 cm in the control to 0.8 cm in the test.

In subsequent work, McCalla and Duley (1949) found in greenhouse studies that mulching of soil from the Agronomy Farm at Lincoln, Nebraska with wheat straw at the rate of 2 to 4 tons per acre reduced the percentage germination of corn grains from 92% in the control soil to 44% in the test.

Evenari (1949) gave a thorough summary of research concerning the production by seed plants of seed germination inhibitors. Only a few of his original findings will be mentioned here. He found that bulb juice of *Allium cepa* and *A. sativum* contains such inhibitors, as does the root sap of *Armoracia rusticana*, the tuber sap of *Brassica caulocarpa*, and the fruit juice of *Citrus aurantium*, *C. limonia*, and *C. maxima*. He stressed the widespread presence of potent seed germination inhibitors in various species of the Cruciferae and pointed out that evidence indicates that mustard oils are the chief inhibiting substances in such cases. Evenari pointed out that when a portion of an orange or lemon peel is put in a large petri dish in which a small petri dish containing 50 wheat grains on moist filter paper is placed, germination of the wheat grains is completely inhibited indicating that a volatile inhibitor is produced by the peels. He gave considerable evidence that the volatile inhibitor is an essential oil.

Curtis and Cottam (1950) presented strong evidence that the fairy-ring pattern of the prairie sunflower, *Helianthus rigidus* (*H. scaberrimus*), is due to autotoxic effects of that species. This possibility was mentioned earlier by Cooper and Stoesz (1931), but without much substantiation. Curtis and Cottam found a large reduction in plant numbers and inflorescences in the center of the clone, and control of soil types and fertilizer content did not alter the results. When prairie sunflower plants were grown in soil from which all roots and rhizomes were removed, the plants were normal and flowered well. They concluded that inhibition resulted from decay of dead plant parts.

Keever (1950) studied the causes of plant succession in revegetating old fields in the piedmont region of North Carolina. She observed that *Erigeron canadensis* disappears very rapidly from such fields after the first year of abandonment, and subsequently found that decaying roots of plants of this species inhibit growth of seedlings of the species. For reasons that are not clear, Keever inferred that this inhibition was not important as a cause of succession.

Bonner (1950) reviewed some of the evidence concerning the role of toxic substances in the interactions of higher plants and concluded that association or nonassociation of different species as a result of specific chemical compounds secreted by them may be of common occurrence.

Deleuil (1950, 1951a,b) presented excellent evidence that the virtual absence of annual plants in the Rosmarino-Ericion in Provence, France is due to the production of toxins by the shrubby dominants.

He found that seeds of several annual plants which do not occur in the Rosmarino-Ericion germinated normally in garden soil watered with water that had previously percolated through soil from the shrubland, but the seedlings subsequently wilted and died. However, seedlings growing from similar seeds planted in the same kind of garden soil and irrigated with water that had not previously passed through soil from the shrubland continued to grow and develop normally. He found also that extracts of macerated roots of characteristic species from the shrubland inhibited growth and killed annual plants when the extracts were used to water test plants growing in garden soil.

Grümmer (1955) reviewed much of the previous work on allelopathy and suggested a system of naming inhibitory compounds on the basis of the types of plants that produce them and the types of plants affected, as described in Chapter 1.

Guyot (1957) attributed mosaiclike dominance patches of different species in old-field successional communities of southern France to allelopathic influences of the dominant species in each patch. He and his associates had previously carried out experiments that led to this conclusion (Guyot *et al.*, 1951).

Patrick and Koch (1958) reported that substances capable of markedly inhibiting the germination of tobacco seeds and the respiration and growth of tobacco seedlings were obtained after residues from timothy, corn, rye, or tobacco plants were allowed to decompose in soil.

Mergen (1959) reported that succession appeared to be remarkably slow in tree-of-heaven, *Ailanthus altissima,* stands, with virtually pure stands remaining for long periods of time. He found that alcohol extracts of the rachis, leaflets, and stem of the tree-of-heaven caused rapid wilting of other plants of the species when applied to the cut surface of the stems. Similar results occurred when these extracts were applied to 35 species of gymnosperms and 11 species of angiosperms. The only species not adversely affected was *Fraxinus americanus.* Approach grafting of *Ailanthus* with several species gave results similar to those with extracts.

It has been known for many years that the yield of flax is much reduced when even a relatively small percentage of flaxweeds, *Camelina alyssum,* is growing among the flax plants. Grümmer and Beyer (1960) found no toxic root excretions, but leachates of the leaves proved to be very inhibitory to flax plants. Using artificial rain, flax plants in close proximity to *Camelina* plants produced 40% less dry matter than control plants in which the same amount of water was applied directly to the soil instead of allowing it to fall on the leaves and drip off on the soil.

Börner (1960), Woods (1960), and Garb (1961) wrote reviews of previous work on allelopathy, all from somewhat different viewpoints.

Jameson (1961) found some 20 species of native trees, shrubs, forbs, and grasses in northern Arizona which inhibited growth of wheat radicles. Several species of *Juniperus, Quercus,* and pinyon pine (*Pinus edulis*) were among the group and most exhibited pronounced inhibitory activity in the field.

Ahshapanek (1962) found that extracts of six different parts of buffalo-bur, *Solanum rostratum,* were inhibitory to many assay seedlings including buffalo-bur. Autotoxicity was pronounced because this species was found to be greatly inhibited when grown in soil in which plants of the species had grown previously. These results apparently explain why buffalo-bur, which is present in virtually a solid stand in a disturbed area during 1 year, may be almost entirely absent the next year, even though very few plants of other species are present.

This brings me to the present decade during which research on allelopathy has expanded rapidly and which will be covered in considerable detail in later chapters.

II. HIGHER PLANTS VERSUS MICROORGANISMS

It was many years after the first written suggestions were made concerning allelopathic interactions between higher plants before anyone suggested that higher plants may produce chemical inhibitors of microorganisms. The expression "higher plants" has been used with many meanings, but I am using it here to refer to all plants other than the microorganisms in order to simplify terminology. In other words, I am considering all algae, fungi (including slime molds), and bacteria as lower plants and microorganisms. I am considering all other plants as higher plants, including species of the following phyla: Bryophyta, Psilophyta, Lycophyta, Sphenophyta, Filicophyta, and Spermatophyta.

Livingston (1905) in his classic work on the toxic effects of water from sphagnum bogs used an undesignated species of the algal genus, *Stigeoclonium,* as his bioassay organism to determine the presence of toxins in various water samples.

Leather (1911) reported low nitrification under perennial grass.in India, indicating an inhibition of the nitrifying bacteria by certain perennial grass species. The general topic of inhibition of nitrification by certain types of vegetation will be discussed thoroughly in a later chapter.

Russell (1914) found that cropped soil had a much lower nitrate content than uncropped similar soil and suggested that this was due to interference by crop plants with nitrate production. Lyon *et al.* (1923), on the other hand, attributed the lower nitrate content under plants to an increased uptake by microorganisms stimulated by root excretions with high C/N ratios.

Starkey (1929) suggested that root exudates of plants may be important to the biological balance of organisms in the soil. Becker *et al.* (1951) fully agreed with Starkey's view.

Richardson (1935, 1938) reported that the level of ammonium nitrogen was several times greater than the level of nitrate nitrogen in grassland soils at Rothamsted, again suggesting an interference with production of nitrate from ammonium nitrogen.

McKnight and Lindegren (1936) and Walton *et al.* (1936) reported that vapors from crushed garlic, *Allium sativum*, are bactericidal to *Mycobacterium cepae*. Later, Cavallito and Bailey (1944) and Cavallito *et al.* (1944, 1945) isolated and identified the active toxin as allicin.

Thorne and Brown (1937) found that most legume-nodule bacteria (*Rhizobium*) investigated by them were able to grow in freshly expressed juices of their host plants, but such juices were bactericidal to other species of root-nodule bacteria.

Waksman (1937) discussed soil deterioration from the viewpoint of soil microbiology and suggested that the effects of root exudates on microorganisms might be of great importance, especially in forest stands where one crop is grown continuously.

Apparently, the first person to survey a large group of higher plants for antibacterial substances was Osborn (1943). He investigated effects of water extracts of 2300 different species and varieties of green plants (mostly flowering plants) against two species of bacteria, *Staphylococcus aureus* and *Escherichia coli*, using the diffusion technique on solid media. He found 63 genera, belonging to 28 families, which inhibited the growth of at least one of the bacteria. All species tested of the family Ranunculaceae were very inhibitory to both bacterial species, and most test species of the following families were moderately inhibitory to both species: Amaryllidaceae, Annonaceae, Cruciferae, Flacourtiaceae, Liliaceae, Moraceae, and Rosaceae.

In a series of papers beginning in 1944, Lucas and his colleagues reported on effects of water and ethanol extracts of many plant parts of an enormous number of species of seed plants against several species of bacteria (Lucas and Lewis, 1944; Gottshall *et al.*, 1949; Lucas *et al.*, 1951, 1955; Frisbey *et al.*, 1953, 1954). In the initial paper, Lucas and Lewis (1944) reported the effects of extracts of several plants against *Staphylococcus aureus, Escherichia coli, Phytomonas phaseoli,* and *Phytomonas campestris*. The last two are plant pathogens, and these were the only bacterial species tested that have any significance in basic ecology. All subsequent papers emphasized effects of plant extracts on *Mycobacterium tuberculosis* and other bacteria of interest in human ailments. Eleven hundred species of seed plants were tested, and 16.3% had specific activity against *Mycobacterium tuberculosis* only. Thirty-four percent of all species tested were inhibitory to *M. tuberculosis*, and 13.5% were inhibitory only to species other than *M. tuberculosis*.

Seegal and Holden (1945) reported that extracts of *Anemone pulsatilla* and an unnamed species of buttercup (*Ranunculus*) inhibited growth of *Mycobacterium tuberculosis* and the fungus, *Monilia albicans*. Later, Baer *et al.* (1946) found that anemonin and protoanemonin are antibacterial substances produced by *Anemone pulsatilla*.

Hayes (1947) tested water extracts of many species of plants against four species of bacteria, two of which are plant pathogens. The plants included algae, lichens, liverworts, lycopods, horsetails, ferns, and seed plants. Many species were found to be inhibitory to one or more of the bacteria.

Theron (1951) found that the rate of nitrification in a South African grassland soil was lessened by a perennial grass crop, and Eden (1951) reported that grassland (patana) soils in Ceylon are extremely low in nitrate and that the low nitrification rate lasts for several years after breaking the land for tea cultivation.

Stiven (1952) tested aqueous root extracts of several species of grasses and forbs from a climax grassland in the Transvaal Highveld (South Africa) against four species of bacteria: *Escherichia coli, Bacillus subtilis, Staphylococcus aureus* (Oxford strain), and *Streptococcus haemolyticus*. A bunchgrass, *Trachypogon plumosus*, was found to be very inhibitory to all four bacterial species. Three forbs were found to be inhibitory to at least some of the bacteria, and one of these, *Pentanisia variabilis* (Rubiaceae), showed marked activity against two of the bacterial species and slight activity against two others.

Dommergues (1952, 1954, 1956) studied the effects of forest cover in Madagascar on the activity of different physiological groups of microorganisms. He compared this activity to microbiological activity in cultivated soils and found the following: (1) ammonification is much more active in humid tropical forest soils than agricultural; (2) nitrification is very weak in humid tropical forest soils with no more than 10 to 100 nitrifiers per gram of soil; (3) the concentration of aerobic cellulose-decomposing bacteria and fungi is much lower in humid forest soils than in good agricultural soils; and (4) nitrification is higher in dry tropical forest soils than in humid tropical forest soils.

Mills (1953) reported that *Pennisetum purpureum, Chloris* sp., and *Paspalum* sp. drastically reduced the rate of nitrification in crop lands in Uganda, Africa.

Berlier and his associates (Jacquemin and Berlier, 1956; Berlier *et al.*, 1956) found that the activity of nitrifying bacteria in savanna and forest-covered soils of the Ivory Coast of Africa was very low and that it increased on clearing and burning. Nye and Greenland (1960) reviewed work in many African areas and vegetation types and reported that little if any nitrate nitrogen is found in the soil where the dominant vegetative cover is a grass, regardless of other conditions.

Ferenczy (1956) reported that the seeds or fruits of many species of higher plants contained antibacterial and antifungal compounds. This important finding will be discussed in more detail in a later chapter.

In the late 1950's and early 1960's, many investigators presented evidence that the resistance of plants to infection by fungal, bacterial, and viral diseases may be associated with the production by resistant varieties of inhibitors of the pathogens (Schaal and Johnson, 1955; Kúc, *et al.*, 1956; Kúc, 1957; Cadman, 1959; Byrde *et al.*, 1960; Condon and Kúc, 1960; Cruickshank and Perrin, 1960; Hughes and Swain, 1960; Farkas and Kiraly, 1962). This subject is obviously of great importance in agriculture and in natural ecosystems and will be discussed in some detail later.

Nickell (1960) thoroughly reviewed the work on the antimicrobial activity of vascular plants. He reported 157 families of vascular plants that have been found to produce phytoncides, and an extremely long list of species.

Bowen (1961) found that seeds of *Centrosema pubescens* and *Trifolium subterraneum* were inhibitory to *Rhizobium* when the seed coats were sterilized and the seeds placed on petri plates inoculated with *Rhizobium*. Elkan (1961) found that a nonnodulating, near isogenic soybean strain significantly decreased the number of nodules produced on its normally nodulating sister strain when inoculated plants of the two types were grown together in nutrient solution. Nodulation in ladino clover was significantly inhibited also by the mutant soybean. Both results suggested the exudation by the roots of the non-nodulating strain of substances inhibitory either to *Rhizobium* or to the nodulating process or both.

Meiklejohn (1962) reported that grassland soils in Ghana contain few ammonia oxidizers and very few or no nitrite oxidizers. She found that none of the grassland samples taken after the start of the rainy season contained any nitrite oxidizers.

This brings us to the present decade again, and the later research on phytoncides will be discussed in later chapters. It is obvious, in reviewing most of the work on this subject done before 1963, that most of the effort has gone into research that was concerned with inhibition of possible human pathogens. This was true particularly of the large screening projects. The research on inhibitors of the nitrifiers, nitrogen-fixers, decomposers, and plant pathogens certainly does have significance in agriculture and basic ecology.

III. MICROORGANISMS VERSUS HIGHER PLANTS

As I previously mentioned, only a relatively small amount of research has been done on the chemical inhibition of higher plants by microorganisms, except for the specialized field of plant pathology. There is no question that many (if not most) pathogenic microorganisms bring about abnormal symptoms in the host plants through the production of toxins, but this topic will not be discussed to any appreciable extent. For this reason, the subject will be covered up to the present date in this chapter and will be discussed only briefly in some other chapters.

When Konishi (1931) used 4-week-old liquid cultures of the alfalfa *Rhizobium* and *Bacterium coli* (apparently *Escherichia coli*) which were grown together to inoculate tubes containing alfalfa, *Medicago sativa*, plants in agar, the *Bacterium coli* inhibited or completely prevented nodule formation. *Bacillus fluorescens* and *Bacterium aerogenes* slightly inhibited nodulation in similar experiments. The design of the experiments was such that it was not possible to tell whether the inhibition of nodulation was due to the inhibition of *Rhizobium*, to some more direct effect on the nodulation process, or to both.

Martin and his colleagues investigated the effects of citrus trees on the fungal flora of the soil and of certain fungi on the growth of citrus seedlings (Martin, 1948, 1950a,b; Martin *et al.*, 1953; 1956; Martin and Ervin, 1958). *Pyrenochaeta* sp. and an unidentified fungus were found only in old citrus soil, and several species of *Fusarium* were found in much higher numbers in old citrus than in noncitrus soil in early studies. *Thielaviopsis basicola* was identified later from old citrus soils, and it was found to reduce the growth of citrus seedlings greatly, just as old citrus soils do.

After the Lee soybean was released to the public in 1954, it was found that plants of this variety often developed upper-leaf chlorosis. Erdman *et al.* (1956) found that the chlorosis was caused by certain strains of *Rhizobium* in the nodules of afflicted plants. Later, Johnson and Clark (1958) concluded that some growth-damaging or chlorophyll-inhibiting factor is formed in the nodular tissue owing to the presence of the chlorosis-producing strain of *Rhizobium.* Johnson *et al.* (1959) tested aqueous extracts of nodules from soybean initiated by the chlorosis-inducing strain of *Rhizobium* and extracts of nodules from normal green soybean plants against 38 species of seed plants. Most of the species were either made chlorotic, inhibited in growth, or both, by the extract from the nodules on chlorotic plants, whereas the extracts of nodules of normal green plants had no effect.

Ludwig (1957) reported that *Helminthosporium sativum* produces a toxin in culture medium which inhibits its own growth and that of seedlings of several species of seed plants. Its toxic action predisposes the seedlings for infection by the fungus also.

In certain known instances and no doubt in many others, microorganisms are responsible for changing noninhibitory metabolites of higher plants into compounds that are inhibitory to those plants or other plants (Börner, 1959, 1960). This is a very important subject, and it will be developed further in a later chapter.

Ceratocystis ulmi, the causative agent of Dutch elm disease, apparently produces a metal-containing organic compound that ties up adenosine triphosphate (ATP), thus blocking the source of energy for the water-lifting mechanism in the tree (Anonymous, 1962).

In a group of 91 fungi isolated from a plot in Nebraska farmed by the subsurface tillage method to keep stubble mulch on the soil surface, 14 of the fungi reduced germination to 50% or less in corn soaked in a potato dextrose broth in which the fungi had grown (Norstadt and McCalla, 1963). One fungus, *Penicillium urticae,* produced a toxin that severely stunted the growth of corn even in soil culture. The toxin was identified as patulin. McCalla and Haskins (1964) discussed numerous soil fungi that have been demonstrated to produce various types of growth defects in higher plants.

Heilman and Sharp (1963) described a probable inhibition of some liverworts and mosses by a lichen, and this is one of a very few projects concerned with allelopathic effects against nonvascular plants other than microorganisms. Randon (1966) found that an extract of the lichen, *Rocelle fucoides*, was inhibitory to the germination of several kinds of seeds.

Twelve of twenty isolates of the fungus, *Cylindrocarpon radicicola*, produced nectrolide (Brefeldin A), an antibiotic produced also by *Penicillium brefeldianum* (Evans *et al.*, 1967). A low concentration (6 μg/ml) completely arrested growth of blackbutt, *Eucalyptus pilularis*, and even 2–4 μg/ml caused severe stunting and blackening of the roots. Thus, nectrolide is a potent marasmin as well as an antibiotic.

White and Starratt (1967) isolated a phytotoxic compound from cultures of the pathogenic fungus *Alternaria zinniae* and named it zinniol ($C_{15}H_{22}O_4$).This toxin causes severe shrivelling of stems of plants, browning of leaf veins, and chlorosis of surrounding leaf tissue. It also, inhibits seed germination and has weak inhibitory activity against bacteria and fungi.

Rhizobitoxine, a chlorosis-producing compound produced by certain strains of *Rhizobium japonicum*, is very effective as a weed killer (Anonymous, 1969). The minute amount of 3 ounces/acre has been shown to be effective as a toxin against several weed seedlings.

Hattingh and Louw (1969b) found that a strain of *Pseudomonas* (designated as W78) isolated from the rhizoplane of clover, *Trifolium repens*, markedly inhibited the growth and development of inoculated or uninoculated clover in agar or sand culture. Moreover, soil suspensions (1000-fold dilution of soil) caused a similar inhibition. It was suggested that the inhibition by *Pseudomonas* was possibly due to the production by the bacterium of 2,4-diacetyl phloroglucinol because the investigators had previously found this bacterium to produce that toxin.

Leelavathy (1969) studied the effects of rhizosphere fungi on seed germination and decided there were only weak effects on a few seeds. In my opinion, however, the techniques used were poor and the experiments badly designed.

It was previously pointed out that certain compounds produced by higher plants have to be acted upon by microorganisms before phytotoxins are produced (Börner, 1959, 1960). Phlorizin is one such compound, and it is known to be degraded to phloretin, phloroglucinol, phloretic acid, and *p*-hydroxybenzoic acid by nonsterile soil (Börner, 1959), certain strains of *Venturia inaequalis* (Holowczak *et al.*, 1960), and species of *Aspergillus* and *Penicillium* (Towers, 1964). Minamikawa *et al.* (1970) reported that this ability to degrade phlorizin is a common feature of fungi. They demonstrated also that cell-free preparations from *Aspergillus niger* are able to catalyze the hydrolysis of phloretin, the first compound produced in the degradation of phlorizin to phloroglucinol and phloretic acid. They isolated the enzyme involved, found that it showed a rather broad substrate specificity, and that some other C-acylated phenols related to phloretin were hydrolyzed also. They found also that the enzyme is inducible, being produced only in the presence of phlorizin or phloretin. This discussion indicates again that there is not always a clear-cut distinction between the various types of phytotoxins as classified by Grümmer (1955) and summarized in Chapter 1 of this book.

IV. MICROORGANISMS VERSUS MICROORGANISMS

There is much published material on this subject of antibiotics, but most of it is related to medical applications and will not be discussed here. There is a rather limited amount of research on this subject related to agriculture, horticulture, or basic ecology; therefore, as with the previous topic of marasmins, most of the pertinent research up to the present will be described here and the subject will not be discussed to any appreciable extent in subsequent chapters, except for antibiosis between algae in connection with algal succession.

Way (1847) was intrigued by the fairy rings of toadstools and speculated that they might result from the production of autotoxins that prevented the mycelium of the fungus from growing in a given portion of the soil after the toxin level reached a certain amount.

Livingston (1905) was interested in the toxic properties of sphagnum bog water. He found that water from the true peat bogs elicited pronounced morphological changes in an alga, *Stigeoclonium,* which he used as a test organism. He did not discover whether the toxins were produced by higher plants in the bogs, by microorganisms, or by both. It is logical to assume on the basis of other research that at least some of the inhibitors may have been produced by microorganisms.

Greig-Smith (1912, 1917) became very interested in the relationship between microorganisms in the soil and soil fertility. In the course of his investigations, he demonstrated that certain microorganisms in the soil were inhibitory to some of the soil bacteria. In a study of ammonification of manure in soil, Conn and Bright (1919) found certain microorganisms in the soil which were antagonistic to other soil microorganisms also.

Fisher *et al.* (1922) investigated the accuracy of the plating method of estimating the density of bacterial populations, and in the course of

d in cultivated garden soil. Mallik (1966) found that soils from
cultivated fields in Minnesota were very inhibitory to the
ation of spores of *Fusarium gramineum*, a common root rot
n, and somewhat inhibitory to germination of the spores of
m moniliforme, an associative organism in the corn root rot
According to Mallik, the presence of this toxic factor is of
al significance in growth and survival of root pathogenic or-
. Nobody knows what is responsible for the widespread fung-
soil, but Lockwood (1959) suggested that diffusible toxins pro-
y Streptomyces spp. might be an important cause. If so, this
e an extremely important type of antibiosis in agriculture,
ure, and natural ecosystems.

othrudu (1955) investigated varieties of pigeon pea, *Cajanus*
esistant and susceptible to wilt caused by *Fusarium udum*.
to 33% of the rhizosphere microorganisms isolated from the
variety strongly inhibited *Fusarium udum*, whereas most
ates from the susceptible variety were not inhibitory to the
he active organisms were all species of *Streptomyces*. Jack-
) gave much evidence for the ecological importance of anti-
tween soil microorganisms, and thus this appears to be an
fruitful area for future research.

this investigation came to the conclusion that certain microorganisms
apparently inhibited others.

Millard and Taylor (1927) concluded from their studies that the
reason green manuring helped inhibit the scab disease of certain
plants was that it promoted antagonisms between the scab-causing
organism and other microorganisms.

Konishi (1931) isolated several bacteria from soil which were inhibitory to various species of *Rhizobium*, and generally these were
aerobic rod-shaped, gram positive, and non-spore-forming. He ex-
perimented with several species of known bacteria also and found that
two common soil bacteria, *Bacillus subtilis* and *Bacillus megaterium*, inhibited *Rhizobium* from both alfalfa (*Medicago*) and pea
(*Pisum*) nodules.

Waksman (1937, 1947) did a tremendous amount of work on antibiotics, and he stressed the importance of these compounds in basic
ecology as well as in medicine.

Pratt (1940) and Pratt and Fong (1940) presented evidence that *Chlorella vulgaris* cells produce and liberate into the external medium a
substance that retards the growth and multiplication of this alga.
Lucas (1947) reviewed the literature on ecological effects of external
metabolites with emphasis on the algae and concluded that micro-
planktonic organisms do produce substances externally, either during
life or in death, which assist some and hinder others of their fellows in
their growth. Rice (1954) confirmed and expanded the results of Pratt
and his colleagues. Rice found that *Chlorella vulgaris* (Chloro-
phyceae) and *Nitzschia frustulum* produce antibiotics that inhibit
themselves and each other. Later, Proctor (1957) grew five common
species of freshwater algae in the ten possible two-membered combinations and found that no two species grew as well together as each
did alone. *Chlamydomonas reinhardi* was found to be particularly
inhibitory to *Haematococcus pluvialis*.

Saunders (1957) reviewed the literature concerning the production
by phytoplankton of inhibitors of all levels of plants and even of animals. Vacca and Walsh (1954), Chesters and Stott (1956), and Sieburth
(1959) reported the production of antibacterial inhibitors by various
algae, and Burkholder *et al.* (1960) reported the production of antibacterial and antifungal compounds by many marine algae from Puerto
Rico. They tested extracts of 150 marine algae against four laboratory
indicator species, *Staphylococcus aureus, Escherichia coli, Mycobacterium smegmatis,* and *Candida albicans,* and against several isolates
of marine bacteria. Sixty-six kinds of algae demonstrated antibiotic
activity against *Staphylococcus aureus* or other laboratory test organ-

isms, and a few strongly inhibited marine bacteria. Some of the more active algal species from the standpoint of production of antibiotics were *Chondria littoralis, Falkenbergia hillebrandii, Murrayella periclados,* several species of *Wrangelia, Laurencia obtusa,* and *Dictyopteris justii.* The algae, *Dictyopteris plagiogramma* and *Goniaulax tamarensis,* collected from a red tide, were found to have both promoting and inhibitory action against crude populations of marine bacteria in seawater.

Cooper and Chilton (1950) investigated several actinomycetes isolated from sugarcane soils in Louisiana for antibiotic activity against *Pythium arrhenomanes,* the sugarcane root rot fungus. They found several actinomycetes that were antagonistic under laboratory conditions, but obtained no evidence as to whether antibiotics are produced by these organisms under field conditions. If so, such antibiotics against plant pathogens could play very important roles in agriculture and in natural ecosystems.

Iuzhina (1958) reported that many bacteria, fungi, and actinomycetes isolated from soils of the Kola Peninsula in the U.S.S.R. were antibiotic to the growth of *Azotobacter,* a free-living bacterium that adds nitrogen to the soil.

Santos *et al.* (1964) tested extracts of 33 species of Philippine lichens against three gram-positive bacteria, four gram-negative bacteria, one acid-fast bacterium, two yeasts, and two filamentous fungi. Thirty of the extracts inhibited at least one of the test organisms.

Sevilla-Santos *et al.* (1964) tested aqueous extracts of the sporophores of 587 samples of Philippine Basidiomycetes against *Micrococcus pyogenes* var. *aureus* (209P), *Micrococcus pyogenes* (penicillin-resistant strain), *Bacillus subtilis* (FDA 219), *Escherichia coli, Salmonella gallinarum, Pseudomonas aeruginosa,* and *Alcaligenes faecalis.* Five hundred and six of the test extracts inhibited at least one of the test bacteria.

Visona and Pesce (1963) and Visona and Tardieux (1964) performed a series of experiments demonstrating that there are microorganisms in the rhizosphere of red clover, *Trifolium pratense,* and alfalfa, *Medicago sativa,* which are antibiotic to *Rhizobium.* These results supported those of Konishi (1931) obtained many years before.

Neal *et al.* (1964) found that the rhizosphere microfloras of three morphologically different mycorrhizae of Douglas fir, *Pseudotsuga menziesii,* were very different. These variations were attributed to differences in the fungal symbionts making up the different mycorrhizae, but not necessarily to chemicals produced by them. This would be one logical possibility, however.

Craigie and McLachlan (1964) and McL found that the alga, *Fucus vesiculosus,* pro ing substances which are very inhibitory t algae in low concentrations of 25 µg/ml or l

Stillwell (1966) isolated an imperfect fu from yellow birch, *Betula alleghaniensis,* that this fungus inhibited growth of 31 Ba decaying material in coniferous and decid the Dutch elm disease fungus (*Ceratocy* cete, *Phytophthora infestans.* He foun liquid culture, produced a substance *fomentarius,* the fungus most commonly ing branches of yellow birch. He found a inhibited markedly by the presence of yellow birch wood. The amount of decay peeled logs of balsam fir, *Abies balsamea* sion of mycelial fragments of *Cryptospo* tic phenomenon is widespread, it could in the prevention of decay of living tree rate of dead plant parts.

Van der Merwe *et al.* (1967) and Ha lated 1091 bacteria from the rhizoplan *lium repens, T. pratense,* and *T. si* these isolates inhibited the growth of The inhibitory bacteria belonged to t *thomonas, Flavobacterium, Achromo Aerobacter, Bacillus, Streptomyces, Arthrobacter,* and *Brevibacterium.* Th largest number were pseudomonads identified the inhibitor produced *Pseudomonas* sp. (Strain W78), as 2,4-d

Stewart and Brown (1969) reporte *Cytophaga* (N-5), which kills green apparently a new species, and it forn with thin, spreading margins. As it a soluble pigment. The bacterium ly green algae, even when the bacteriu

The occurrence in soil of factors t fungistasis, is apparently widesprea lik, 1966). Dobbs and Hinson found mination of *Penicillium frequentai commune, Cladosporium herbarun*

land a
sever
germi
patho
Fusar
diseas
ecolog
ganism
istasis
duced
could
horticu

Agni
cajan,
Thirtee
resistan
such is
fungus.
son (19
biosis b
extreme

3

Roles of Allelopathy in Phytoplankton Succession

I. INTRODUCTION

The amount of information published on the allelopathic inter-actions between algae is not as great as I feel the importance of the subject warrants. This is the only area, however, in which sufficient research has been done on allelopathic interactions of microorganisms to demonstrate the role of antibiotics in an important basic ecological process or phenomenon. Therefore, I feel the subject warrants a sepa-rate chapter, even though it is brief.

Some of the experiments that will be discussed in this chapter were mentioned briefly in the historical account of research on antibiotics in order to indicate how they fit into the chronological sequence of developments in that research area. They will generally be discussed more fully here, however.

The tremendous fluctuations in abundance of phytoplankton in all kinds of bodies of water have intrigued phycologists, limnologists, and oceanographers for many years (Rice, 1954). Various terms, such as blooms and pulses, have been used to refer to the rapid increases in numbers of phytoplankton above the numbers that previously existed in a given area. Sometimes the blooms are primarily due to the in-crease in numbers of one species of algae and sometimes to increases in numbers of several species. Another striking fact about the blooms is that they often disappear as rapidly as they appear, or even faster.

Many different suggestions have been advanced to explain the abun-dance of each species, the size of the total population, and the succes-sion of important (dominant) species during the growing season (Rice,

1954). Most workers have felt that these conditions and changes are due to variations in physical factors, to a lack of necessary nutrients, or to a combination of these. Some persons have even suggested that the variations in populations are the result of the action of filter-feeding animals (Rice, 1954). A further suggestion was made that the increased population of one species might affect the growth of another or several species by the production of toxins, thus influencing seasonal succession.

II. EVIDENCE FOR IMPORTANCE OF ALLELOPATHY IN SUCCESSION OF PHYTOPLANKTON

Akehurst (1931) was apparently the first scientist, or at least one of the first, to suggest that toxins might be produced by blooms of algae and that these toxins might inhibit some species and not others. He investigated the phytoplankton in several freshwater ponds over a period of several years, and attempted to correlate the fluctuations in populations with chemical and physical factors in the generally accepted fashion at that time. He failed completely in this effort and inferred, therefore, that other kinds of factors must be involved. He suggested that one possibility might be that the phytoplankton produce substances that inhibit the growth of some species of phytoplankton and stimulate the growth of others. Unfortunately, there was little available evidence in 1931 to support Akehurst's suggestion, but his hypothesis did stimulate research along these lines a few years later.

Pratt (1940) investigated the growth and reproduction of the unicellular green alga, *Chlorella vulgaris,* in great detail. He found that the maximum population density attained was independent of the size of the inoculum, that the rate of multiplication throughout the growth period in different cultures varied inversely with the initial density of the population, and that the rate of multiplication as measured by the increase in number of cells/hour/cell decreased during nearly the entire period of growth. He pointed out that these data could be interpreted as evidence for the production of a growth inhibitor by the cells.

Pratt and Fong (1940) designed a number of experiments to test Pratt's hypothesis that *Chlorella vulgaris* produces an autotoxin that limits the size of population it can produce in a given culture. Their procedure involved studying the increases in the populations of cultures in media prepared by adding varying proportions of a medium in which *Chlorella* had previously grown. This would, of course, result in some variations in the total amounts, and possibly the relative proportions, of the various elements in the media. They did several preliminary experiments, therefore, to determine effects of concentrations and relative proportions of the elements in the medium. They found that they could dilute the medium employed to twice its original volume with distilled water or double the concentration of the standard solution without seriously impairing growth. In fact, under the conditions employed, growth was relatively unaffected by changes in the total salt concentration of the nutrient solution from 0.01 to 0.1 mole/liter. They found also that growth of *Chlorella* was unaffected by changes in the salt proportions within relatively broad limits.

The test media were made by adding uniform quantities of salts to each solution consisting of distilled water and sufficient amounts of filtrate of an old culture of *Chlorella* to make concentrations of filtrates varying from 0–90%. The minimum concentration of salts, therefore, was 0.063 *M* in the medium prepared with distilled water, and the possible maximum was 0.12 *M* in the medium prepared with 90% filtrate and 10% distilled water. It was probably never that high, and thus the range of concentrations was within the optimum range of 0.01–0.1 *M* previously mentioned. The pH of each medium was set at 4.45. Three sets of cultures were prepared for each test medium with initial populations of 1, 100, and 1000 cells/mm^3.

It was found that growth of *Chlorella* was inhibited by the presence in the growth medium of filtrate from old *Chlorella* cultures, that the depression of growth increased as the percentage of filtrate in the medium increased, and that, for a given concentration of filtrate in the medium, the growth varied inversely with the initial population of the inoculum.

Similar experiments were performed subsequently, except that the filtrates of previous cultures used to make the test media came from cultures of different ages. The results of this set of experiments indicated that the depression of growth increased with the physiological age of the filtrate used in making the test medium.

In other experiments, it was found that the age of the parent cultures from which inocula for new cultures were withdrawn influenced the early growth rate of the daughter colonies, but had very little, if any, effect on the final populations attained. The early growth rate was somewhat retarded in cultures inoculated with cells taken from relatively old colonies.

Pratt and Fong presented excellent evidence against the possibility that their results might be due to pH changes or to reduction in trace elements. Therefore, they concluded that *Chlorella* cells produce and liberate into the growth medium a substance that retards their growth.

According to T. R. Rice (1954), Rodhe (1948) found that the planktonic alga, *Asterionella formosa,* had a lower rate of division when cultured in the presence of *Chlorella* than when grown alone.

Additional research (T. R. Rice, 1954) was conducted on possible allelopathic effects of *Chlorella.* Two species of freshwater algae were used in these experiments, *Chlorella vulgaris* and *Nitzschia frustulum* (Bacillarieae), because he was curious as to whether a species could influence its own growth as well as growth of another species. First a medium in which each of these two rather different species could grow well had to be devised. The growth curves, daily division rates, and effects on pH of the culture medium were determined each day for a 7-day period with pure cultures of each of the species. Next, growth curves and daily division rates were determined for each species, and the pH of the medium each day was determined when the species were grown in mixed culture. *Chlorella* grown in mixed culture attained a population size only 60% of that attained when grown alone under the same conditions and in the same medium (Fig. 2), and

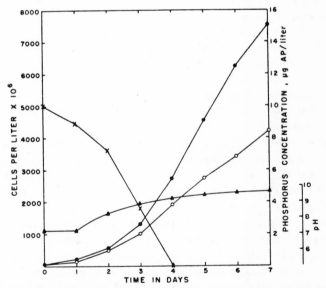

Fig. 2. Comparison of growth curves of *Chlorella* in *Chlorella* culture and in mixed culture with *Nitzschia* prepared with standard culture medium. Closed circles represent growth curve in *Chlorella* culture; open circles, growth curve in mixed culture; ×, phosphorus concentration; triangles, pH. (From T. R. Rice, 1954.)

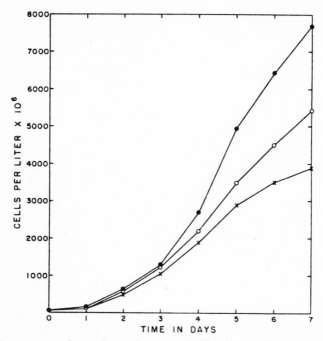

Fig. 4. Comparison of typical growth curves of *Chlorella* in culture medium prepared with Norit-washed and autoclaved *Chlorella*- and *Nitzschia*-conditioned medium, with *Chlorella*-conditioned medium, and with *Nitzschia*-conditioned medium. Closed circles represent growth curve in culture medium prepared with Norit-washed and autoclaved *Chlorella*- and *Nitzschia*-conditioned medium; open circles, growth curve in culture medium prepared with *Chlorella*-conditioned medium; ×, growth curve in culture medium prepared with *Nitzschia*-conditioned medium. (From T. R. Rice, 1954.)

Nitzschia after 5 days in the pond water, which was Berkefeld filtered only, was 70% of that obtained in the conditioned pond water medium that had been washed with Norit A and autoclaved. Rice inferred from these data that a substance was present in the pond water which inhibited the growth of both *Chlorella* and *Nitzschia*. According to Rice, Lefevre *et al.* (1948) grew several species of algae in media prepared with filtered medium in which *Pandorina* had previously grown and they found that the majority divided poorly and that some shrank in size and died.

Pratt (1942, 1944, 1948) named the inhibitory substance from *Chlorella* chlorellin and determined a number of its properties. Chlorellin is soluble in 95% ethanol, ether, and petroleum ether and is more readily extractable from aqueous alkaline solution than from acid solution. It diffuses through a collodion membrane indicating that its mole-

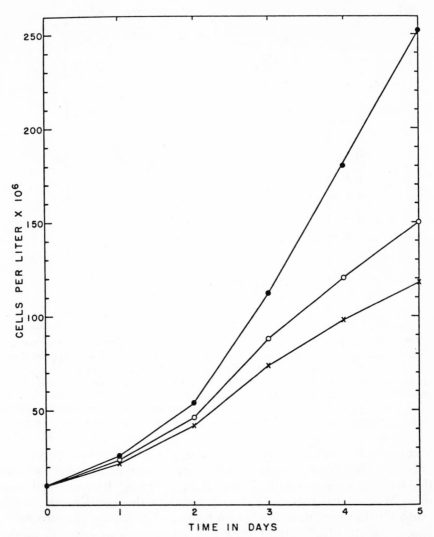

Fig. 5. Comparison of typical growth curves of *Nitzschia* in culture medium prepared with Norit-washed and autoclaved *Nitzschia*- and *Chlorella*-conditioned medium, with *Nitzschia*-conditioned medium, and with *Chlorella*-conditioned medium. Closed circles represent growth curve in culture medium prepared with Norit-washed and autoclaved *Nitzschia*- and *Chlorella*-conditioned medium; open circles, growth curve in culture medium prepared with *Nitzschia*-conditioned medium; ×, growth curve in culture medium prepared with *Chlorella*-conditioned medium. (From T. R. Rice, 1954.)

TABLE 1

Populations of *Chlorella* and *Nitzschia* Obtained in Culture Medium Prepared from *Pandorina*-Conditioned Pond Water [a,b]

	Chlorella		*Nitzschia*	
Culture medium	Initial population	Population after 7 days	Initial population	Population after 5 days
Pandorina-conditioned pond water				
Berkefeld-filtered	70	6450	10	195
Berkefeld-filtered, Norit-washed, and autoclaved	70	7930	10	280
Control				
Distilled water with standard culture nutrients	70	7690	10	264

[a] Modified from Rice (1954).
[b] Data given in 10^6 cells/liter.

cules are probably less than 15 Å in diameter. It is destroyed by heat. Pratt also studied a number of factors that affect the production and accumulation of chlorellin. Apparently, the substance has not yet been identified.

According to Saunders (1957), Lefevre and his colleagues (Lefevre *et al.*, 1948; Lefevre, 1950, 1952) performed many experiments in both field and laboratory relating to the effect of certain species of algae on other species of algae. They reported that algae produce substances in culture medium which may be algastatic, algacidal, or algadynamic, and they felt that the relative proportion of these substances is what determines their overall effect. They proposed, as a general conclusion from their research, that when a species of alga multiplies abundantly in natural waters, it secretes substances in sufficient amounts to inhibit the development of other algae present, which eventually die except for a few individuals in each species resistant to the inhibitors. As soon as the dominant alga disappears, perhaps due to autotoxins, the antibiotic action ceases and the resistant individuals of other species multiply rapidly.

Proctor (1957) performed an excellent series of experiments that did a great deal toward strengthening the evidence for the widespread inhibition of phytoplankton by other phytoplankton. He tested seven species of phytoplankton for production of antibiotics effective against algae. In initial experiments, he tested the relative growth of five algal species grown in the ten possible two-membered culture combinations, and he found that one species failed to grow in three of the ten combinations and that very little growth of one species occurred in three other combinations (Table 2). One or both species were inhibited in all combinations. It was particularly striking that *Anacystis nidulans* almost completely prevented the growth of all four other test species. *Chlamydomonas reinhardi* completely prevented the growth of *Haematococcus pluvialis,* causing the latter to form resting spores or generally to die. Proctor decided to do detailed studies with these two species because of the pronounced inhibition and because the two species could be distinguished readily even under low magnification.

TABLE 2

The Relative Growth of Five Different Algae Grown in Ten Possible Two-Membered Cultures [a,b]

Two-membered cultures	Relative growth
Scenedesmus quadricauda	25
Chlorella vulgaris	100
Chlamydomonas reinhardi	25
Chlorella vulgaris	75
Chlamydomonas reinhardi	87
Scenedesmus quadricauda	12
Haematococcus pluvialis	20
Chlorella vulgaris	100
Haematococcus pluvialis	29
Scenedesmus quadricauda	38
Haematococcus pluvialis	0
Chlamydomonas reinhardi	100
Anacystis nidulans	100
Chlorella vulgaris	5
Anacystis nidulans	100
Scenedesmus quadricauda	10
Anacystis nidulans	100
Chlamydomonas reinhardi	0
Anacystis nidulans	100
Haematococcus pluvialis	0

[a] From Proctor (1957).
[b] Growth of the algae in single-membered cultures under the same conditions is taken as 100%.

Proctor did a series of experiments with cell-free media conditioned by the previous growth of *Chlamydomonas*, using procedures very similar to those used by T. R. Rice (1954) and described previously in this chapter. He found *Haematococcus* actually grew better in a medium conditioned for only 1–2 days by the growth of *Chlamydomonas*, but growth of *Haematococcus* was markedly inhibited by a medium conditioned for 4–6 days by growth of *Chlamydomonas* and with the pH set at 8.5. The same medium was considerably less inhibitory when the pH was set at 7.5. The toxin from *Chlamydomonas* was relatively heat stable, as indicated by the fact that the conditioned medium could be autoclaved for 10–15 minutes without any appreciable loss in inhibitory activity. Autoclaving for even 2 hours lowered the inhibitory activity by only approximately 50%.

In subsequent experiments, Proctor (1957) boiled the inhibitory cell-free conditioned medium and allowed the steam to pass through a water-cooled condenser column packed with glass wool or beads. A substance collected on the column and packing as a yellowish-white film or as droplets. This material was insoluble in water, but dissolved slowly in a basic aqueous solution. It was very toxic to *Haematococcus* cells, completely killing them within 24 hours after inoculation into a medium to which the material from the condenser was added. Much larger amounts of the toxin were obtained when conditioned medium containing *Chlamydomonas* cells was boiled in a similar apparatus.

Proctor inferred from several lines of evidence that the inhibitor, or inhibitors, produced by *Chlamydomonas* was probably a long-chain fatty acid or several such fatty acids. He did not attempt to identify any of these compounds from *Chlamydomonas* cells or from the conditioned medium, but he did a lot of experiments on the effects of six saturated and two unsaturated fatty acids under various pH conditions on the growth of six species of algae, including *Haematococcus*. He found that all of the fatty acids tested were inhibitory to *Haematococcus* in dilute concentrations of 5 mg/liter or less at a pH of 8.2. All test species were inhibited by all fatty acids in at least some concentration, but some required concentrations were relatively high. Oleic, palmitic, and linoleic acids were the most inhibitory generally to all species of the compounds tested. Lowering the pH lowered the inhibitory effects of the fatty acids, and this agreed with the results concerning the inhibitory material from *Chlamydomonas*.

T. R. Rice (1954) suggested ". . . that substances originating from phytoplankton may have one of the following effects upon the growth rate of some species of phytoplankton: (1) they may be necessary for any growth, (2) they may stimulate growth, or (3) they may inhibit growth.

If these assumptions are correct, it can be seen that the seasonal fluctuations in total phytoplankton numbers and in the numbers of each
species, as well as a definite succession of species, may in part be
dependent upon the phytoplankton itself."

As early as 1947, Lucas concluded the following based on his careful
review of the literature.

> That microplanktonic organisms do produce substances externally, either
> during life or death, which assist some and hinder others of their fellows in
> their growth is now confirmed. One point, however, can scarcely be empha-
> sized too strongly: since planktonic organisms do produce such substances,
> then only those forms which are unharmed by them can continue to live and
> develop unaffected in association with the forms producing them. It may be
> that some benefit from such associations, but if they are not at least tolerant,
> then they must either migrate or slowly succumb. Only those which are
> tolerant, too, can succeed after the production of such substances, whilst
> such tolerant forms must quickly be overtaken in the succession by any forms
> which have developed favourable adaptations to the conditons. Both in evo-
> lution and in seasonal ecology these arguments seem certain, and mere tole-
> ration seems biologically improbable.

The evidence for the production in culture media of inhibitors of
phytoplankton by other phytoplankton is very positive and in-
disputable, in my opinion. There is some evidence that a similar situation prevails in natural bodies of water also, although it is more
difficult to get firm evidence in such situations because of the complexity of the habitat. One species of algae seldom, if ever, exists alone
in natural bodies of water, although blooms are generally dominated
by one species (T. R. Rice, 1954). Another difficulty in investigating
production of inhibitors by phytoplankton in natural bodies of water is
that the water contains, in addition to inorganic nutrients, many organic
materials obtained from soil, animals, and other plants, in addition to
any produced by phytoplankton. Despite the lack of completely desirable confirmatory evidence from natural bodies of water, I feel the
overall evidence is excellent that fluctuations in numbers of phytoplankton and succession of species with time is controlled, at least in
part, by allelopathic interactions.

4

Roles of Allelopathy in
Old-Field Succession

I. INTRODUCTION AND OLD-FIELD SUCCESSION IN CENTRAL OKLAHOMA AND SOUTHEAST KANSAS

Plant succession and its causes have been topics of interest to ecologists for many years, as indicated in the two previous chapters. Most investigators have attributed the causes of succession to changes in physical factors in the habitat, availability of essential minerals, differences in seed disperal and seed production, competition, or combinations of these. Cowles (1911) was very energetic in his attempts to explain the causes of plant succession, and he emphasized the production of toxins by plants as a possibly important factor in succession. His suggestion was based entirely on the work of others, however. Numerous investigators have attributed succession of phytoplankton primarily to allelopathy, as indicated in the previous chapter.

Many of my students and I have been interested in various types of changes associated with plant succession in revegetating old fields that have been abandoned from cultivation because they are no longer profitable for farming owing to low fertility. Moreover, we have been interested in the causes of succession. This chapter is primarily a synthesis of our research during the past decade relating allelopathy to old-field succession.

Booth (1941a) found that succession in abandoned fields in central Oklahoma and southeast Kansas included four stages: (1) pioneer weed, (2) annual grass, (3) perennial bunch grass, and (4) true prairie. The weed stage lasted only 2 to 3 years. The annual grass stage lasted from 9 to 13 years and was dominated by triple awn grass, *Aristida oligantha*. The perennial bunch grass stage was dominated by little bluestem, *Andropogon scoparius,* and this stage was still present 30 years after abandonment. This was the oldest abandoned field studied by Booth so he was not able to ascertain how long a period is required for the return of the true prairie, which in central Oklahoma is dominated by little bluestem, big bluestem (*A. gerardi*), switch grass (*Panicum virgatum*), and Indian grass (*Sorghastrum nutans*).

In a study in the southern Great Plains, Savage and Runyon (1937) found that none of the abandoned fields possessed a cover comparable in composition with the climax of the region, even after 40 years. Tomanek *et al.* (1955) reported that the climax composition had not been attained in a field in central Kansas that had been abandoned for 33 years. I have studied old fields abandoned over 30 years that still have almost a pure stand of *Aristida oligantha* (E. L. Rice, unpublished).

My students and I have become interested, therefore, in two major problems concerning old-field succession: (1) why the weed stage is replaced so rapidly by a small depauperate species such as *Aristida oligantha* when the weed stage is dominated by such robust plants as *Helianthus annuus, Ambrosia psilostachya, Erigeron canadensis, Chenopodium album, Sorghum halepense, Digitaria sanguinalis, Bromus japonicus,* etc.; and (2) why the annual grass (*Aristida oligantha*) and perennial bunch grass stages remain so long before the true prairie returns.

II. ALLELOPATHY AND THE RAPID DISAPPEARANCE OF THE PIONEER WEED STAGE

The usual generalized explanation for the successional changes is that each stage increases the supply of minerals and organic matter and improves soil structure and water relationships, thus making the listed conditions more conducive to the incoming than the outgoing species. Such a generalized theory has never explained why the first stage is replaced so rapidly by *Aristida oligantha* because I have obtained considerable evidence that *A. oligantha* thrives under conditions of low fertility and low water supply which will not support most of the species in the pioneer weed stage (Rice, 1971b). Preliminary studies in my laboratory indicated that some pioneer weed species from stage 1 produce substances inhibitory to their own seedlings and seedlings of other species in that stage, but not to *Aristida oligantha.* I hypothesized, therefore, that several species of stage 1 eliminate the species of that stage and that *A. oligantha* invades after that because it is not inhibited by the substances that are toxic to the pioneer species. Moreover, it is able to grow in soil that is still so low in minerals that it will not support the species that come in still later in succession. Several of my graduate students and I have designed and carried out experiments to test the validity of this hypothesis.

A. Inhibition by Johnson grass, *Sorghum halepense*

One of the earliest species we investigated in relation to my hypothesis was Johnson grass, *Sorghum halepense*. Under certain conditions, when Johnson grass is prominent in a cultivated field before abandonment, it remains an important species in the early stages of succession. It occurs often in almost pure stands for protracted periods, suggesting that perhaps something more than an excellent ability to compete for light, minerals, and water might be involved. Preliminary work indicated that extracts of the rhizomes of Johnson grass and the soil in the rhizosphere of that species were inhibitory to the growth of the primary root of rice seedlings (Abdul-Wahab, 1964). More comprehensive experiments were run subsequently to determine the ability of Johnson grass to inhibit several species of plants with which it is associated in abandoned fields (Abdul-Wahab and Rice, 1967). Initial experiments in this series consisted of testing aqueous extracts for inhibition of germination of seeds and seedling growth of several pioneer weed species from old fields. Extracts were prepared by boiling 10 gm fresh weight of Johnson grass leaves or rhizomes for 5 minutes in distilled water, grinding in a Waring blender for 10 minutes, allowing to stand for 30 minutes, and filtering through Whatman No.1 paper with a Büchner funnel. The volume of the extract was made up to 100 ml with distilled water.

Two hundred seeds each of seven species of plants were germinated at room temperature (about 24°C) for 5 days in the dark in petri plates on filter paper saturated with a solution consisting of a 1:5 ratio of nutrient solution (Hoagland and Arnon, 1950) to rhizome or leaf extract of Johnson grass. Controls were run with a 1:5 ratio of nutrient solution to distilled water. Both rhizome and leaf extracts caused a statistically significant reduction in percentage of germination in four of the seven species tested. Germination of seeds of two species, including *Aristida oligantha*, the dominant of the second stage of succession, were only slightly inhibited, and there was no effect on one species. Leaves and rhizomes had virtually the same inhibitory effect on germination.

Seedlings of eight species of plants were grown in quartz sand for 2 weeks in a complete nutrient solution. They were then transferred to vials containing a 1:5 ratio of nutrient solution to plant extract and were allowed to grow for 10 days in a photoperiod of 16 hours at 27°C, and a night temperature of 20°C. Controls were run with a 1:5 ratio of nutrient solution to distilled water under the same conditions. Both rhizome and leaf extracts significantly reduced the oven-dried weight of the seedlings of all species except one. These results indicated that experiments of a more ecologically meaningful nature were in order.

A series of experiments was designed to determine the effects of decaying tops and rhizomes of Johnson grass in soil on the germination of seeds and seedling growth of several species of plants often associated with Johnson grass in the first stage of old-field succession. We determined the amount of plant material that would be added to soil by the death of all the Johnson grass about the time of its peak standing crop in an old field by collecting the tops and rhizomes to a depth of approximately 17 cm (the depth of plowing). The air-dried weights were found to be 3.65 tons of leaves and culms per acre and 2.4 tons of rhizomes per acre. Using the accepted figure of 2,000,000 lb/acre as the weight of soil to the depth of plowing, this amounted to 1.85 gm of leaves and culms per 454 gm of soil, and 1.2 gm of rhizomes per 454 gm of soil to the depth of plowing. These data were used in determining the effects of decaying Johnson grass plant materials.

Seeds of Johnson grass and six species of plants often associated with Johnson grass were germinated in pots containing soil mixed with either 1.85 gm of air-dried leaves and culms per 454 gm of soil, 1.2 gm of air-dried rhizomes per 454 gm of soil, or 1.85 gm of washed, air-dried peat moss per 454 gm of soil for controls. The percentage of germination was determined for 1 week, and the oven-dried weights of the seedlings were taken after 3 weeks. This experiment was repeated (experiment No. 2, Tables 3 and 4). In another experiment, pots containing either Johnson grass plant materials or peat moss mixed with soil in the proportions described above were allowed to stand for 6 months with occasional watering, after which the same species used in the other two experiments were planted. The percentage of germination was determined for 1 week, and the oven-dried weights of the seedlings were taken after 4 weeks.

Decaying Johnson grass plant materials appeared to exert at least some inhibitory activity on seed germination of most of the seven species (Table 3). Both decaying rhizomes and leaves exhibited considerable inhibitory activity against seed germination of *Amaranthus retroflexus* and *Sorghum halepense*. In general, decaying rhizomes

TABLE 3

**Percent Germination of Seeds of Different Species of Plants
in Decaying Johnson Grass Material** [a]

Plants	Experiment No.	Germination (%)		
		Control	Rhizome	Leaf
Amaranthus	1	90	60	57
retroflexus	2	63	33	59
	3 [b]	57	17	50
Setaria	1	53	53	40
viridis	2	40	33	40
Digitaria	1	60	60	47
sanguinalis	2	56	36	53
Aristida	1	40	10	20
oligantha	2	64	59	59
	3 [b]	86	69	86
Bromus	1	90	83	90
tectorum	2	86	64	86
	3 [b]	90	76	76
Bromus	1	97	73	90
japonicus	2	89	59	89
	3 [b]	92	92	90
Sorghum	1	60	53	43
halepense	2	53	33	33
	3 [b]	56	30	36

[a] From Abdul-Wahab and Rice (1967).
[b] Plant material mixed with soil and left to be decayed for 6 months.

inhibited seed germination more than decaying leaves. Both decaying rhizomes and leaves significantly inhibited seedling growth in soil of all species except *Aristida oligantha,* the dominant of the second successional stage (Table 4). Even this species was inhibited significantly by material left to decay for 6 months. There was a significant difference also between the inhibitory effects of decaying rhizomes and the effects of decaying leaves in most experiments against all species except *Bromus japonicus.* The decaying leaves were most inhibitory against the majority of the test species including Johnson grass seedlings. The inhibitory activity of Johnson grass plant materials that were allowed to decay for 6 months was generally more pronounced than recently added material on seedling growth.

In order to determine the effects of root and rhizome exudates of Johnson grass on seedling growth, roots of 14-day-old seedlings of *Amaranthus retroflexus, Setaria viridis,* and *Bromus japonicus* were placed in glass vials through which culture solution was circulated.

TABLE 4

Effect of Decaying Johnson Grass Material on Growth of Species of Plants Often Associated with Johnson Grass [a]

Plants	Experiment No.	Oven-dried weight (mg)		
		Control	Rhizome	Leaf
Amaranthus	1	86.2	8.6 [c,d]	51.7 [c,d]
retroflexus	2	85.0	7.1 [c,d]	48.0 [c,d]
	3 [b]	250.0	110.0 [c,d]	178.5 [c,d]
Aristida	1	13.7	12.6 [d]	7.4 [c,d]
oligantha	2	14.0	12.0	8.5
	3 [b]	50.5	23.0 [c,d]	37.0 [c,d]
Bromus	1	13.9	8.5 [c]	7.8 [c]
japonicus	2	19.3	10.3 [c]	10.0 [c]
	3 [b]	55.5	31.0 [c]	37.5 [c]
Bromus	1	10.7	9.0 [c,d]	7.3 [c,d]
tectorum	2	22.5	11.5 [c,d]	16.0 [c,d]
	3 [b]	72.0	43.5 [c]	40.5 [c]
Digitaria	1	58.3	24.4 [c,d]	6.7 [c,d]
sanguinalis	2	60.0	23.0 [c]	6.9 [c]
	3 [b]	482.0	190.0 [c]	277.0 [c]
Setaria	1	42.0	6.9 [c]	6.1 [c]
viridis	2	74.7	8.5 [c]	41.2 [c]
	3 [b]	328.0	124.0 [c,d]	261.5 [c,d]
Sorghum	1	70.1	46.2 [c,d]	16.0 [c,d]
halepense	2	195.0	70.5 [c]	66.1 [c]
	3 [b]	272.0	138.0 [c]	173.0 [c]

[a] Modified from Abdul-Wahab and Rice (1967).
[b] Plant material mixed with soil and left to be decayed for 6 months.
[c] Dry weight significantly different from the control.
[d] Significant difference between rhizome and leaf treatments.

The vials for the control plants were connected to a pot containing just quartz sand, and the test vials were connected to a pot containing quartz sand in which Johnson grass was growing. A mineral solution was allowed to drip from a supply reservoir into the pot containing Johnson grass or into the control pot. These solutions were allowed to pass through the vials by gravitational force and then into collecting reservoirs. The solutions were then pumped back to the supply reservoirs so the cycle could continue over a 4-hour period each day.

The oven-dried weights of the plants were determined after 10 days' growth, and we found that the exudate caused a significant reduction in growth of *Amaranthus retroflexus* and *Setaria viridis,* but not of *Bromus japonicus.*

It is clear from the results described above that Johnson grass produces a toxin or toxins that are exuded from living roots and rhizomes and released by decay of tops and rhizomes. It is also clear that these toxins are inhibitory to seed germination and seedling growth of several pioneer species of weeds from revegetating old fields, and that they are generally less toxic to *Aristida oligantha*, the dominant of the second stage of succession. An important point that should always be kept in mind is that even a temporary slowing of germination or seedling growth can cause a seedling to have a pronounced disadvantage in ordinary competition with seedlings that develop rapidly. In other words, competition serves as a feedback mechanism to accentuate allelopathic effects.

Chlorogenic acid, *p*-coumaric acid, and *p*-hydroxybenzaldehyde were the main plant inhibitors present in the leaf and rhizome extracts.

B. Inhibition by Sunflower, *Helianthus annuus*

The annual sunflower, *Helianthus annuus,* is often the most prominent plant in the initial weed stage of many revegetating old fields, and initial tests indicated that aqueous extracts of various organs of sunflower were allelopathic to several test species often associated with sunflower in revegetating fields. For these reasons, the potential allelopathic effects of *Helianthus annuus* were investigated in considerable detail (Wilson and Rice, 1968).

A field near Norman, Oklahoma, abandoned for 1½ years after having last been cultivated in wheat, was selected as a study site. In this and other fields of the same stage, definite zones of reduced growth of some associated species were seen around sunflowers. To quantify these observations, all the plants within a 0.25 m² quadrat frame, laid around the base of the sunflowers, were clipped and separated as to species. Clippings were repeated 0.5 and 1 m from the same plants using the same size quadrats. The series of quadrats was placed in a predetermined direction, and the last quadrat of each series did not lie within 1 m of adjacent sunflowers. Five quadrat series were clipped every 2 weeks for 5 months, June through October in 1966 and 1967. The oven-dried weights of *Erigeron canadensis* and *Rudbeckia hirta* were significantly lower in the quadrat around the sunflower than at 1 m away (Table 5). *Haplopappus ciliatus* and *Bromus japonicus* had lower mean oven-dried weights near the sunflowers than at 1 m away, but the reduction was not statistically significant. *Croton glandulosus*

TABLE 5

Results of Field Clippings of Species Associated with *Helianthus annuus* [a]

Species	No. of sunflowers sampled	Mean oven-dried weight in gm/0.25 m^2 Quadrats [b]			Fs
		A	B	C	
Erigeron canadensis	100	7.64	10.78	26.97	21.8 [c]
Rudbeckia hirta	100	0.23	0.51	0.63	12.5 [c]
Haplopappus ciliatus	100	5.38	8.06	11.88	1.7
Bromus japonicus	75	1.74	2.96	4.52	2.8
Croton glandulosus	100	5.50	9.27	2.22	2.9

[a] From Wilson and Rice (1968).
[b] Quadrat A includes the sunflower plant; quadrat B extends 0.5 m from quadrat A; quadrat C extends 0.5 m from quadrat B.
[c] Significant difference among quadrats (Anova test).

expressed a different pattern because its mean oven-dried weight increased in the middle quadrat, but decreased in the outermost quadrat.

Soil samples collected at 0.25 and 1 m from the sunflower plants were compared for certain selected mineral and physical properties. The properties compared were pH, organic carbon, total phosphorus, and total nitrogen. There were no significant differences in the pH or mineral content, and thus these factors were apparently not responsible for the vegetation patterns that developed around the sunflower plants.

Experiments were designed to determine, therefore, if the vegetative patterns around sunflower plants in the field were the result of allelopathy. Soil minus litter was removed from beneath sunflowers and placed in 4-inch glazed pots. Soil 1 m away from the same sunflowers was removed in a similar way and used as control soil. The soil collections were made in July during active growth of *H. annuus* and in October after the accumulation of *H. annuus* debris; the two collections were treated as separate experiments. Seeds of the test species were placed in their respective pots and allowed to germinate. After germination, the five largest plants in each pot were grown for 2 more weeks and compared on an oven-dried weight basis (Table 6).

The July soils from beneath sunflower significantly reduced the oven-dried weights of sunflower, *Erigeron canadensis, Rudbeckia hirta, Digitaria sanguinalis,* and *Amaranthus retroflexus* (Table 6). Dry weights of these same species, plus the seedlings of *Haplopappus ciliatus* and *Bromus japonicus,* were significantly reduced in the soils of the October collection. *Croton glandulosus* and *Aristida oligantha* were not inhibited by the July or October soil collections. Both soil collections reduced the germination percentage appreciably of all species except *Digitaria sanguinalis, Aristida oligantha,* and *Croton glandulosus* in July.

Thus, the soil experiments indicated that substances do get into soil from sunflower plants and have a differential effect on the growth of associated species; there is a greater phytotoxicity in the soils after

TABLE 6

Effects of Field Soils Previously in Contact with Sunflower Roots on Germination and Growth [a]

Test species	Date soil taken	Mean dry weights of seedlings (mg)		Germination [c]
		Control [b]	Test	
Helianthus	July	24	15 [d]	63
annuus	Oct.	28	18 [d]	48
Erigeron	July	19	2 [d]	29
canadensis	Oct.	24	3 [d]	41
Rudbeckia	July	14	6 [d]	78
hirta	Oct.	9	5 [d]	62
Digitaria	July	28	16 [d]	94
sanguinalis	Oct.	24	12 [d]	86
Amaranthus	July	50	12 [d]	83
retroflexus	Oct.	50	8 [d]	64
Haplopappus	July	12	9	64
ciliatus	Oct.	16	11 [d]	72
Bromus	July	11	10	79
japonicus	Oct.	34	16 [d]	66
Croton	July	28	27	89
glandulosus	Oct.	26	24	76
Aristida	July	9	10	91
oligantha	Oct.	9	12 [d]	96

[a] Modified from Wilson and Rice (1968).
[b] Control soils were from same field as test soils but not from around sunflower plants.
[c] Expressed as percent of the control.
[d] Weight significantly different from that of the control.

accumulation of debris than during the active growth of the
sunflowers. *Erigeron canadensis* and *Rudbeckia hirta* exist as winter
annuals in these abandoned fields, and during the later winter months
zones of inhibition around dead sunflower stalks are expressed
through these two species. The greater phytotoxicity of the soils after
accumulation of debris may help explain these zones of inhibition, as
well as give insight into the carry-over of allelopathy from season to
season.

Experiments were planned next to determine how the toxins from
sunflower enter the soil. The possible methods would be by diffusion
of volatile materials, decay of dead sunflower organs, exudates from
roots, and leachates from living or dead organs during rains. To test
the inhibitory capacity of decaying sunflower leaves, 25 test seeds
were placed in 4-inch glazed pots containing 1 gm air-dried sunflower
leaf powder in the test pots and 1 gm air-dried peat moss in control
pots per 454 gm of a mixture consisting of two-thirds soil to one-third
sand. The amount of sunflower leaves used is a realistic figure based
on quadrat sampling for the amount of air-dried sunflower leaves
present per 454 gm of soil to the depth of plowing (top 17 cm) in a
stand of sunflowers. The plants were cultured under greenhouse conditions with equal volumes of distilled water. After germination was
completed, the plants were thinned to the 5 largest plants per pot,
grown for an additional 2 weeks, and then compared on an oven-dried
weight basis.

Decaying sunflower leaves had an inhibitory effect on the germination of *Helianthus annuus, Erigeron canadensis, Amaranthus
retroflexus,* and *Haplopappus ciliatus* (Table 7). There was no effect
on percentage germination of *Rudbeckia hirta* and the three grasses
tested: *Bromus japonicus, Digitaria sanguinalis,* and *Aristida oligantha.* Growth of the seedlings of *Aristida oligantha* was stimulated
by decaying sunflower leaves, whereas that of all other species was
significantly reduced.

The effects of *Helianthus annuus* root exudate on the test species
were investigated using an experimental design modified from Martin
and Rademacher (1960a). Test species were grown in quartz sand for
14 days with nutrient solution. The sunflowers for these tests were
brought into the greenhouse from the field when approximately 2–3
feet high and planted in quartz sand in 4-inch glazed pots. The experimental design was arranged to eliminate competition for light,
minerals, and water between the sunflowers and the test species. Pots
containing the 14-day-old test seedlings and pots containing
sunflowers were placed on alternate steps of a modified staircase and

TABLE 7

Effects of Decaying Sunflower Leaves on Growth of Seedlings and Germination [a]

Test species	Experiment No.	Mean dry weight of seedlings (mg)		Germination [b]
		Control	Test	
Helianthus	1	44	22 [c]	52
annuus	2	36	21 [c]	40
Erigeron	1	54	19 [c]	87
canadensis	2	32	16 [c]	71
Rudbeckia	1	17	3 [c]	95
hirta	2	12	2 [c]	81
Digitaria	1	126	16 [c]	106
sanguinalis	2	97	11 [c]	97
Amaranthus	1	78	12 [c]	56
retroflexus	2	91	16 [c]	32
Haplopappus	1	13	8 [c]	71
ciliatus	2	26	10 [c]	64
Bromus	1	47	17 [c]	97
japonicus	2	39	15 [c]	94
Aristida	1	15	21	97
oligantha	2	19	23	102

[a] Modified from Wilson and Rice (1968).
[b] Expressed as percent of the control.
[c] Dry weight significantly different from control.

connected with glass tubing sprayed with aluminum paint to keep down the growth of algae. A control series consisting of pots of test species only was placed on the staircase adjacent to the test series. Complete nutrient solution was pumped from the reservoir at the bottom of each series to a reservoir at the top of each series where it dripped from pot to pot down the staircase for recirculation 4 hours daily. The mineral supply and water were replenished daily. This method excluded all mutual effects except the interaction of root exudates. The term exudate has been used in a very broad sense here to refer to any substance that gets into the substrate directly from the roots of the inhibitory plants, which results from the breakdown of cells that are sloughed off the roots, or from the action of microorganisms on substances that get out of the roots in any way.

Growth of *Helianthus annuus, Erigeron canadensis, Rudbeckia hirta, Digitaria sanguinalis,* and *Amaranthus retroflexus* was significantly reduced by root exudate of sunflower after 14 days on the staircase (Table 8). The exudate did not significantly reduce the oven-

TABLE 8

Effects of Sunflower Root Exudate on Seedling Growth [a]

Test species	Experiment No.	Mean dry weight (mg)	
		Control	Test
Helianthus	1	44	32 [b]
annuus	2	58	40 [b]
Erigeron	1	53	36 [b]
canadensis	2	59	45 [b]
Rudbeckia	1	36	18 [b]
hirta	2	33	14 [b]
Digitaria	1	53	39 [b]
sanguinalis	2	43	25 [b]
Amaranthus	1	71	23 [b]
retroflexus	2	64	15 [b]
Haplopappus	1	63	53
ciliatus	2	48	42
Bromus	1	63	61
japonicus	2	54	52
Croton	1	34	32
glandulosus	2	47	46
Aristida	1	99	95
oligantha	2	96	91

[a] Modified from Wilson and Rice (1968).
[b] Dry weight significantly different from control.

dried weights of *Haplopappus ciliatus, Bromus japonicus, Croton glandulosus,* or *Aristida oligantha.*

To investigate the allelopathic nature of *Helianthus annuus* leaf leachate, a fine mist of cistern water was sprayed over mature sunflower plants. The leachate collected in this manner was used to water pots containing a mixture of two-thirds soil and one-third sand and 25 seeds each of one of the test species. Control pots of each species received equal volumes of cistern water that had not passed over the sunflower leaves. After germination was completed, the plants were thinned to the five largest plants per pot, the plants were grown for an additional 2 weeks, and compared on an oven-dried weight basis. *Helianthus annuus* leaf leachate reduced the percentage germination of *H. annuus* and *Amaranthus retroflexus,* but the germination of most other species was not greatly affected (Table 9). The leachate significantly reduced the oven-dried weight of seedlings of *Erigeron canadensis, Rudbeckia hirta, Digitaria sanguinalis, Amaranthus retroflexus,* and *Haplopappus ciliatus,* but did not affect *Helianthus annuus, Bromus japonicus, Croton glandulosus,* or *Aristida oligantha* (Table 9). The leaf leachate experiments were first attempted using quartz sand as the substrate for the test species, but under these conditions the leaf leachate was not phytotoxic. When a mixture of two-thirds soil to one-third sand was used as the substrate, however, the reported results were obtained. This suggests that the colloidal material of the soil may play a role in accumulating these phytotoxins to a toxic level.

Toxins produced by the sunflower are probably responsible for the spatial patterns of associated species in the field because strong correlations existed between those species found to be inhibited by the sunflower in laboratory experiments and those apparently inhibited by sunflower in the field.

The sunflower is very inhibitory to its own seedlings and to seedlings of several other species from stage 1 of old-field succession, but not to the seedlings of *Aristida oligantha*, the dominant of the second successional stage. The only statistically significant effect on *A. oli-*

TABLE 9

Effects of Sunflower Leaf Leachate on Germination and Seedling Growth [a]

Test species	Experiment No.	Mean dry weight of seedlings (mg)		Germination [b]
		Control	Test	
Helianthus	1	47	41	78
annuus	2	48	37	63
Erigeron	1	137	75 [c]	103
canadensis	2	147	50 [c]	89
Rudbeckia	1	73	23 [c]	106
hirta	2	60	30 [c]	91
Digitaria	1	37	8 [c]	95
sanguinalis	2	26	15 [c]	91
Amaranthus	1	228	80 [c]	75
retroflexus	2	206	72 [c]	68
Haplopappus	1	16	6 [c]	127
ciliatus	2	29	17 [c]	92
Bromus	1	73	72	102
japonicus	2	60	51	97
Croton	1	73	67	92
glandulosus	2	82	80	81
Aristida	1	15	12	104
oligantha	2	22	24	101

[a] Modified from Wilson and Rice (1968).
[b] Expressed as percent of the control.
[c] Dry weight significantly different from the control.

gantha, in fact, was a stimulation in growth due to soil collected in October.

C. Inhibition by Crabgrass, *Digitaria sanguinalis*

Digitaria sanguinalis is often a very important species in old fields during the first year after abandonment. Initial experiments using aqueous extracts of various organs of crabgrass demonstrated that the species is quite toxic to several associated species from old fields. A project was undertaken, therefore, to determine the allelopathic potential of crabgrass using experiments on decaying material and root exudates similar to those employed with *Helianthus* (Parenti and Rice, 1969).

Field measurements indicated that thick stands of crabgrass in the field average over 1 gm of air-dried weight of tops and roots per 454 gm of soil to the depth of plowing. Seeds of crabgrass and of four other species usually associated with it in old fields were planted in soil containing 1 gm of air-dried whole plant material per 454 gm of soil or 1 gm of washed air-dried peat moss per 454 gm of soil for controls. Unlike the results with decaying Johnson grass or sunflower, decaying crabgrass did not inhibit seed germination or seedling growth of any species in any experiment.

In two experiments on effects of root exudates of crabgrass designed as was indicated for sunflower, all test species were significantly inhibited in both experiments except one (Table 10). Even *Aristida oligantha* was inhibited by the root exudate of crabgrass.

Crabgrass is a very important species during the first year of the weed stage (stage 1), and the pronounced inhibition of seedlings of several important species of that stage by root exudate of crabgrass probably helps eliminate some of the pioneer species. This may be true particularly in the case of *Amaranthus retroflexus.* This species is markedly inhibited by crabgrass as well as by *Helianthus annuus* and *Sorghum halepense* (Abdul-Wahab and Rice, 1967; Wilson and Rice, 1968), and it disappears from old fields during the first year. Crabgrass is one of the first species of the weed stage to be lost, also, and this is probably due to the pronounced sensitivity of its seedlings to inhibitors produced by other important pioneer species (Abdul-Wahab and Rice, 1967; Wilson and Rice, 1968).

The failure of *Aristida oligantha* to invade old fields immediately after abandonment has always been somewhat of a mystery because the seeds are widely dispersed (Rice *et al.,* 1960) and the plants are

TABLE 10

Effects of Crabgrass Root Exudate on Six-Week-Old Plants [a]

Plant name	Experiment No.	Mean oven-dried weight (gm) with S.E.	
		Control	Test
Amaranthus	1	9.49 ± 0.96	5.45 ± 0.56 [b]
retroflexus	2	9.45 ± 0.84	5.32 ± 0.51 [b]
Ambrosia	1	4.98 ± 0.50	4.32 ± 0.62
elatior	2	4.83 ± 0.27	4.33 ± 0.45
Aristida	1	4.26 ± 0.30	2.18 ± 0.25 [b]
oligantha	2	4.32 ± 0.30	2.35 ± 0.32 [b]
Bromus	1	11.51 ± 0.79	7.80 ± 1.21 [b]
japonicus	2	11.57 ± 0.75	8.00 ± 1.00 [b]
Helianthus	1	8.05 ± 0.75	4.05 ± 0.74 [b]
annuus	2	8.23 ± 0.61	3.95 ± 0.52 [b]

[a] Modified from Parenti and Rice (1969).
[b] Dry weight significantly different from the control.

able to grow well in the infertile soil. A possible explanation may be that crabgrass keeps it out, because the root exudate of *Digitaria* was very inhibitory to the seedlings of *A. oligantha*. This was unlike the situation in other pioneer species because they inhibited species of stage 1 and not *A. oligantha* in most tests. The rapid disappearance of crabgrass from the weed stage would prevent it from having any effect on the invasion of *A. oligantha* after 2 or 3 years of abandonment.

Three inhibitors, chlorogenic, isochlorogenic, and sulfosalicyclic acids, were identified in whole plant extracts. Sulfosalicylic acid was found only in fresh extracts, however.

D. Inhibition by Western Ragweed, *Ambrosia psilostachya*

Western ragweed is a characteristic species found in the first stage of old-field succession, and it persists through the later stages with less cover. Neill and Rice (1971) did a comprehensive study of chemical interactions between western ragweed and numerous associated species chiefly in relation to patterning of vegetation, but partially in relation to succession also. The experiments performed were similar to those of Wilson and Rice (1968) described above, so only the pertinent results will be given here.

Soil collected adjacent to western ragweed plants in the field in July was generally either stimulatory to growth of associated pioneer species from stage 1 of succession or had no effect. On the other hand, soil collected similarly in January was usually inhibitory to seedling growth of the same species or had no effect. *Aristida oligantha* was not affected by soil collected on either date.

Seed germination of two species and seedling growth of three species (total of six stage 1 species tested) were significantly inhibited by 1 gm of decaying leaves of western ragweed per 454 gm of soil, if the leaves had previously overwintered on the parent plant. *Aristida oligantha* was significantly inhibited also.

Leaf leachate of western ragweed inhibited growth of some pioneer species when it was used to water seedlings growing in soil. One of six stage 1 species was significantly stimulated by the leachate, as was *Aristida oligantha*.

Five of six stage 1 species were significantly inhibited in growth by root exudate of western ragweed. *Aristida oligantha* was stimulated significantly in one experiment and inhibited significantly in another.

Western ragweed probably helps eliminate *Amaranthus retroflexus, Bromus japonicus, Erigeron canadensis,* and *Haplopappus ciliatus* from the first stage of old-field succession. On the other hand, *Aristida oligantha,* the dominant of the second successional stage, is generally either not affected by western ragweed or it is stimulated.

E. Inhibition by *Euphorbia supina*

Euphorbia supina is sometimes a common species in revegetating old fields (Drew, 1942). Often it is prominent only in limited parts of such old fields. Brown (1968) found in some initial experiments that aqueous extracts of this species were very inhibitory to most test species, which included several cultivated plants in addition to *Bromus japonicus* and *Aristida oligantha*.

In subsequent experiments using procedures similar to those of Wilson and Rice (1968), Brown found that the root exudate of *Euphorbia supina* was very inhibitory to seedling growth of *Erigeron canadensis,* but was not inhibitory to *Bromus japonicus* and *Helianthus annuus*. It was slightly inhibitory to *Aristida oligantha* also.

Decaying whole plant material at the rate of 1 gm air-dried weight per 180 gm of soil caused a statistically significant inhibition of seedling growth of *Bromus tectorum,* whereas the same amount caused a slight stimulation of growth of *Bromus japonicus*. Three-tenths and 0.1 gm per 180 gm of soil caused a statistically significant stimulation in growth of the latter. Growth of *Aristida oligantha* was not affected by either concentration.

Overall, it seems likely that *Euphorbia supina* would exert sufficient allelopathic activity against some pioneer weeds to speed their elimination from stage 1. It appears that the inhibitory effect against *Aristida oligantha* is slight enough that it would not retard the entry of *A. oligantha* into the old fields after most of the pioneer species have been eliminated.

I found that another species of *Euphorbia,* which is often prominent in the pioneer weed stage of some old fields, *E. corollata,* produces gallic acid and tannic acid in large amounts (Rice, 1965a), and Olmsted and Rice (1970) found that both of these compounds are very inhibitory to species from stage 1 but not to *Aristida oligantha.*

F. Effects of Identified Plant Inhibitors on Species from First Two Stages of Old-Field Succession

Several phenolic compounds were identified as the plant inhibitors produced by the allelopathic species Johnson grass, sunflower, crabgrass, *Euphorbia corollata,* and *Euphorbia supina* (Rice, 1965a; 1969; Abdul-Wahab and Rice, 1967; Wilson and Rice, 1968; Parenti and Rice, 1969). The next logical step seemed to be to test the pure compounds against species from the first stage of succession and *Aristida oligantha,* the dominant of the second stage (Floyd and Rice, 1967; Olmsted and Rice, 1970).

Six phenolic inhibitors were selected for testing against *Amaranthus retroflexus* and *Bromus japonicus* from stage 1, and *Aristida oligantha* (Olmsted and Rice, 1970)). The six inhibitors involved were chlorogenic acid, *p*-coumaric acid, gallic acid, *p*-hydroxybenzaldehyde, isochlorogenic acid, and tannic acid. Seedlings of the three test species were grown for 12 days in sand culture for use as test plants. The seedlings were selected for uniform size and transferred to 40-ml plastic vials containing the test or control solutions in which the roots were immersed. Each test vial contained 30 ml of the inhibitor solution consisting of 10^{-3}, 10^{-4}, 10^{-5}, 10^{-6}, or a 10^{-7} M concentration of the appropriate chemical in distilled water and 6 ml of Hoagland's nutrient solution (Hoagland and Arnon, 1950), giving an effective inhibitor concentration of 0.83 times the molar value. The control vials contained 30 ml distilled water and 6 ml nutrient solution. The pH of all solutions was adjusted to 5.8.

The plants were grown for 12 days in a growth chamber on a

16-hour photoperiod at 29.5°C and an 8-hour dark period at 21°C. The plants were placed in previously weighed aluminum vials, oven-dried for 48 hours at 105°C, placed in a desiccator for 24 hours, and the weights recorded for statistical analysis.

At least one concentration of all six inhibitors caused a statistically significant inhibition of both species from stage 1, except for p-coumaric acid, which inhibited only *Amaranthus retroflexus*. The highest concentration of p-coumaric acid did appear to inhibit *Bromus japonicus* also, but the reduction in growth was not statistically significant. No toxin was inhibitory to *Aristida oligantha* in the concentrations tested. The only statistically significant effect on *A. oligantha* was a stimulation of growth by the 0.83×10^{-4} M concentration of chlorogenic acid (Table 11). The results with chlorogenic acid were fairly representative of the kinds of results obtained with other inhibitors, except for stimulation of *A. oligantha*.

It seems clear from the evidence presented that several important species in the first stage of old-field succession in central Oklahoma produce toxins that are inhibitory to several other species from that stage and sometimes to themselves, but are generally not inhibitory to *Aristida oligantha* in most tests. Moreover, this evidence is strongly supported by tests with pure compounds of the identified inhibitors. Present evidence supports the hypothesis, therefore, that the species of stage 1 are eliminated rapidly because toxins produced by several of them are inhibitory to species of stage 1 but not to *Aristida oligantha*, the dominant of stage 2. Moreover, *A. oligantha* is able to grow well and reproduce in soil that is still so low in minerals that it will not support species coming in later in succession.

III. ALLELOPATHY AND THE SLOWING OF SUCCESSION STARTING WITH STAGE 2

A. Introduction

The very slow invasion of abandoned fields by climax grasses, even when such species completely surround the fields, has always been quite puzzling. Rice *et al.* (1960) found that viable fruits of one of the climax species in central Oklahoma, little bluestem, are not commonly dispersed much over 6 feet from the parent plant. Even this movement would accomplish a much faster invasion of old fields than

TABLE 11

Effect of Different Concentrations of Chlorogenic Acid on Seedling Growth [a]

| Species | Experiment | | Mean oven-dried weight (mg) | | | | |
		Control	0.83 ×10⁻⁷ M	0.83 × 10⁻⁶ M	0.83 × 10⁻⁵ M	0.83 × 10⁻⁴ M	0.83 ×10⁻³ M
Amaranthus	1	90.1	76.6 [b]	78.0 [b]	77.5 [b]	75.7 [b]	41.3 [c]
retroflexus	2	78.8	68.4 [b]	67.3 [b]	67.2 [b]	64.7 [b]	30.9 [c]
Aristida	1	31.2	30.4	29.8	30.2	35.8 [c]	31.6
oligantha	2	32.9	33.2	32.0	32.0	37.9 [c]	32.1
Bromus	1	28.4	25.6	25.9	24.4	28.9	16.6 [c]
japonicus	2	28.5	25.9	24.2	24.4	30.6	16.2 [c]

$M = \frac{0.83 \times 10^{-7} M}{}$

[a] Modified from Olmsted and Rice (1970).
[b] Differs from respective control mean at 5% level or better.
[c] Differs from all other means in respective series at 5% level or better.

occurs. Apparently, ecesis fails to occur often even when the fruits of the climax species are present.

Investigations by Daniel and Langham (1936), Finell (1933), Chaffin (no date), and Harper (1932) indicated that old fields in Oklahoma were generally low in nitrogen and phosphorus. Rice *et al.* (1960) studied the nitrogen and phosphorus requirements of three species that come in at different stages of succession in revegetating old fields starting with stage 2. They found the apparent order of the three species based on increasing requirements for nitrogen and phosphorus to be as follows: (1) triple awn grass, (2) little bluestem, and (3) switchgrass. This is the relative order in which the three species invade abandoned fields. It certainly appears, therefore, that the relative requirements for nitrogen and phosphorus are of considerable importance in determining the order of establishment of various species of plants in abandoned fields in central Oklahoma. If so, any factors that would regulate the rate of formation or accumulation of available nitrogen or phosphorus in such an area would affect the rate of succession.

Sources of nitrogen gain in an abandoned field that is not fertilized would include nitrogen-fixation by lightning; nitrogen-fixation by blue-green algae; nitrogen-fixation by free-living bacteria, such as *Azotobacter* and *Clostridium;* and nitrogen-fixation symbiotically by *Rhizobium*. Organic nitrogenous compounds must be continuously decomposed to ammonium nitrogen, since available nitrogen in the soil at any time is rarely sufficient to support the vegetation throughout a growing season. Many types of microorganisms are involved in ammonification, however, so the only significant limiting factor in this process would probably be the amount of organic nitrogenous compounds present. The rate of nitrogen-fixation regulates the rate of increase of organic nitrogenous compounds in soils low in total nitrogen and thus regulates the amount of available nitrogen. Therefore, factors affecting the survival or metabolism of any of the nitrogen-fixing organisms would probably affect competition between plants with different nitrogen requirements, and thus the rate of succession in infertile old fields.

Several investigators demonstrated that certain microorganisms in the soil are inhibitory to *Azotobacter* and *Rhizobium* (Konishi, 1931; Iuzhina, 1958; Van der Merwe *et al.*, 1967). Others found that seeds and other plant parts were inhibitory to *Rhizobium* (Thorne and Brown, 1937; Bowen, 1961; Fottrell *et al.*, 1964), and Elkan (1961) reported that a non-nodulating soybean strain significantly decreased the number of nodules produced on its normally nodulating almost isogenic sister strain when inoculated plants of the two types were grown together in nutrient solution. Beggs (1964) reported on a spectacular practical problem resulting from the failure of oversown, inoculated white clover, *Trifolium repens,* to nodulate properly and become established in large areas of *Nasella* (Agrostideae) and *Danthonia* (Aveneae) grasslands in the province of Marlborough in New Zealand. Many types of fertilization were tried, including the addition of all likely trace elements, with no improvement in nodulation and establishment. Often no nodules formed at all, and those that did appeared to be ineffective as suppliers of nitrogen. Treatment of test plots with formalin, the turf killer sodium dichloropropionate, or trichloroacetate, resulted in excellent nodulation and establishment of the white clover. Beggs concluded that the failure of clover to nodulate in untreated areas was due to some growth-inhibitory factor or factors in the soil probably produced by certain soil microflora. He pointed out, however, that it is very difficult (or well-nigh impossible) to separate turf-killing effects from possible control of growth inhibitors such as fungi. He emphasized that fertilizer experiments in areas where moisture was abundant indicated that competition between higher plants in the traditional sense was probably not involved. The results of the experiments described suggest that the failure of white clover to nodulate in the untreated grasslands might have been due to inhibitors produced directly by the grasses.

The various types of evidence presented above caused me to hypothesize that perhaps the low nitrogen-requiring early plant invaders of abandoned fields may produce inhibitors of the nitrogen-fixing bacteria and blue-green algae. This would give such plants a selective advantage in competition over plants with higher nitrogen requirements, and could conceivably slow down plant succession.

B. Inhibition of Nitrogen-Fixing Bacteria

Twenty-four species of plants of some importance in revegetating old fields were tested for inhibitory activity against one strain of *Azotobacter chroococcum,* one of *A. vinelandii,* one of *Rhizobium leguminosarum,* and one of *Rhizobium* sp. (Rice, 1964, 1965b,c).

The same media were used for the maintenance of stock cultures of the bacteria and for all tests of inhibition. The mannitol medium described in "Manual of Microbiological Methods" (Society of American Bacteriologists, 1957, p. 109) was used for *Azotobacter.* The pH was adjusted to 8.2. A yeast extract–mannitol medium (Society of American Bacteriologists, 1957, p. 113) was used for *Rhizobium*. The same media were used for liquid inocula and solid plates. Fifteen grams of Bacto-Agar were added per liter if a solid medium was desired. In all solid media the agar was melted before setting the pH to prevent a rather large drop in pH while autoclaving. All stock cultures and test plates were kept at 30°C, which comparative tests showed was near optimum for all strains.

For all tests of antibacterial activity, extracts were made by grinding 10 gm fresh weight of plant material in 100 ml of deionized water in a Waring blender and filtering through Whatman No. 1 paper with a Büchner funnel. All of the general screening tests were made with fresh extracts.

The extracts were tested for antibacterial activity by the diffusion technique on solid media (Vincent and Vincent, 1944). Filter-paper disks (about 13 mm diameter) saturated with a given inhibitory extract were used for most tests. This method gave zones of a more consistent size than adding known amounts of extracts to porcelain peni-cylinders. This result is in agreement with Vincent and Vincent (1944). Approximately 0.1 ml of extract was required to saturate a disk.

Two-tenths of a milliliter of a 24-hour liquid culture of *Azotobacter* or *Rhizobium* was used in seeding the test plates. The test disks were added immediately, and zones of inhibition were measured after 3 days.

Extracts of various organs of the test plants were investigated for inhibitory activity, and extracts of at least one organ of each of twelve species exhibited considerable activity against most of the test bacteria (Rice, 1964, 1965b,c). The inhibitors produced were found to be relatively stable against autoxidation and decomposition by microorganisms (Rice, 1964). Extracts of some inhibitory plants were found to retard nodulation of inoculated legumes in soil, and living plants of some species were found to reduce the amount of nodulation of inoculated legumes when growing with the legumes in sand culture (Rice, 1964). *Ambrosia psilostachya, Aristida oligantha, Bromus japonicus, Digitaria sanguinalis, Euphorbia supina,* and *Helianthus annuus* were among the species that were found to be very inhibitory to the nitrogen-fixing bacteria, and these species are some of the most prominent ones in the first two stages of succession in our old fields. *Euphorbia supina,* however, is more likely to be important in localized areas and not of general distribution. According to Russell and Russell (1961), by far the most important source of addition of nitrogen to unfertilized areas is symbiotic nitrogen-fixation. It was decided, therefore, to investigate further the effects of the six species listed above on the nodulation and nitrogen-fixing ability of legumes (Rice, 1968, 1971b).

Very young seedlings of *Ambrosia psilostachya* and *Helianthus annuus* were transplanted from a field near Norman into a 2:1:1 mixture of prairie loam soil, river sand, and rotted peat in 4-inch glazed pots (one per pot). Three and one-half weeks later, red kidney bean seeds were treated with the appropriate Nitragin inoculum, five seeds were planted per pot in the control pots, and three seeds were planted in each of the other pots. The bean plants were thinned to one per pot, except in the control pots where two plants were left in order to keep the total plant mass about the same in all pots. Nodules were counted and fresh weights were taken 32 days after the beans were planted.

There was a highly significant reduction in nodule number on the bean plants growing with *H. annuus* compared with the control number, but there was no change in number on the bean plants growing with *A. psilostachya*. The nodules on the control plants were a bright pinkish color, whereas the nodules on the test bean plants were small and grayish in color, even when growing with *A. psilostachya* where the number was not reduced. Moreover, the control plants were dark green in color, while the test bean plants were yellowish. The average fresh weight of the test bean plants was less than that of the controls, and the primary leaves generally abscissed early. It has been recognized for many years that nodules of legumes have to contain hemoglobin in order to be effective in nitrogen-fixation (Alexander, 1961), and the test bean plants growing with both *H. annuus* and *A. psilostachya* appeared to be nitrogen deficient. This experiment indicated that living sunflower plants inhibit nodulation of legumes in soil under some conditions, and suggested that both *H. annuus* and *A. psilostachya* interfere with the nitrogen-fixing ability of the nodules.

There were pronounced tumors at the bases of the hypocotyls of the bean plants growing with *H. annuus* similar to those produced after application of 2,4-dichlorophenoxyacetic acid or other related growth substances. The tumors plus other symptoms indicated that some kind of chemical was entering the bean plants as a result of association with the inhibitor plants.

Owing to the fact that the bean plants growing with *A. psilostachya* appeared to be nitrogen deficient, even though there was no change in nodule number, and the nodules were small and gray, the experiment was repeated with that species. Mulder (1954) reported that inoculated, molybdenum-deficient *Trifolium repens, T. pratense,* and *Medicago sativa* plants had more nodules than control plants, and the nodules were smaller and yellow or brown-gray instead of pink as on the controls. Becking (1961) observed a similar effect of molybdenum deficiency on size and number of nodules in alder (*Alnus glutinosa*). The experiment with *Ambrosia psilostachya* was expanded, therefore, to determine if the change in nodule size and color on bean plants growing with *A. psilostachya* was due to a deficiency of Mo or other trace elements resulting from the presence of the inhibitor plant in the same pot with the legume.

Very young seedlings of *A. psilostachya* were transplanted as before from a field into a similar substrate and similar pots (one per pot). As soon as the *A. psilostachya* plants were well established, inoculated red kidney bean seeds were planted in all the pots. The bean plants were thinned to two per pot in the control sets and one per pot in the test series with *A. psilostachya*. At the time beans were planted, the controls were divided into three sets. Set A received no further treatment, set B had 1 ppm of molybdenum (based on weight of soil in pot) added in solution as 85% molybdic acid, and set C had 2 ml of Hoagland and Arnon's (1950) supplementary trace solution (B, Mn, Zn, Cu, Mo) added per pot. The test pots were divided into three sets also, with one set receiving no further treatment, the second set receiving 1 ppm of Mo, and the third set receiving 2 ml per pot of the supplementary trace solution. The bean plants were watered when needed with distilled water and allowed to grow under greenhouse conditions until 28 days from the time of planting. The bean plants were harvested, weighed, and the number of nodules was counted on each plant. The nodules were picked from ten randomly selected control plants (from set A without added trace elements) and from ten randomly selected plants growing with *A. psilostachya* without added trace elements. The hemoglobin was extracted with pyridine containing a small amount of sodium hydrosulfite, and the heme content was determined quantitatively according to the method of Virtanen *et al.* (1947) as an indication of the relative amount of hemoglobin present.

There was a highly significant reduction in nodule number in all test sets as compared with all control sets (Table 12), but there were no significant differences in nodule numbers between test sets. The nodules in all test sets were minute and gray in color in contrast to the large bright pink nodules on the control plants in all sets. It appears, therefore, that the change in size and color of the nodules on bean plants growing with *A. psilostachya* was not due to a deficiency of molybdenum or other trace elements. According to Bould and Hewitt (1963), 1 ppm of added molybdenum should have been sufficient for adequate plant growth even if the soil had none in the beginning. The bean plants growing with *A. psilostachya* appeared to be very nitrogen deficient, and the heme content of the nodules on test plants was found to be significantly reduced (Table 12), indicating that the hemoglobin content was greatly lowered. The heme content per nodule on the test plants was 27.1% lower than in the control plants, in addition to the nodule number being greatly reduced on the test plants. Stewart (1966) and Virtanen *et al.* (1947) reported that the amount of nitrogen fixed is directly proportional to the hemoglobin content of the nodules. There is little doubt, therefore, that the test plants in the present experiment fixed much less nitrogen than the control plants owing to their lowered nodule numbers and reduced hemoglobin content per nodule. The average fresh weight of the test bean plants in all sets was significantly lower than the average weights of plants in all the control sets (Table 12), which may have been due at least in part to a reduced amount of nitrogen fixed.

It is possible that the inhibition of nodulation of legumes by living inhibitor plants, when the inhibitor plants and legumes are growing in

TABLE 12

Effects of Living *Ambrosia psilostachya* Plants on Nodulation of Red Kidney Bean Plants Growing with Them in Soil [a]

Treatment	No. of bean plants	Average fresh weight (gm) of bean plants with S.E.	Average nodule No. with S.E.	Average μg heme per plant with S.E.
Control A (beans only)	30	27.2 ± 0.9	303.4 ± 23.5	224.0 ± 23.9
Control B plus 1 ppm Mo	30	26.7 ± 1.1	412.9 ± 31.0 [c]	—
Control C plus trace solution	30	25.3 ± 0.9	364.8 ± 19.4 [c]	—
Ambrosia psilostachya	40	14.0 ± 0.6 [b]	223.4 ± 13.6 [d]	130.8 ± 14.1 [c]
A. psilostachya plus 1 ppm Mo	40	13.1 ± 0.6 [b]	218.6 ± 13.6 [d]	—
A. psilostachya plus trace solution	38	13.7 ± 0.6 [b]	236.3 ± 11.6 [d]	—

[a] From Rice (1968).
[b] Difference from each control mean significant at better than 0.001 level.
[c] Difference from control A significant at 0.05 level or better.
[d] Difference from each control mean significant at 0.01 level or better.

the same pots, may be due to competition for minerals, water, light, or a combination of these factors. Experiments were designed, therefore, to eliminate competition for the above factors and to determine if exudates of species previously found to be inhibitory to *Rhizobium* would affect nodulation of inoculated legumes. The same type of setup was used as previously described for allelopathic studies of root exudates of sunflower. The solution used was Hoagland and Arnon's No. 1 solution with one-tenth the usual amount of nitrogen. The solution was replenished daily to maintain the desired water and mineral levels. The pumps were run 2½ hours/day.

The six inhibitor species under study were tested against three species of legumes, red kidney beans, *Lespedeza stipulacea* (Korean lespedeza), and *Trifolium repens* (white clover). Red kidney beans were used because they are easily grown in the laboratory, grow rapidly, and nodulate well. Korean lespedeza is the most common legume found in our abandoned fields. It is introduced, of course, as are most of the common plants in such areas. White clover is found fairly often in our abandoned fields also, in addition to being a very common lawn plant.

The inhibitor species were grown from seeds collected from fields near Norman or were transplanted as young seedlings from the fields. They were grown in washed flint-shot sand in 4-inch glazed pots. The inhibitor plants were kept on a complete Hoagland and Arnon's solution until they were well established, after which they were thinned usually to two per pot. Just prior to assembly of the circulating apparatus, the inhibitor pots were thoroughly leached with distilled water. At that time the legume seeds were inoculated with the appropriate Nitragin inoculum and planted in flint-shot sand in 4-inch glazed pots. The apparatus was then assembled in the greenhouse, and after establishment, the legumes were thinned to either two plants per pot in the case of the beans, or four plants per pot for Korean lespedeza and white clover. The bean plants were harvested 3–4 weeks after planting, whereas the white clover and Korean lespedeza plants were harvested 5–6 weeks after planting. Fresh weights were taken, and the nodules were counted.

The exudates of all inhibitor species reduced the average nodule number on all three legume species (Table 13). In all but two experiments the reduction was highly significant statistically. In some instances there was almost a complete inhibition of nodulation. The nodules on the test legumes generally lacked the bright pink color of those on control plants. In all experiments except two, there was a significant reduction in fresh weight of the legumes because of the

TABLE 13

Effects of Root Exudates of Inhibitor Species on Nodulation of Legumes [a]

Inhibitor species	Average nodule No. with S.E.					
	Red kidney bean		Korean lespedeza		White clover	
	Control	Test	Control	Test	Control	Test
Forbs						
Ambrosia psilostachya	180.6 ± 10.0	62.1 ± 3.8 [b]	8.1 ± 0.3	3.9 ± 0.2 [b]	8.2 ± 0.6	4.3 ± 0.4 [b]
Euphorbia supina	198.4 ± 11.2	181.4 ± 16.4	14.0 ± 0.5	6.5 ± 0.5 [b]	5.5 ± 0.3	4.2 ± 0.4 [b]
Helianthus annuus	298.6 ± 17.4	22.5 ± 2.8 [b]	17.0 ± 1.5	2.3 ± 0.6 [b]	6.5 ± 0.6	0.4 ± 0.1 [b]
Grasses						
Aristida oligantha	214.3 ± 12.3	145.5 ± 7.7 [b]	6.4 ± 0.2	5.5 ± 0.3 [b]	11.1 ± 0.7	4.3 ± 0.4 [b]
Bromus japonicus	129.8 ± 5.1	127.7 ± 5.5	9.9 ± 0.3	6.5 ± 0.3 [b]	5.9 ± 0.8	2.3 ± 0.4 [b]
Digitaria sanguinalis	174.1 ± 7.7	109.2 ± 6.3 [b]	14.1 ± 0.6	8.3 ± 0.5 [b]	19.5 ± 1.0	3.5 ± 0.4 [b]

[a] Modified from Rice (1968).
[b] Difference from corresponding control significant at the 0.01 level or better.

exudate from the inhibitor species. At least part of the poor growth probably was due to the low supply of nitrogen available to those plants that did not nodulate well because the culture solution used had only one-tenth the usual amount of nitrogen in a complete Hoagland and Arnon's solution. There may possibly have been a direct effect of the exudate on the growth of the legumes in addition to the effect on nodulation.

Based on clip quadrats in field stands of the inhibitor species, it was determined that a mature stand of *H. annuus* or *A. psilostachya* produces more than 1 gm air-dried weight of leaves per pound of soil (454 gm) to the depth of plowing. The other four species under study were found to produce considerably over 1 gm air-dried weight of whole plant material per pound of soil to the same depth. It was decided, therefore, to determine what effect 1 gm of air-dried, ground plant material of each species would have on the nodulation of inoculated plants of red kidney bean, Korean lespedeza, and white clover. Only leaves of *H. annuus* and *A. psilostachya* were used, but entire plants of the other four species were used.

In each experiment involving red kidney bean plants, a sufficient amount of a 3:2 mixture of prairie loam soil and river sand was prepared to fill fifty 4-inch glazed pots. Air-dried inhibitor plant powder was added to half the soil–sand mixture at the rate of 1 gm of powder per pound of mixture. Milled peat was added to the rest of the soil–sand mixture at the rate of 1 gm per pound of the mixture for control pots. In each case the powder was thoroughly mixed with the soil–sand substrate before filling the 25 test and 25 control pots. Seeds of red kidney bean were inoculated with the appropriate Nitragin inoculum and planted in all the pots. The pots were watered when needed with distilled water and were kept in a growth chamber at a day temperature of 85°F, with a light intensity of about 2000 ft-c and a night temperature of 70°F. A 16-hour photoperiod was used in all experiments. When the bean plants were established, they were thinned to two plants per pot in control and test series. The bean plants were allowed to grow for 1 month from the time of planting, at which time they were harvested, fresh weights were taken, and the nodules were counted.

The same general procedure was used in experiments with Korean lespedeza and white clover, except only 14 control and 14 test pots were used. After establishment of the plants, they were thinned to four plants per pot. Plants of these species were allowed to grow for 6–7 weeks, after which they were harvested, fresh weights were taken, and the nodules were counted.

Decaying material of all the forbs reduced the average nodule number on all three legume species in all experiments except one (Table 14). The reduction was highly significant statistically in all experiments except two. Moreover, the nodules were often smaller and lacked the bright pink color of the control nodules. The decaying material from the grass species did not reduce the nodule number significantly in any experiment, despite the fact that exudates of all the grass species significantly reduced the nodule numbers of most of the test legumes (Table 14). Decaying material of *Bromus japonicus* even resulted in a significant increase in the nodule number of bean plants. The failure of decaying grass plants to reduce the nodule number of inoculated legumes as effectively as did decaying material of the three forbs is probably related to the differences in bacterial inhibitors in the two groups of plants (Rice, 1965a,b,c; Rice and Parenti, 1967). In spite of the pronounced reducing effect of the decaying material of the forbs on nodule numbers, the fresh weight of the test plants was significantly reduced in only three experiments.

The data presented above clearly demonstrated that living plants of all six test species definitely inhibit nodulation of heavily inoculated legumes. Both root exudate and decaying material from the three forbs were inhibitory to nodulation, whereas only the root exudate of the three grasses was inhibitory to the process.

Another way in which inhibitors can get out of plants in addition to root exudates and decay of plant parts is by leaching from above-ground parts during rains (Tukey, 1966). Experiments were initiated, therefore, to determine whether nodulation of inoculated legumes is affected by leachates from the foliage of any of the six inhibitor species involved in the previous nodulation experiments. The same three legumes—white clover, Korean lespedeza, and red kidney beans —were employed in this investigation (Rice, 1971a).

The inhibitor species were grown from seeds collected from fields near Norman or were transplanted as young seedlings from the field. They were grown in a soil–sand–peat moss mixture (6:4:1) in 4-inch glazed pots in the greenhouse. The inhibitor plants were allowed to grow until they were well developed vegetatively. To obtain a leachate of the leaves, all pots of a given inhibitor species were arranged alongside a plastic-lined trough with most of the leaves hanging over the trough. A very fine mist of cistern water was sprayed over the leaves and allowed to drip into the trough, after which the leachate was collected in carboys.

At this time the legume seeds were inoculated with the appropriate Nitragin inoculum and planted in pots in the same soil–sand–peat

TABLE 14

Effects of Decaying Material from Inhibitor Species on Nodulation of Legumes [a]

Inhibitor species	Average nodule No. with S.E.					
	Red kidney bean		Korean lespedeza		White clover	
	Control	Test	Control	Test	Control	Test
Forbs						
Ambrosia psilostachya	241.0 ± 11.0	159.6 ± 12.7 [b]	7.5 ± 0.5	3.7 ± 0.3 [b]	93.0 ± 5.7	86.3 ± 6.1
					30.9 ± 2.0	31.0 ± 3.3 [c]
Euphorbia supina	272.8 ± 13.4	190.3 ± 9.4 [b]	20.1 ± 1.0	17.1 ± 0.7 [b]	52.7 ± 4.0	21.8 ± 2.1 [b]
Helianthus annuus	306.4 ± 12.9	186.8 ± 11.3 [b]	14.0 ± 1.3	10.4 ± 1.3	35.9 ± 3.9	17.7 ± 3.8 [b]
	193.9 ± 10.7	82.0 ± 7.3 [b,c]				
Grasses						
Aristida oligantha	237.6 ± 13.4	218.7 ± 14.6	14.0 ± 1.0	16.4 ± 1.1	52.1 ± 3.9	44.7 ± 4.2
Bromus japonicus	254.4 ± 14.0	307.0 ± 14.6 [b]	14.0 ± 1.0	14.0 ± 1.0	93.0 ± 5.7	103.0 ± 6.9
Digitaria sanguinalis	241.0 ± 11.0	257.9 ± 12.2	14.2 ± 0.6	13.0 ± 0.5	28.8 ± 2.9	33.2 ± 2.4

[a] Modified from Rice (1968).
[b] Difference from corresponding control significant at the 0.02 level or better.
[c] Leaf powder 9 months old.

moss mixture as described above. Half of the pots of each species were watered with leachate of the inhibitor species and half with cistern water for controls. All pots were kept in a growth chamber on a 16-hour photoperiod at a temperature of 29.5°C, a light intensity of 2000 ft-c, and a night temperature of 21°C. When the plants were well established, the bean plants were thinned to two per pot, whereas the Korean lespedeza and white clover were thinned to four plants per pot.

The bean plants were allowed to grow for 4 weeks from the time of planting and the clover and lespedeza for 6–7 weeks, at which time they were harvested, fresh weights were taken, and the nodules were counted. In two experiments, the hemoglobin in test and control nodules was extracted, and the heme content was determined quantitatively according to the method of Virtanen *et al.* (1947) as an indication of the relative amounts of hemoglobin present. The pH of the test and control soil was determined at the termination of several experiments. The nodule numbers of red kidney beans and white clover were not significantly reduced by the leachates of any of the inhibitor species. Leachate of *Euphorbia supina* leaves did significantly increase the nodule number of bean plants in one experiment. Leachates of all inhibitors species, except *Ambrosia psilostachya* and *Digitaria sanguinalis,* significantly reduced the nodule number of Korean lespedeza in most experiments.

No significant differences were found in the pH of the test and control soils at the close of any experiment. The fresh weights of the test and control legumes differed significantly in only 2 of the 26 experiments. Both were concerned with Korean lespedeza. *Ambrosia psilostachya* leachate significantly increased the weight of test lespedeza plants, whereas *Helianthus annuus* leachate significantly decreased the weight of test lespedeza plants in one experiment.

In the two experiments in which the hemoglobin content was quantitatively determined in test and control nodules, *Helianthus annuus* leachate reduced the mean hemoglobin content 36% per plant in Korean lespedeza; and *Euphorbia supina* leachate reduced the mean hemoglobin content 24.3% per plant in white clover. It was notable that in the latter experiment the nodule number was not significantly affected by the leachate.

It is significant that the leachates inhibited nodulation in Korean lespedeza because, as previously stated, it is the most important legume in our revegetating old fields. Even though the nodule numbers of the beans and clover were not reduced by the leachates, the nodules on test plants usually appeared to be smaller and gray in color in contrast to the brighter pink nodules on control plants. The hemoglobin content of test nodules was found to be reduced in the only two experiments in which it was quantified. One of these concerned the effect of *Euphorbia supina* on white clover. In this experiment, the nodule number was not significantly affected by the leachate, but, nevertheless, the hemoglobin content was reduced by 24.3% per plant. There is little doubt, therefore, that many of the test plants fixed less nitrogen then the control plants because of a reduced nodule number, a reduced hemoglobin content, or both.

The pH of the soil is known to have a marked effect on the growth of *Rhizobium* and nodulation of legumes (Alexander, 1961). The leachates did not appreciably affect soil pH, however, so they had to exert their effects through another mechanism.

There is no doubt that the combined effects of leaf leachate, root exudate, and decaying material from the inhibitor species on symbiotic nitrogen-fixation by the test legumes would be considerably greater than the individual effects demonstrated.

All six inhibitor species involved in the nodulation experiments were previously found to be inhibitory to free-living nitrogen-fixing bacteria in addition to being inhibitory to *Rhizobium* (Rice, 1964, 1965b,c). Moreover, all six species are very important in the pioneer stages of old-field succession in Oklahoma and adjacent states. It appears likely, therefore, that these species play a prominent role in reducing the rate of addition of nitrogen to abandoned fields and thus slow the rate of succession.

Gallic and tannic acids were found to be produced by several species of *Euphorbia* (Rice, 1965a,b, 1969) and *Rhus copallina* (Nierenstein, 1934). I found these compounds to be very inhibitory to the free-living nitrogen fixer, *Azotobacter*, and to *Rhizobium*. Experiments were performed, therefore, to determine whether these two compounds would inhibit nodulation of legumes, whether they could be extracted from soil under plants which produce them, and whether resistant strains of *Rhizobium* could be selected which would cause effective nodulation in the presence of the inhibitors (Blum and Rice, 1969). Initial experiments in sand culture demonstrated that concentrations of both compounds as low as 10^{-8} M produced highly significant reductions in nodule numbers of heavily inoculated red kidney bean, *Phaseolus vulgaris*, plants. Subsequent experiments using red kidney bean plants in soil indicated that concentrations of 33–400 ppm of tannic acid reduced the mean nodule number, and all reductions were statistically significant except that due to 33 ppm. The amount of hemoglobin was also reduced in each case. Using the best techniques that we were able to devise at the time, we found we had to add at least 400 ppm of tannic acid to the soil before we could recover any immediately after its addition. In spite of this, the nodule number was reduced to some extent even with 33 ppm, indicating that the tannic acid remains biologically active even after being tightly bound in the soil.

Both gallic and tannic acids were recovered from soil under *Euphorbia supina* and *Rhus copallina* in the field. The amount of tannic acid in the top 5 cm of soil under *Rhus copallina* ranged from 600–800 ppm throughout the year, and this inhibitor was found to a depth of 75 cm in the soil indicating that it is stable enough to remain for long periods of time and to leach downward in the soil. Soil taken from under *R. copallina* during all seasons of the year was found to be inhibitory to nodulation (Table 15) and to hemoglobin formation in the nodules (Table 16) of bean plants (Blum and Rice, 1969).

Tannic acid-resistant strains were obtained by growing *Rhizobium phaseoli* in yeast and soil extract–mannitol broth with a $10^{-7} M$ concentration of tannic acid for a 2-week period, at which time they were transferred to a $10^{-6} M$ concentration and subsequently to 10^{-5} and 10^{-4} M concentrations at 2-week intervals. Resistant and nonresistant types were incubated at 31°C for 10 days in yeast and soil extract–mannitol broth to use in inoculation of bean seeds. Red kidney bean seeds inoculated with each type were planted in control soil and similar soil to which 400 ppm of tannic acid was added. Fresh weight, nodule number, and quantity of hemoglobin were determined 4 weeks from the time of planting. The resistant strain was not as effective in nodulation as the nonresistant strain, but it was as effective in the presence of

TABLE 15

Effects of Field Soil from underneath *Rhus copallina* on Nodulation of Bean Plants [a]

Date of soil sample	Control soil [b]		Test soil [b]	
	Mean nodule No.	Mean plant weight (gm)	Mean nodule No.	Mean plant weight (gm)
Sept. 23, 1966	139.2 ± 7.5	12.37 ± 0.48	106.6 ± 6.9 [c]	11.6 ± 0.68
April 26, 1967	163.4 ± 10.7	10.43 ± 0.98	125.5 ± 6.7 [c]	12.4 ± 0.44
June 26, 1967	130.9 ± 8.0	15.70 ± 0.63	107.1 ± 8.2 [c]	12.59 ± 0.67
Oct. 6, 1967	130.9 ± 8.0	15.70 ± 0.63	102.3 ± 7.6 [c]	13.25 ± 0.66

[a] From Blum and Rice (1969).
[b] Each figure represents mean of 20 plants.
[c] Difference from control significant at 0.05 level or below.

TABLE 16

Effects of Soil from under *Rhus copallina* on Hemoglobin Content of Nodules [a]

Date of soil sample	Hemoglobin (μg)			
	Mean total [b] per plant	% Reduction	Mean per nodule	% Reduction
Control	90.9 ± 7.68	—	0.6415 ± 0.062	—
June 26, 1967	57.6 ± 9.48 [c]	36.7	0.4798 ± 0.073	25.21
Oct. 6, 1967	45.7 ± 8.1 [c]	49.8	0.4864 ± 0.095	14.18

[a] From Blum and Rice (1969).
[b] Each figure represents mean of 15 plants.
[c] Difference from control significant at 0.05 level or below.

tannic acid as without it (Table 17). The resistant strain was considerably less effective also in initiating the production of hemoglobin in the nodules (Table 17). Even though the resistant strain was just as effective in the presence of tannic acid as without it, it was no more effective in the soil with tannic acid than the nonresistant strain.

Schwinghamer (1964, 1967) found that strains of *Rhizobium* resistant to antibiotics were less effective in inducing nodulation than the original strains, and he suggested that such reduction in effectiveness was due in part to morphological changes of the bacterial walls. Therefore, even though strains of *Rhizobium* evolve that are resistant to

TABLE 17

Effects of Tannic Acid-Resistant Strains on Nodulation and Hemoglobin Content [a,b]

Series	Mean [c] nodule No.	Plant weight (gm)	Hemoglobin (μg)	
			Per plant	% Reduction
Nonresistant strain, control soil	66.3 ± 4.4	12.61 ± 0.57	90.00 ± 8.4	—
Nonresistant strain, soil with tannic acid	59.2 ± 3.7 [d]	11.75 ± 0.45	79.30 ± 6.7	11
Resistant strain, control soil	51.2 ± 5.3 [d]	12.28 ± 0.53	71.87 ± 10.5	20
Resistant strain, soil with tannic acid	45.5 ± 4.5 [d]	12.65 ± 0.56	66.37 ± 8.1	25

[a] From Blum and Rice (1969).
[b] 400 ppm tannic acid.
[c] Each figure represents mean of 20 plants.
[d] Difference from nonresistant strain in control soil significant at 0.05 level or below.

various inhibitors, their failure to be effective in nodulation and nitrogen-fixation would continue to decrease the amount of nitrogen fixed
in old fields for prolonged periods, thus slowing succession.

C. Inhibition of Nitrogen-Fixing Blue-Green Algae

The ability of certain blue-green algae to fix nitrogen has been
known for many years (Russell and Russell, 1961; Alexander, 1961).
Shields and Durrell (1964) reviewed the literature on soil algae and
indicated the importance and high frequency of blue-green algae on
prairie and desert soils of Oklahoma and the southwestern United
States. Booth (1941b) reported that blue-green algae, primarily *Nostoc*, which is an important nitrogen-fixing genus, may form a 32%
cover between bunches of grass in the third stage of succession.

Many papers have been published concerning the allelopathic effects of seed plants on other seed plants, but there are few papers on
the inhibitory effects of seed plants on soil algae. Livingston (1905)
observed the effect of bog waters on the growth of *Stigeoclonium* sp.,
and he may have been the first to note allelopathic effects of seed
plants on algal growth. Shtina (1960) noted that the rhizosphere of
diseased plants had fewer algae than soil distant from the roots. Gonzalves and Yalavigi (1960) working with cotton, sorghum, and wheat
reported: (1) the number of algal species was greater in rhizospheres
than in control soils; (2) the "rhizosphere effect" varied with the
crop plant (i.e., in addition to the permanent algal inhabitants of the
soil, different species of algae were associated with each crop plant);
and (3) the plant seemed to be more important than the degree of
fertility of the soil in determining the number of algal species in the
rhizosphere. The data from Gonzalves and Yalavigi seem to indicate
that the plant creates a unique and very localized environment that
acts selectively upon the growth of soil algae. If such selective growth
occurs in the rhizosphere of a particular native species, that species
when present as a dominant could have an important ecological role
in succession. Shtina and Gonzalves and Yalavigi referred only to
those algae intimately associated with the roots as rhizosphere algae.

Owing to the importance of nitrogen in succession in infertile old
fields, it seemed desirable to determine if certain species of seed
plants, including species previously found to be inhibitory to nitrogen-fixing bacteria, are inhibitory to potential nitrogen-fixing blue-
green algae. Eight species of seed plants were selected for study, and
these were chosen to represent different stages of old-field succession

(Parks and Rice, 1969). Preliminary experiments involved determination of algal genera in cultures made from soil samples, minus litter, collected immediately adjacent to the stems of the species of seed plants selected for investigation. The samples were collected from the top ½ inch level of sandy loam soils from sites in which each species of seed plant occurred in almost a pure stand. The populations of potential nitrogen-fixing algae were very low in cultures made from soil samples taken near *Chenopodium album, Ambrosia psilostachya, Helianthus annuus, Sorghum halepense,* and *Rhus glabra.*

Soil samples were next collected at intervals of 1 foot for a distance of 3 feet on the north and south sides of sunflower stems that were growing in relatively bare areas of a field plowed a few months previously. Cultures were made again, and after 2 weeks the algal genera were determined. *Anabaena, Nostoc,* and *Schizothrix* (which are usually nitrogen fixers) increased in prominence in the cultures with increase in distance from the sunflower plants. Using a chlorophyll extraction and quantitation procedure (Parks and Rice, 1969) to measure algal growth, it was found that there was virtually no difference in growth on the north and south sides, suggesting that shading was not involved. There was an increase in total algal growth, however, with each increase in distance from the stems of sunflower. Thus, the evidence indicated that *Helianthus* inhibited algal growth, particularly of some of the possible nitrogen-fixing blue-green algae.

Plants of the test species were collected in June from the same fields in which soil samples were collected. These were dried and finely ground after being separated into roots, leaves, stems, etc. Ten test flasks were prepared for each plant part of each species containing 15 ml of modified Bristol's solution (Bold, 1949) and 0.2 gm of ground plant material per flask. All flasks were steamed in an autoclave for 5 minutes at 100°C. This precaution against aerial algal contamination was carried out in all experiments that involved unialgal cultures. A 0.5 ml aliquot of a well-dispersed unialgal culture of *Lyngbya* sp. (Indiana Culture Collection No. 488) was inoculated into each of the test solutions. Ten control cultures, which contained no plant material, were prepared. The cultures were incubated for 10 days under the same conditions employed in the initial experiment, after which they were harvested and analyzed for growth by the chlorophyll extraction procedure. Blanks for the dried plant material were obtained and subtracted from the total chlorophyll a content of the harvested material. Some plant parts significantly stimulated growth of *Lyngbya,* others significantly inhibited growth, and still others had no effect (Table 18). All test plants except *Andropogon scoparius,* a member of the

TABLE 18

Effects of 0.2 gm Dried Plant Parts of Various Seed Plants on Growth of *Lyngbya* sp. (Indiana Culture Collection No. 488) [a,b]

Helianthus annuus	Rhus glabra	Erigeron canadensis	Ambrosia psilostachya	Sorghum halepense	Chenopodium album	Aristida oligantha	Andropogon scoparius
—	—	—	—	Inflorescence, roots	Leaves, roots	Leaves, stems	Roots
Control	Control	Control, stems	Control, stems	Control	Control	Control	Control, leaves and stems
Leaves, roots, stems	Leaves, stems, roots, rhizomes	Leaves, roots	Leaves, roots, rhizomes	Leaves, rhizomes, stems	Stems	Roots	—

[a] From Parks and Rice (1969).

[b] Plant parts listed above upper dotted line significantly stimulated growth compared with the control; those below the bottom dotted line significantly reduced growth (Anova test).

climax prairie, possessed at least one plant part which was inhibitory to growth of *Lyngbya*.

A similar experiment was conducted involving *Anabaena* sp. (Indiana Culture Collection No. B380), a possible nitrogen-fixing species. Results were somewhat similar to those with *Lyngbya* (Table 19). At least one plant part of all species, including *Andropogon scoparius,* significantly inhibited growth of *Anabaena*. The inhibition of this possible nitrogen-fixing alga by the roots of *A. scoparius* was especially interesting, and may help explain in part why the bunch grass stage of old-field succession dominated by *Andropogon scoparius* remains for such a long time.

The experiment with *Anabaena* was repeated using 0.1 gm plant material in the test solutions. The 50% reduction in amount of plant material reduced the concentration below the inhibitory level for many plant parts. However, the leaves of *Helianthus annuus* and *Ambrosia psilostachya,* stems of *Chenopodium album,* and all plant parts of *Rhus glabra* were still inhibitory to growth of *Anabaena*. The remaining plant parts, except the leaves of *Erigeron canadensis,* were stimulatory. The striking effect of dried material of *Rhus glabra* and *Chenopodium album* on the growth of *Anabaena* correlated very well with the results obtained with cultures made from soil samples.

Leaf leachate of one species was inhibitory to both *Anabaena* and *Lyngbya,* and root exudates of several species were inhibitory to the growth of possible nitrogen-fixing blue-green algae.

Eight phenolic inhibitors previously found to be produced by plants involved in this study and to be inhibitory to seed plants and bacteria (Rice, 1965a,b,c; Abdul Wahab and Rice, 1967; Wilson and Rice, 1968; Olmsted and Rice, 1970) were tested against pure cultures of *Lyngbya* and *Anabaena*. The eight phenolics were chlorogenic acid, *p*-coumaric acid, gallic acid, *p*-hydroxybenzaldehyde, isochlorogenic acid, α-naphthol, scopoletin, and tannic acid.

The cultures were incubated for 7 days under the same conditions employed in the experiments on surface soils, after which they were analyzed by the chlorophyll extraction technique. All phenolic compounds tested were inhibitory to the growth of *Anabaena* and *Lyngbya* in concentrations of $0.66 \times 10^{-3}\,M$. Tannic acid was the only compound inhibitory to *Lyngbya* in a concentration of $0.66 \times 10^{-5}\,M$, whereas chlorogenic acid, *p*-coumaric acid, gallic acid, α-naphthol, and tannic acid were significantly inhibitory to the growth of *Anabaena* at this concentration. Tannic acid was inhibitory to *Anabaena* even at the $0.66 \times 10^{-7}\,M$ concentration. These experiments indicated that *Anabaena* sp., a possible nitrogen-fixing species, was much more

TABLE 19

Effects of 0.2 gm Dried Plant Parts of Various Seed Plants on Growth of *Anabaena* sp. (Indiana Culture Collection No. B380) [a,b]

Helianthus annuus	*Rhus glabra*	*Erigeron canadensis*	*Ambrosia psilostachya*	*Sorghum halepense*	*Chenopodium album*	*Aristida oligantha*	*Andropogon scoparius*
Stems	—	Stems	Stems	Inflorescence, roots, leaves	Leaves	Leaves, stems	—
Control	Control	Control	Control	Control	Control, roots	Control	Control, stems and leaves
Leaves, roots	Leaves, stems, roots, rhizomes	Leaves, roots	Leaves, roots, rhizomes	Stems, rhizomes	Stems	Roots	Roots

[a] From Parks and Rice (1969).
[b] Plant parts listed above upper dotted line significantly stimulated growth compared with the control; those below the bottom dotted line significantly reduced growth (Anova test).

sensitive to some of the known phenolic inhibitors than *Lyngbya* sp., a non-nitrogen-fixing species.

Blum and Rice (1969) found almost 46,000 ppm of tannic acid in duff under *Rhus copallina* in fall samples and 600–800 ppm in the top 5 cm of soil under this species in the field. Moreover, they found that 30 ppm added to soil originally free of tannic acid greatly reduced the nodule number of heavily inoculated bean plants growing in the soil. A $0.66 \times 10^{-5} M$ solution of tannic acid contains about 10 ppm of that compound and a $0.66 \times 10^{-7} M$ solution contains about 0.1 ppm of tannic acid. Both of these concentrations were highly inhibitory to *Anabaena* sp., and a $0.66 \times 10^{-5} M$ solution was highly inhibitory to *Lyngbya* sp. Analyses in this laboratory of various plant parts of *Rhus glabra* and soil under this species have indicated that all contain high amounts of tannins also. All the phenolics tested against *Anabaena* and *Lyngbya* were previously shown to be produced by various test species involved in the present experiments and to get out of the plants in various ways. It appears possible and perhaps even likely, therefore, that the variations in field populations of algae near certain plants were due, at least in part, to the presence in the soil of various phenolic inhibitors.

Certain weeds from stage 1 of old-field succession and *Aristida oligantha* from stage 2 were inhibitory in several ways to the possible nitrogen-fixing soil algae, whereas *Andropogon scoparius* from stage 3 and the climax was not inhibitory in most tests. These results complement the previous findings of similar inhibitions of nitrogen-fixing bacteria and the inhibition of effective legume nodulation by many of the same species. The combined effects may result in a slowing of the rate of addition of nitrogen to infertile old fields and, thus, the slowing of succession. This could certainly explain why the intermediate stages remain so long.

IV. GENERAL CONCLUSIONS

The evidence presented above suggests that the rapid disappearance of the pioneer weed stage in infertile revegetating old fields in central Oklahoma and southeast Kansas is due to allelopathic interactions of the pioneer weeds. In other words, they eliminate themselves through the production of toxins. *Aristida oligantha,* the dominant of the second stage, is not inhibited generally by the same toxins and is able to grow in the still infertile soils that will not yet support species that invade in the later stages of succession. Therefore, *A. oligantha* invades starting stage 2.

Many plants of stage 1 and *A. oligantha* are inhibitory to nitrogen-fixing bacteria, to nodulation of legumes, and to nitrogen-fixing blue-green algae. Consequently, the soils that are very low in nitrogen at the time of abandonment remain low in nitrogen for a prolonged period. Therefore, those plants that have higher nitrogen requirements are not able to compete in the infertile soils with the low-nitrogen-requiring early invaders. This results in a slowing of succession during the intermediate stages. Eventually conditions improve for the later invaders, and, once they are able to invade, *A. oligantha* is not able to compete with the more robust subclimax and climax species and thus is eliminated.

In the eastern part of Oklahoma and throughout the eastern United States broomsedge, *Andropogon virginicus,* invades old fields 3–5 years after abandonment and remains for many years, sometimes in almost pure stands (Rice, 1972). Based on my past experience in the field of allelopathy, I hypothesized that *A. virginicus* might produce chemicals inhibitory to other higher plants and to nitrogen-fixing bacteria. Experiments were designed to test this hypothesis (Rice, 1972).

Aqueous extracts of fresh roots and shoots of *Andropogon virginicus* (broomsedge) were found to be inhibitory to the growth of seedlings of *Amaranthus palmeri, Bromus japonicus, Aristida oligantha,* and *Andropogon scoparius.* The first two species are often important in the pioneer stage of old-field succession in eastern Oklahoma; *Aristida* is prominent in the second stage; and *Andropogon scoparius* is important later in succession including the climax *Quercus stellata–Quercus marilandica* savanna. Sterile dilute extracts of roots and shoots of broomsedge were inhibitory to two test species of *Azotobacter* and to two species of *Rhizobium.* Small amounts of decaying shoots of broomsedge (1 gm per 454 gm of soil) were very inhibitory to the growth of the four test species of seed plants listed above and to *Amaranthus retroflexus,* another species often important in the first stage of succession. Similar amounts of decaying material in soil also significantly inhibited growth and nodulation of the two most important species of legumes in old-field succession in eastern Oklahoma: *Lespedeza stipulacea* and *Trifolium repens.* Broomsedge is known to compete vigorously and to grow well on soils of low fertility; therefore, the inhibition of nodulation of legumes could help keep the nitrogen supply low and give broomsedge a selective advantage in competition over species that have higher nitrogen requirements. The combined interference of broomsedge against other species resulting from competition and allelopathy could help explain why it invades old fields in 3 to 5 years after abandonment from cultivation and remains so long in almost pure stands.

5

Inhibition of Nitrification by Vegetation; Increases during Succession and Pronounced Inhibition by Climax Ecosystems

I. GENERAL EVIDENCE FOR CHEMICAL INHIBITION OF NITRIFICATION BY VEGETATION

A. In Grasslands

Russell (1914) reported that cropped soil had a much lower total nitrate content than uncropped similar soil even when the amount taken up by plants was included, and suggested that the lower amount was due to a diminished production in the presence of plants. Lyon *et al.* (1923) performed a series of experiments in which they found that maize, wheat, and oats markedly depressed nitrate production. Data from one of their experiments with maize and wheat are shown in Table 20. They suggested that the reason for the lower total nitrates recovered from the soil and plants was that the plants liberate carbonaceous matter into the soil, which may favor the development of nitrate-consuming organisms in the soil. They further suggested that the nitrates are converted by these microorganisms into other compounds and that differences in the composition of the exudate from the roots of plants might account for the differences they cause in the disappearance of nitrates. They stated that plants high in nitrogen

TABLE 20

**Estimate of Nitrate Nitrogen Produced between Planting
and Three Different Stages of Growth** [a]

Kind of plants	Period of growth (days)	Nitrate nitrogen in soil (mg)	Nitrogen in plants (mg)	Nitrate nitrogen formed (mg)
None	57	4311.2	0.0	4311.2
Maize	57	3715.5	525.0	4240.5
Wheat	57	759.2	2300.0	3059.2
None	77	7517.8	0.0	7517.8
Maize	77	1277.4	3230.0	4507.4
Wheat	77	382.2	3750.0	4132.2
None	119	9898.9	0.0	9898.9
Maize	119	246.0	6560.0	6806.0
Wheat	119	1913.1	5520.0	7433.1

[a] Modified from Lyon et al. (1923). Journal of American Society of Agronomy **15**:457–467.

might liberate substances less rich in carbohydrates, which might be less encouraging to the nitrate-consuming bacteria. They found that addition to soil of ground organic matter containing different percentages of nitrogen resulted in differences in the amounts of nitrates that could subsequently be leached from the soil. No data were given, however, on amounts of ammonium nitrogen in the various soils to determine if nitrification may have been reduced, and no tests were run to determine if the various types of organic matter may have contained different amounts of substances inhibitory to the nitrifying bacteria.

Richardson (1935, 1938) did a very comprehensive study of the nitrogen cycle in grassland soils at Rothamsted Experimental Station in England. He found that the level of ammonium nitrogen was several times greater generally than the level of nitrate nitrogen, and that the ratio of ammonium to nitrate nitrogen increases with the age of the sward (Table 21). He reported also that the grasses and other plants absorb the ammonium nitrogen as readily as nitrate, and that much of the nitrogen is taken up as ammonia.

Theron (1951) investigated problems arising in South Africa when grasses were used as a means of rehabilitating wornout soils. Normally, a luxuriant growth of grass takes place during the first season after the sward is established, but growth soon deteriorates, and, by the third or fourth season, the sward is so poor that it hardly affords any grazing and appears to be valueless as a rebuilder of soil. The

TABLE 21

Age and Mineral Nitrogen Equilibria of Grassland Soils [a]

Soil	Years under grass	Depth of sample (cm)	Mean ammonia (mg N/kg)	Mean nitrate (mg N/kg)
Hoos field	<1	20	1.07	0.53
Stackyard	2	20	2.16	1.05
Great field	59	10	4.67	1.32
Park grass	>200	20	5.44	1.14

[a] From Richardson (1938). Reproduced by permission of Cambridge University Press.

growth of the grass can be increased again either by plowing the soil or by the application of nitrogenous fertilizers. In any event, the sequence is soon repeated. Theron found ample quantities of nitrates in the soil solution during the period of luxuriant growth, but in the intervening periods of poor growth, little or no nitrate was found. Exchangeable ammonia was still present in small quantities.

Theron ran numerous lysimeter experiments in which some lysimeters contained crop plants, some contained a local perennial grass species, and some were left fallow. Examples of his usual results were those obtained using annual millet as the crop plant and *Hyparrhenia* sp. as the perennial grass. Comparatively large quantities of nitrogen were mineralized during the first year in all three types of lysimeters. Under the millet, virtually a steady state was reached with respect to both yield and to the nitrogen lost to the crop and the percolate that year. The nitrate in the percolate of the cropped soil had cyclic changes associated with the growth and maturation of the millet (Table 22). By the time the second crop had matured in February 1949, the nitrate content had fallen to a very low concentration. However, it again increased to a high value during the ensuing winter, with 27.1 ppm being present in the percolate in November 1949. Virtually no nitrates were found in the percolate of the perennial grass plots at any time after the first year of growth. In the fallow soil, nitrogen was freely mineralized consistently. These results illustrated the very important point that nitrification took place actively from the second season on throughout the entire winter in the cropped and fallow soil, but not in the soil under perennial grass, even though the grass was dormant from May to September. According to Theron, the soil remained equally moist in all plots, and other external conditions were the same.

TABLE 22

Concentration of Nitrate in Parts Nitrogen per Million Percolate [a,b]

Date	Annual millet	Perennial grass	Fallow
2/1/49	2.1	0.0	39.7
3/15/49	8.0	0.5	32.6
4/4/49	11.3	0.0	28.6
5/3/49	14.0	0.3	30.2
6/15/49	19.2	0.0	28.7
7/21/49	18.9	0.0	21.4
9/7/49	23.3	0.4	23.2
10/7/49	23.5	0.0	20.9
11/16/49	27.1	0.0	21.2
12/20/49	16.9	0.0	20.4
1/13/50	0.6	0.0	17.1
1/31/50	0.0	0.0	18.0
2/14/50	0.0	0.0	17.8
3/6/50	0.5	0.0	19.4
6/18/50	0.9	0.0	20.9
5/10/50	1.9	0.0	20.7
6/24/50	4.4	0.0	21.8

[a] Modified from Theron (1951). Reproduced by permission of Cambridge University Press.

[b] The second crop was harvested on February 28, 1949; the third crop was planted on October 20, 1949 and harvested on March 7, 1950.

Theron argued very emphatically that the continued low concentration of nitrate in the percolate under perennial grass was not due to the consumption of nitrate by microorganisms stimulated by carbonaceous matter from the roots of the grass, as suggested by Lyon *et al.* (1923). He felt that this explanation was untenable for the following reasons. (1) The amount of carbonaceous material required to bring about the results was too great to be excreted by the roots of the grass. (2) Nitrate reappeared in the cropped soil immediately after the maturity and death of the crop and continued high until growth of the subsequent crop, even though the total supply of carbonaceous material from the dead roots was higher than at any other time. (3) Nitrate did not appear in the soil under grass even when the roots were dormant and could not likely have excreted sufficient carbonaceous material for nitrates to be reassimilated by microorganisms even if they did when the roots were active. (4) When such carbonaceous material is added to a soil, not only the nitrates but also the ammonia is reassimilated by microorganisms. Actually, although one finds little or no nitrate under grass, ammonium nitrogen is generally present in larger amounts than are usually present in cultivated soil. Theron grew sunflowers in small quantities of soil and found that ammonia accumulates in the soil when the plants are maturing, even though it is entirely absent during the early stages of growth.

Theron concluded, therefore, that perennial grasses and other actively growing plants interfere only with nitrification and not with ammonification. He concluded further that the inhibition of nitrification is probably due to bacteriostatic excretions by living roots, and suggested that only very minute quantities of the inhibitors would probably be necessary to inhibit the rather sensitive nitrifying bacteria.

Eden (1951) found that grassland (patana) soils in Ceylon are extremely low in nitrate, and the low nitrification lasts for several years after breaking the land for tea cultivation. This is the time when one would normally expect an increase in nutrients from decomposing vegetation.

In a study of the rate of nitrification in soils taken from plant communities representing various stages of secondary grassland succession on the Transvaal Highveld in South Africa, Stiven (1952) found that soils taken from the *Trachypogon plumosus* grassland climax community showed a consistent lag in production of nitrate. When *T. plumosus* plants with their surrounding soil cores were placed in pots and the aerial parts of the plants were removed, little regeneration of the top occurred. Little or no nitrate was found in water that percolated through the soil, and no weeds seemed to grow in the pots. Stiven hypothesized that the roots were secreting toxic materials that inhibited the activity of the nitrifying bacteria. He found that distilled water extracts of the roots were very inhibitory to *Escherichia coli*, *Bacillus subtilis*, *Staphylococcus aureus* (Oxford strain), and *Streptococcus haemolyticus*, but he did not test the extract against the nitrifiers, probably because of the difficulty of culturing them.

Mills (1953) reported that fallow soil in Uganda, Africa may have nitrate accumulations as high as 200 ppm (even 300 ppm in the top 2.5 cm), 10 ppm on shaded and/or mulched soil, and something in between in cropped soil. After resting 3 years under a sward of elephant grass, *Pennisetum purpureum*, *Chloris*, or *Paspalum*, the nitrate content down to 183 cm was found to be virtually zero. After the area was opened up, the rate at which nitrate accumulation occurred in the surface horizons varied with the species of grass previously present. It accumulated very slowly in *Paspalum* plots, slightly faster in *Chloris* plots, and still faster in elephant grass plots. The rate was still slow in the elephant grass plots.

Greenland (1958) found almost no nitrate throughout the year in permanent grassland plots at Ejura in Ghana, Africa. On the other hand, he found that the amounts of nitrate under temporary or successional grass plots were greater than under the climax grasses, but lower than in cropland. He pointed out that the cause of low nitrate levels was not likely due to nitrate absorption, because he had found that little microbial nitrate absorption takes place under crops. In addition, soil samples taken from the permanent grassland plots showed a high rate of nitrification in spite of a very high carbon/nitrogen ratio of over 20. Greenland concluded, therefore, that the low level of nitrate under grassland was due to suppression of mineralization caused by an excretion of the plant roots that is toxic to the nitrification process.

Nye and Greeland (1960), in reviewing many African areas and vegetation types, reported that, irrespective of the C/N ratio of the soil, its pH, or moisture regime, very little, if any, nitrate nitrogen is found in the soil while the dominant vegetative cover is a grass.

Meiklejohn (1962) found that grassland soils in Ghana contain few ammonia oxidizers and very few or no nitrite oxidizers, and she stated that the lack of available nitrogen in Ghana grassland soils seems to be due mainly to the absence of bacteria able to oxidize nitrite to nitrate. In a later project near Salisbury, Rhodesia, she reported that soils under native grass contained very few nitrifiers, but that the same soils, when cleared and planted with crops, contained many more nitrifiers (Meiklejohn, 1968). Soils under improved grass pastures and under two legumes contained about 100 times as many nitrifiers as soils under native grass.

Boughey *et al.* (1964) reported that two species of *Hyparrhenia,* grasses abundant in the Rhodesian high-veld savanna, secrete a toxin that suppresses the growth of nitrifying bacteria. In the same year, I reported that numerous species of herbaceous plants important in old-field succession in Oklahoma inhibit the growth and nitrifying ability of the nitrifiers (Rice, 1964). The only climax species which I studied, *Andropogon scoparius* and *Erigeron strigosus,* showed little activity against the nitrogen-fixing bacteria, but both were very inhibitory to the nitrifiers. Munro (1966a,b) found that root extracts of several climax species from the Rhodesian high veld were more inhibitory to nitrification than several seral species investigated.

Warren (1965) found that the populations of nitrifiers in the climax purple veld of South Africa were much lower than in successional stages. During the greater part of the year, the nitrite oxidizers were almost completely absent in the purple-veld soil, and were only slightly higher in *Hyparrhenia* soils. Moreover, there was a gradual decrease in nitrite and nitrate with succession.

Neal (1969) investigated the effects on nitrification *in vitro* of aqueous root extracts of six climax grass species and eight species of grasses or forbs that increase in importance on or invade overgrazed grasslands in Alberta, Canada. Inhibitors of both *Nitrosomonas,* which oxidizes ammonium nitrogen to nitrite, and *Nitrobacter,* which oxidizes nitrite to nitrate, were found in root extracts of grasses and forbs that commonly increase on or invade overgrazed grasslands. *Stipa comata* was the only climax grass that inhibited nitrification appreciably. In general, *Nitrobacter* was inhibited more than *Nitrosomonas.*

Moore and Waid (1971) did an elegant series of experiments on the effects of exudates of ryegrass (*Lolium perenne*), wheat (*Triticum aestivum*), Cos lettuce (*Lactuca sativa*), salad rape (*Brassica napus* var. *arvensis*), and onion (*Allium cepa*), on nitrification in a clay loam soil from a cultivated site at the University Farm at Reading, England. The experimental procedure in each experiment was as follows. (1) The soil was percolated intermittently for 28–30 days with ammonium and nutrient solutions until nitrification proceeded at a steady rate. (2) The soil was percolated intermittently for a desired experimental period with ammonium solution and a solution that had previously percolated through quartz chips containing the living roots of the test species. (3) Control soil was percolated intermittently during the experimental period with ammonium solution only. (4) The leachates of the test and control soil were collected at regular intervals and analyzed immediately for ammonium, nitrite, and nitrate. (5) The amounts of ammonium disappearing from and nitrate appearing in the solutions that had leached through the soil columns were calculated. Corrections were made for retention in the plant containers and additions of nitrate from the plant containers and the nutrient solution. Results were expressed on a rate per day basis. Modifications of this procedure were used also in which various stages were repeated on a cyclic basis.

Moore and Waid found that all test species reduced the rate of nitrification, but the effects of rape and lettuce were only temporary. Ryegrass root exudates had the most pronounced and persistent effects and reduced the rate of nitrifiation up to 84% (Fig. 6). The control rate remained virtually constant over an 80-day experimental period, after equilibrium was reached (Fig. 7). Wheat root exudate caused a pronounced and persistent decrease in rate over the 80-day experimental period also (Fig. 8), as did onion root exudate. As neither

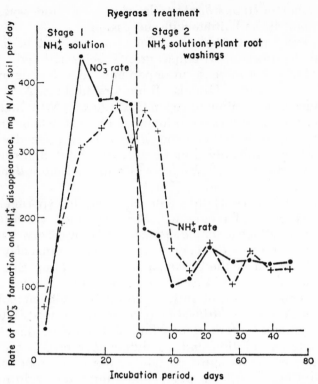

Fig. 6. Influence of washings of living ryegrass roots on rate of ammonium disappearance and nitrate formation in a clay loam. (From Moore and Waid, 1971. Reproduced by permission of Microforms International Marketing Corporation.)

microbial immobilization of inorganic nitrogen nor denitrification appeared to be taking place in the presence of the root exudates, they concluded that the exudates contained inhibitors which retarded nitrification in some way.

B. In Forests

There is less evidence concerning inhibition of nitrification by forest vegetation, and again, as with the research on inhibition of nitrification by grasses, much of it has been done in Africa. Dommergues (1954) did a microbiological study of five forest soil types from central and eastern Madagascar. He found that ammonification was higher and nitrification was lower in the forest soils than in cultivated soils. In a subsequent study of dry tropical forest soils in Senegal, Dommergues (1956) stated that nitrification in dry tropical forest soils is more active than in dense, humid forest soils. Nevertheless, nitrification increases greatly in the dry forest soils on clearing and cultivating.

Jacquemin and Berlier (1956) reported that the nitrifying power in forest-covered soils of the lower Ivory Coast of Africa was low, and that it increased on clearing.

Berlier *et al.* (1956) compared the biological activity of forest and savanna soils on the Ivory Coast and found that the nitrifying activity in savanna soils was practically zero, or, in other words, still lower than in the forest soils. Ammonification was higher also in the forest soils than the savanna soils.

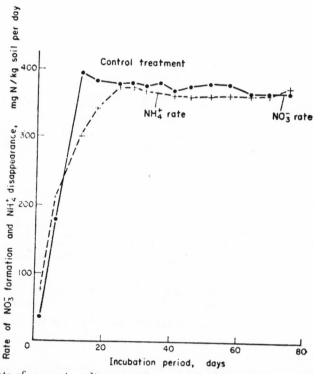

Fig. 7. Rate of ammonium disappearance and nitrate formation in same type of clay loam used for experiment shown in Fig. 6 but without addition of washings of plant roots. (From Moore and Waid, 1971. Reproduced by permission of Microforms International Marketing Corporation.)

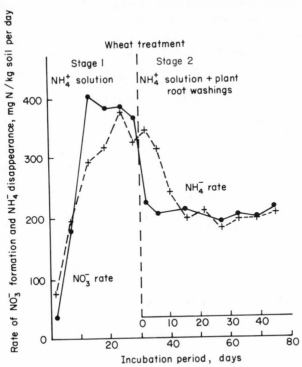

Fig. 8. Influence of washings of living wheat roots on rate of ammonium disappearance and nitrate formation in a clay loam. (From Moore and Waid, 1971. Reproduced by permission of Microforms International Marketing Corporation.)

Nye and Greenland (1960) reported that in the moist evergreen forest covered soils of Africa the numbers of nitrifiers are exceptionally low. In contrast to the low rate of nitrification in such soils, ammonification proceeds rapidly. In Finland, Viro (1963) reported that most of the available nitrogen in the humus layer from stands in which spruce was dominant—pure pine and pure spruce stands—was ammonium nitrogen, with the amount of nitrate nitrogen being very low. Data cited by Russell and Russell (1961) and Weetman (1961) indicate that the rate of nitrification is generally very low under spruce and several other conifers and generally also in forest with a mor type of mulch.

Smith *et al.* (1968) found an 18-fold increase in *Nitrosomonas* and a 34-fold increase in *Nitrobacter* after clear-cutting a forest ecosystem in Connecticut. They felt that the evidence indicated that the pronounced increase in numbers of nitrifiers was due, not to changes in physical conditions, but to elimination of uptake of nitrate by the vegetation, or to a reduction in production of substances inhibitory to the autotrophic nitrifying population. Likens *et al.* (1969) reported a 100-fold increase in nitrate loss in the same ecosystem after cutting.

II. THEORETICAL BASIS FOR SELECTIVE PRESSURE AGAINST NITRIFICATION

Because of my early training in plant physiology, I started my initial work on the role of allelopathy in succession in infertile old fields with the idea that nitrification is essential to make nitrogen available for the growth of plants (Rice, 1964). If so, inhibition of nitrification would give pioneer plants with low nitrogen requirements a selective advantage in competition with the later invaders, which have higher nitrogen requirements (Rice *et al.*, 1960) and thus slow succession. In the course of my investigations, I found that pioneer species did inhibit the nitrifying bacteria in addition to being very inhibitory to nitrogen-fixing bacteria. I decided, however, to test two climax species, *Andropogon scoparius* and *Erigeron strigosus*, against nitrification and nitrogen-fixing bacteria. I found that these climax species were very inhibitory to nitrification, but hardly had any effect on the nitrogen-fixing bacteria (Rice, 1964). These results caused me to carefully reevaluate the necessity of nitrification for the growth of plants.

My first thoughts concerned the known physical facts concerning ammonium and nitrate ions in soil. The ammonium ion is positively charged and is, therefore, adsorbed on the negatively charged colloidal micelles, thus preventing leaching below the depth of rooting due to percolating water. On the other hand, the nitrate ions are negatively charged and are repelled by the colloidal micelles in the soil. Thus, they readily leach below the depth of rooting or are easily carried away in surface drainage. It would appear from these facts that inhibition of nitrification would therefore help to conserve nitrogen.

If plants take up nitrate ions, they have to reduce these ions to nitrite and then to ammonium ions before this nitrogen can react with α-ketoglutaric acid and other keto acids in the formation of amino acids and subsequently of other nitrogenous organic compounds. The reduction of nitrate ions to ammonium ions requires energy, and thus inhibition of nitrification would conserve energy.

The conservation of energy and of nitrogen resulting from nitrification inhibition would appear to be strong forces during succession and in the evolution of ecosystems toward the selection of plant species that inhibit nitrification. If nitrification is inhibited, this would mean that ammonium nitrogen would be the chief form of available nitrogen in later successional stages and in climax ecosystems. The next item of importance, therefore, is concerned with the present status of evidence as to the ability of plants to use ammonium nitrogen, especially noncrop plants.

There is growing evidence concerning plants of every level of complexity that many species, and probably most, can use ammonium nitrogen as effectively or more so than nitrate nitrogen (Allison, 1931; Addoms, 1937; Tam and Clark, 1943; Cramer and Myers, 1948; Cain, 1952; Swan, 1960; Oertli, 1963; Pharis *et al.*, 1964; Nielsen and Cunningham, 1964; McFee and Stone, 1968; Ferguson and Bollard, 1969; Shen, 1969; Gamborg and Shyluk, 1970; Moore and Keraitis, 1971; Christersson, 1972; Gigon and Rorison, 1972; Weissman, 1972). Thus, the inhibition of nitrification makes good biological sense.

III. SPECIFIC EVIDENCE FOR INCREASES IN INHIBITION OF NITRIFICATION DURING SUCCESSION AND IN CLIMAX ECOSYSTEMS

On the basis of the evidence presented in Sections I and II, it was hypothesized that inhibition of nitrification increases during succession and is high in climax ecosystems. Experiments were performed to test the hypothesis (Rice and Pancholy, 1972).

Three stands representing two stages of old-field succession and the climax were selected in each of the following vegetation types in Oklahoma: oak–pine forest, post oak–blackjack oak forest, and tall-grass prairie. Stands in the tall-grass prairie area were located near Norman in Cleveland and McClain Counties, the post oak–blackjack area stands in Hughes County southeast of Wetumka, and the oak–pine stands in Latimer County north of Wilburton. Average annual precipitation in the study areas varied from 44 inches in the oak–pine area, to 38 inches in the post oak–blackjack area, and to 33 inches in the tall-grass prairie area (Gray and Galloway, 1959). The oak–pine plots are located in the Enders–Conway–Hector soil association (Gray and Galloway, 1959) in the Ultisols order (Gray and Stahnke, 1970); the post oak–blackjack plots in the Darnell–Stephenville association (Gray and Galloway, 1959) in the Alfisols order (Gray and Stahnke, 1970), and the tall-grass prairie plots in the Renfrow–Zaneis–Vernon association (Gray and Galloway, 1959) in the Mollisols order (U.S. Department of Agriculture, 1960).

All plots had a sandy loam soil except the first successional stage in the tall-grass prairie area, which had a sandy clay loam soil (Rice and Pancholy, 1972). Moreover, the pH was virtually the same in all three plots of each vegetational type. The amount of organic carbon often varied considerably in the different plots, with the only consistent trend in relation to succession occurring in the tall-grass prairie plots.

The first successional stage investigated (P_1) was in the first year after abandonment from cultivation in the oak–pine and tall-grass prairie areas and in the second year in the post oak–blackjack area. All P_1 plots were in the pioneer weed stage of succession—stage 1 of Booth (1941a; Rice and Pancholy, 1972). The second successional stage (P_2) was in the sixth year after abandonment in the tall-grass prairie area and was dominated by *Aristida oligantha,* which represented stage 2, the annual grass stage, of Booth. The P_2 plot in the post oak–blackjack area was in the eighth year after abandonment and was dominated by *Ambrosia psilostachya, Andropogon virginicus, Aristida oligantha,* and *Lespedeza stipulacea.* The P_2 plot in the oak–pine area was abandoned from cultivation for 25 years and was dominated by *Andropogon virginicus;* a few pine and oak seedlings were present. The chief criteria used in selecting the P_2 plots were availability and a stage of succession somewhere between the pioneer stage and the climax. The climax prairie (P_3) was dominated by *Andropogon gerardi* and *A. scoparius* with *Panicum virgatum* and *Sorghastrum nutans* as important secondary species. The climax post oak–blackjack oak stand was dominated by *Quercus marilandica* and *Q. stellata* with ground cover primarily of *Andropogon scoparius.* The climax oak–pine stand was dominated by *Pinus echinata* and *Quercus stellata.* This stand had virtually no herbaceous ground cover. There were a few very small and sparse patches consisting of *Andropogon gerardi, A. scoparius, Desmodium laevigatum,* and *Tephrosia virginiana.*

Starting in March, 1971, ten evenly distributed soil samples were taken from the 0–15 cm and ten from the 45–60 cm level in each plot every other month for a full year. These were analyzed for ammonium nitrogen by steam distillation with MgO (Bremner, 1965) and for nitrate nitrogen by a specific ion electrode after extracting the soil with distilled water (1:2 ratio of soil:water) for 1 hour with occasional stirring.

Starting in April 1971, eight evenly distributed soil samples were taken from the 0–15 cm level in each plot every other month for a year. These were analyzed for numbers of *Nitrosomonas* and *Nitrobacter* by the most probable number (MPN) method of Alexander and Clark (1965) using white porcelain trays and dimethyl α-naphthylamine and sulfanilic acid reagents instead of the Griess–Ilosvay reagent (Society of American Bacteriologists, 1957, p. 153).

The amount of ammonium nitrogen was lowest in the first successional stage, intermediate in the second successional stage, and highest in the climax stand (Figs. 9, 10, and 11 and Table 23). Moreover,

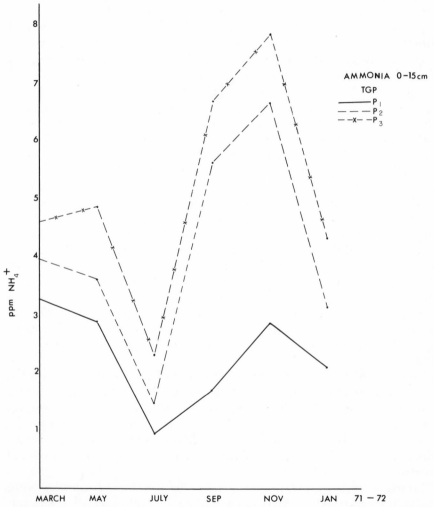

Fig. 9. Amounts of ammonium nitrogen in top 15 cm of soil in relation to old-field succession in tall-grass prairie area of Oklahoma. P_1 is first successional stage, P_2 is an intermediate successional stage, and P_3 is climax. Each point is average of ten analyses. (Data from Rice and Pancholy, 1972.)

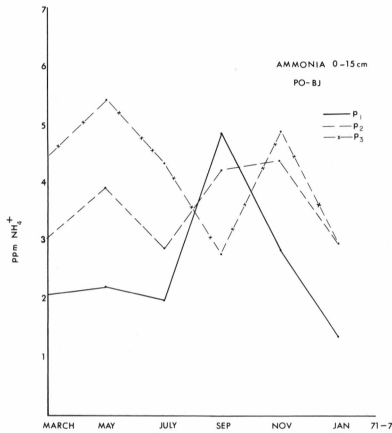

Fig. 10 Amounts of ammonium nitrogen in top 15 cm of soil in relation to old-field succession in post oak–blackjack oak area of Oklahoma. Symbols as in Fig. 9 (Data from Rice and Pancholy, 1972.)

the differences in amounts between P_1 and P_2, P_2 and P_3, and P_1 and P_3 were generally statistically significant. This trend was remarkably consistent throughout all sampling periods, all vegetation types, and both sampling levels in the soil.

The amount of nitrate was highest in the first successional stage, intermediate in the second successional stage, and lowest in the climax stand in both sampling levels, all vegetation types, and virtually all sampling periods (Figs. 12, 13, and 14 and Table 23). The chief exceptions occurred in the 45–60 cm level in the oak–pine area in March and September. Again, the differences between P_1 and P_2, P_2 and P_3, and P_1 and P_3 were usually statistically significant.

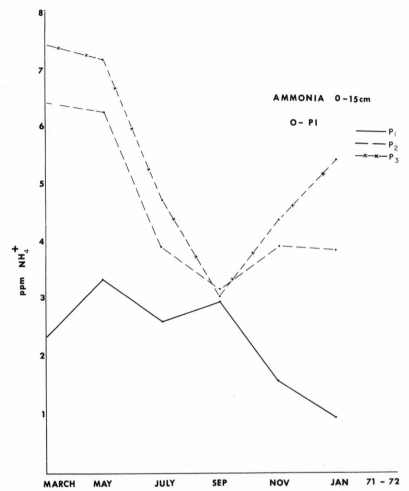

Fig. 11. Amounts of ammonium nitrogen in top 15 cm of soil in relation to old-field succession in oak–pine area of Oklahoma. Symbols as in Fig. 9. (Data from Rice and Pancholy, 1972.)

The consistently high amounts of ammonium nitrogen and very low amounts of nitrate in the climax stands throughout all vegetation types, all sampling periods, and both sampling levels were particularly striking.

The numbers of *Nitrosomonas* per gram of soil were highest in the first successional stage, intermediate in the second successional stage, and lowest in the climax throughout all sampling periods and all vegetation types (Figs. 15, 16, and 17). The one exception was in the tall-grass prairie area in the month of April when numbers were lower than usual in the P_1 and P_2 plots.

The numbers of *Nitrobacter* per gram of soil were generally considerably higher in the first and second successional stages than in the climax (Figs. 18, 19, and 20). In the post oak–blackjack and oak–pine areas, the number in the first successional stage was highest, with the second successional stage generally having an intermediate number. In the prairie area, the first and second successional stages generally had similar numbers of *Nitrobacter*. The particularly striking feature

TABLE 23

Amounts of Ammonium and Nitrate Nitrogen in 45–60 cm Level of Research Plots [a,b]

Date	ppm NH_4^+ at 45–60 cm			ppm NO_3^- at 45–60 cm		
	P_1	P_2	P_3	P_1	P_2	P_3
		Tall-grass prairie				
March 1971	1.37	3.40 [c]	4.12 [d]	4.63	3.68 [c]	1.16 [d,e]
May 1971	1.47	1.89 [c]	2.48 [d,e]	2.49	2.08 [c]	1.36 [d,e]
July 1971	0.76	0.97	1.27	2.67	2.12 [c]	1.44 [d,e]
Sept. 1971	3.32	5.51	5.67 [d]	2.66	2.25 [c]	1.49 [d,e]
Nov. 1971	3.18	5.39 [c]	5.60 [d]	0.85	0.31 [c]	0.13 [d]
Jan. 1972	1.88	2.95	2.75 [d]	1.06	0.92	0.18 [d,e]
		Post oak–blackjack oak				
March 1971	1.65	4.54 [c]	5.19 [d,e]	2.08	1.63 [c]	0.94 [d]
May 1971	0.80	1.12	2.65 [d,e]	1.98	1.40	1.18 [d]
July 1971	0.87	1.26	2.14 [d,e]	2.18	1.66 [c]	0.96 [d,e]
Sept. 1971	3.64	3.01	2.79	2.08	1.63 [c]	0.80 [d,e]
Nov. 1971	1.78	2.95 [c]	3.22 [d]	0.54	0.45	0.22 [d]
Jan. 1972	0.93	1.20	1.55 [d]	0.88	0.64 [c]	0.60 [d]
		Oak–pine				
March 1971	2.79	5.23 [c]	7.06 [d,e]	2.23	1.00 [c]	2.23 [e]
May 1971	1.99	5.37 [c]	6.05 [d]	2.08	1.82	1.58 [d]
July 1971	1.89	3.46 [c]	4.20 [d,e]	2.19	2.12 [c]	1.06 [d,e]
Sept. 1971	1.05	1.57	2.10 [d]	0.00	0.37	0.00
Nov. 1971	1.33	1.61	1.82 [d]	1.39	1.28	0.39 [d,e]
Jan. 1972	0.98	1.31	2.01 [d,e]	0.14	0.06	0.04

[a] From Rice and Pancholy (1972).

[b] Each number is average of ten analyses.

[c] Difference between P_1 and P_2 significant at 0.05 level or better.

[d] Difference between P_1 and P_3 significant at 0.05 level or better.

[e] Difference between P_2 and P_3 significant at 0.05 level or better.

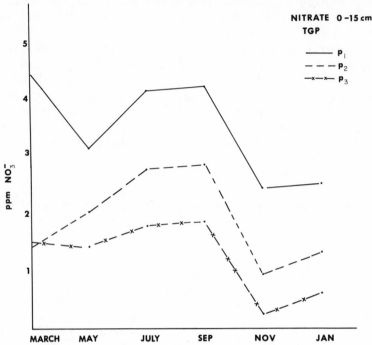

Fig. 12. Amounts of nitrate nitrogen in top 15 cm of soil in relation to old-field succession in tall-grass prairie area of Oklahoma. Symbols as in Fig. 9. (Data from Rice and Pancholy, 1972.)

was the very low number of *Nitrobacter* that occurred in the climax stands in all vegetation types and all sampling periods with the exception of the June period in the tall-grass prairie. The number was often zero.

The inverse correlation between the amount of nitrate and the amount of ammonium nitrogen in all plots was striking. The amount of ammonium nitrogen increased from a low in the first successional stage to a high in the climax, whereas the amount of nitrate decreased from a high in the first successional stage to a low value in the climax. When the additional fact is considered that the counts of nitrifiers were high in the first successional stage and low in the climax, the obvious inference is that the nitrifiers were inhibited in the climax plots so that the ammonium nitrogen was not oxidized to nitrate as readily as in the successional stages. It was obvious from the general soil data (Rice and Pancholy, 1972) that the low rates of nitrification in the climax plots were not due to pH or textural differences. Moreover, the lack of definite trends in amounts of organic carbon in relation to succession in the oak–pine and post oak–blackjack areas indicated that the quantity of organic carbon was not responsible for the low rate of nitrification in the climax plots.

Data from all vegetation types investigated strongly supported our original hypothesis that many soils under climax vegetation are low in nitrate because of an inhibition of nitrification by climax plant species. Moreover, our data definitely indicated that inhibition of nitrification starts during old-field succession and increases in intensity as succession proceeds toward the climax. Data obtained during a second growing season were similar to those reported here, and thus supported the same conclusions (Rice and Pancholy, 1973).

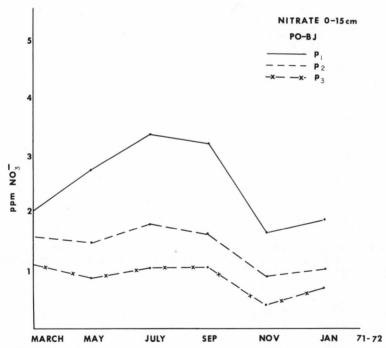

Fig. 13. Amounts of nitrate nitrogen in top 15 cm of soil in relation to old-field succession in post oak–blackjack oak area of Oklahoma. Symbols as in Fig. 9. (Data from Rice and Pancholy, 1972.)

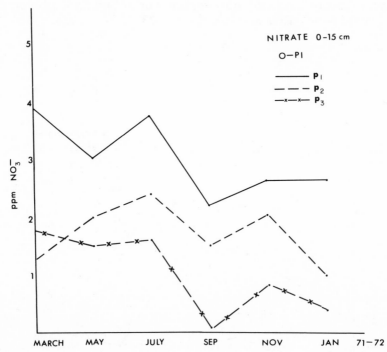

Fig. 14. Amounts of nitrate nitrogen in top 15 cm of soil in relation to old-field succession in oak–pine area of Oklahoma. Symbols as in Fig. 9. (Data from Rice and Pancholy, 1972.)

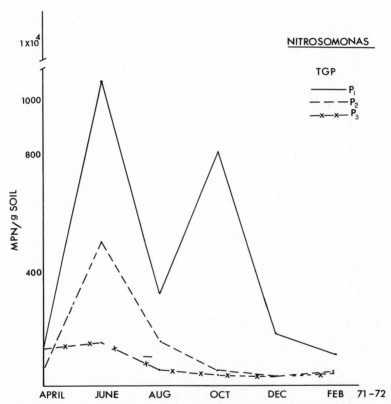

Fig. 15. Numbers of *Nitrosomonas* in top 15 cm of soil in relation to old-field succession in tall-grass prairie area of Oklahoma. MPN, most probable number. Other symbols as in Fig. 9. Each point is average of four analyses. (Data from Rice and Pancholy, 1972.)

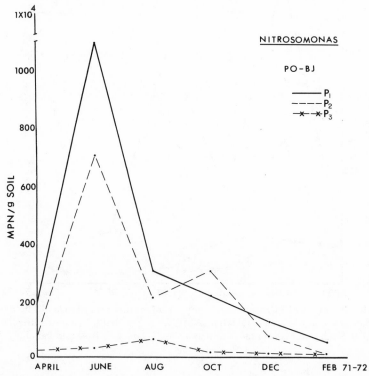

Fig. 16. Numbers of *Nitrosomonas* in top 15 cm of soil in relation to old-field succession in post oak–blackjack oak area of Oklahoma. Symbols as in Figs. 9 and 15. (Data from Rice and Pancholy, 1972.)

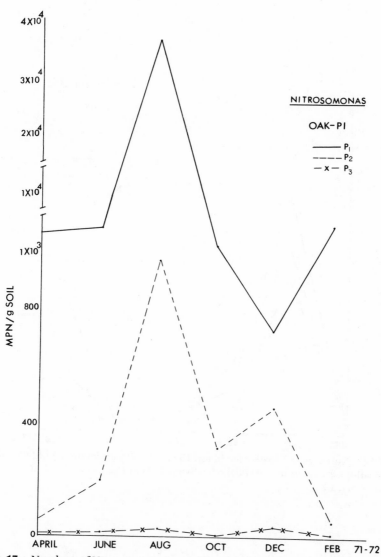

Fig. 17. Numbers of *Nitrosomonas* in top 15 cm of soil in relation to old-field succession in oak–pine area of Oklahoma. Symbols as in Figs. 9 and 15. (Data from Rice and Pancholy, 1972.)

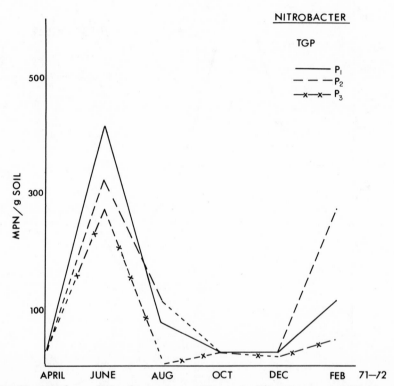

Fig. 18. Numbers of *Nitrobacter* in top 15 cm of soil in relation to old-field succession in tall-grass prairie area of Oklahoma. Symbols as in Figs. 9 and 15. (Data from Rice and Pancholy, 1972.)

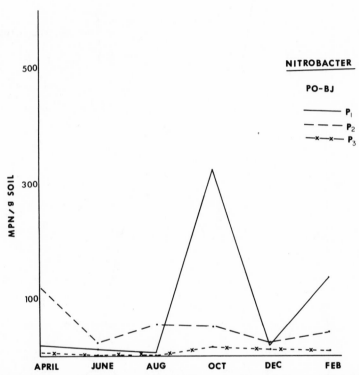

Fig. 19. Numbers of *Nitrobacter* in top 15 cm of soil in relation to old-field succession in post oak–blackjack oak area of Oklahoma. Symbols as in Figs. 9 and 15. (Data from Rice and Pancholy, 1972.)

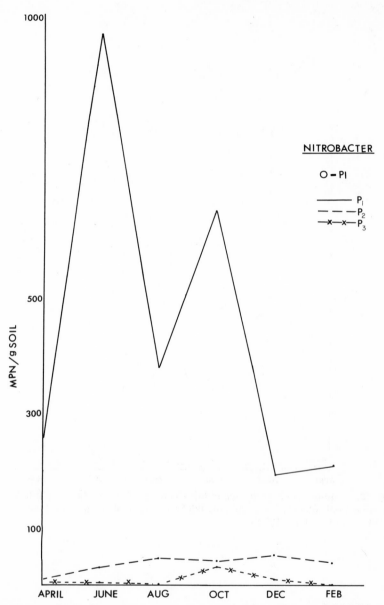

Fig. 20. Numbers of *Nitrobacter* in top 15 cm of soil in relation to old-field succession in oak–pine area of Oklahoma. Symbols as in Figs. 9 and 15. (Data from Rice and Pancholy, 1972.)

IV. CONCLUSIONS

The evidence from many geographic areas and vegetation types indicate that inhibition of nitrification by vegetation is a widespread phenomenon. It appears that inhibition of nitrification increases with the progress of succession toward the climax, and is particularly strong in climax ecosystems. I feel this may be almost a universal occurrence in climax ecosystems owing to selection pressures resulting from the conservation of energy and nitrogen.

It appears likely also that the greater inhibition of nitrification in the later stages of old-field succession aids in the buildup of available nitrogen in the form of ammonium nitrogen, which finally enables the higher nitrogen-requiring climax species to invade.

6

Roles of Allelopathy in Fire Cycle in California Annual Grasslands

I. GENERAL DISCUSSION OF FIRE CYCLE

According to Muller *et al.* (1968), there are large areas of a dense shrubby sclerophyllous vegetation called chaparral in hills and mountains of California. This chaparral is characterized by deep-rooted species and has many aspects depending on topography, parent material, and depth of soil accumulation. Some areas consist of complex mixtures of many species and some may have virtually a pure stand of one species. These investigators pointed out that common species in the chaparral are *Adenostoma fasciculatum*, *Arctostaphylos* spp., *Ceanothus* spp., *Cercocarpus betuloides*, *Dendromecon rigida*, *Heteromeles arbutifolia*, *Lepechinia calycina*, *Pickeringia montana*, *Prunus ilicifolia*, *Quercus dumosa*, *Rhus ovata*, and *Salvia mellifera*. All of these may occur in a relatively small area in many different combinations. *Umbellularia californica* may occur in association with the chaparral along drainage ditches, and *Artemisia californica* is common in some disturbed areas. According to Muller *et al.* (1968), these are not typically chaparral species. Horton and Kraebel (1955) reported that chaparral dominated by chamise, *Adenostoma fasciculatum*, is one of the most abundant associations in the southern California mountains below an elevation of 6000 feet. They occur principally on south-facing slopes, but occasionally on north-facing ones. Chamise chaparral varies from dense stands of chamise and ceanothus, *Ceanothus* spp., to open stands of chamise and black sage, *Salvia mellifera*. According to Horton and Kraebel, the most commonly associated species are hoaryleaf ceanothus (*Ceanothus crassifolius*) and several species of manzanita (*Arctostaphylos* spp.), *Salvia*, and *Eriogonum*.

Fires are frequent in the chaparral, and shrubs commonly found there have certain characteristics enabling them to survive the fires. Some regenerate rapidly from underground rhizomes and burls, some have rapid seed germination after the fires, and some have both characteristics. A few species are killed by fire and seedlings of these species are usually more abundant after fires than seedlings of sprouting species (Horton and Kraebel, 1955).

In the southern California chaparral, fire usually consumes the crowns of the vegetation in addition to the litter on the ground, and many branches an inch or more in diameter are left as snags (Horton and Kraebel, 1955). The soil may be covered with ashes or the ashes may be sparse, as is usual in the chamise chaparral.

The climate in the chamise chaparral area is a Mediterranean one with a rainy season in winter and spring and a long, dry summer and fall (McPherson and Muller, 1969). Fires occur most often in the dry season and little or no plant growth occurs until the next rainy season begins. At that time new growth begins from underground parts of some shrubs and seeds of many shrubs germinate rapidly and in great profusion. McPherson and Muller (1969) stated that they have never found seedlings of several shrubs, such as chamise and black sage, except following fire or disturbance involving removal of the shrubs.

Seeds of herbaceous species germinate in large numbers also following the start of the rainy season after a fire has occurred (Horton and Kraebel, 1955; McPherson and Muller, 1969). This is particularly striking because mature chaparral usually has few or no herbaceous species. Herbaceous plants are definitely the most prominent in the first growing season following a fire, and these consist of annual herbs, biennials, bulb-forming perennials, and short-lived subshrubs. In the second growing season following a fire, weedy, introduced herbaceous species appear, and a rapid decrease in numbers and vigor of herbs begins after the second growing season (McPherson and Muller, 1969). McPherson and Muller cited a study by Sampson (1944) in which he found that the herb population declined in the fifth growing season to about 25% of the first-year maximum. Seven to nine years after a fire, only a very few seeds of herbaceous species germinated. Subshrubs achieved their maximum prominence during the third and fourth seasons and then slowly declined. By about 12 years after a fire very few herbaceous plants or subshrubs remained.

A very similar cycle was found after fires in the chamise chaparral (Horton and Kraebel, 1955). These workers found that shoots from surviving root crowns of the dominant shrubs often reached almost their maximum height in 5 years and most reached maximum height in at least 10–15 years. Seedlings of these species attained almost maximum height in 20 years. In general, the chaparral regains almost the same composition and appearance in 10–15 years after a fire as it had before.

It appears that the herbs coming in during the first year arise from seeds that have remained dormant since the preceding fire, except for the perennials that arise from bulbs. Some of the most common annual plants that appear in the first growing season after a fire are species of *Brassica, Bromus, Chorizanthe, Cryptantha, Emmenanthe, Festuca, Lotus, Oenothera, Phacelia,* and *Pterostegia* (Horton and Kraebel, 1955). Common herbaceous perennials are species of *Brodiaea, Chlorogalum, Convolvulus, Eriophyllum, Gnaphalium, Hazardia, Lupinus, Nama, Penstemon,* and *Scutellaria* (Horton and Kraebel, 1955; Muller *et al.*, 1968). Species of some of these genera and numerous species of other genera become very important in the second to fifth years after a fire. Horton and Kraebel found that the annual grass species, *Bromus rubens, B. tectorum,* and *Festuca megalura,* were somewhat slower to develop in importance after fire than many native annuals. The greatest abundance of these annual grasses was reached in the third to fifth year after a fire.

There has been much speculation as to the reasons for the rapid appearance of annual and perennial herbs after a fire and their disappearance after the revival of the shrubs. Most speculation has involved all types of competitive activities by the dominant shrubs (Muller *et al.*, 1968). Observations by Dr. C. H. Muller were not adequately explained by the idea of competitive suppression of the herbs by the shrubs. This caused him, many of his students, and some of his colleagues to become engaged in a long series of well-conceived, well-planned, and well-executed experiments to elucidate the reasons for the fire cycle (Muller *et al.*, 1964, 1968; Muller and Muller, 1964; C. H. Muller, 1965, 1966, 1969, 1970; W. H. Muller, 1965; Muller and del Moral, 1966; McPherson and Muller, 1969; Chou and Muller, 1972).

II. EVIDENCE FOR ROLE OF ALLELOPATHY

A. Chemical Inhibition by *Salvia* and *Artemisia*

Muller *et al.* (1964) became intrigued with the striking patterns of vegetation in and around patches of *Salvia leucophylla* and *Artemisia californica* in the California annual grasslands (Fig. 21). Vir-

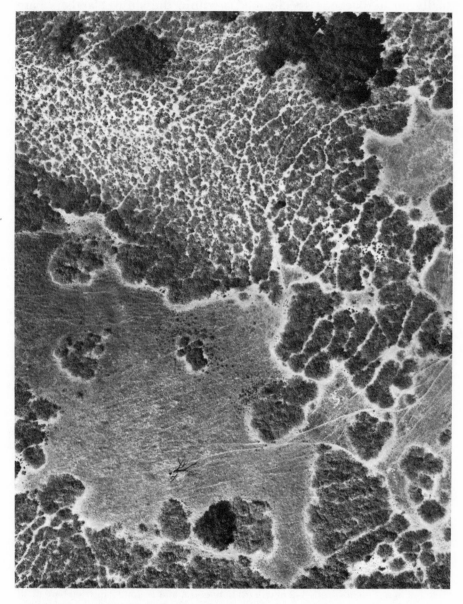

Fig. 21. Aerial photograph of intermixed *Salvia leucophylla* and *Artemisia californica* invading annual grassland in the Santa Ynez Valley, California. This pattern is widespread on Zaca clay soils. (From Muller, 1966.)

tually no herbaceous species occur within the shrub stands, a bare
zone approximately 1–2 m wide occurs around the stands, a zone
about 3–8 m wide containing stunted plants of *Bromus mollis, Erodium cicutarium,* and *Festuca megalura* occurs around the bare zone,
and this is surrounded by normal grassland (Fig. 22). The grassland
consists chiefly of *Avena fatua, Bromus mollis, B. rigidus, B. rubens,
Erodium cicutarium,* and *Festuca megalura* (Muller, 1966).

The zonation did not appear to be correlated in any way with edaphic factors because the shrub thickets spread onto the deeper soils of
grasslands even though they often center on areas of shallow, rocky
soil (Muller, 1966). Trenches dug across contact zones revealed no
recognizable soil differences between adjacent shrub and grass areas.
The inhibition extended far beyond the range of the shrub roots also.
Soil analyses indicated that no consistent differences in mineral content or physical factors occurred in the different zones (Muller, 1966).
There was no evidence of salinity stress in any of the zones. Results

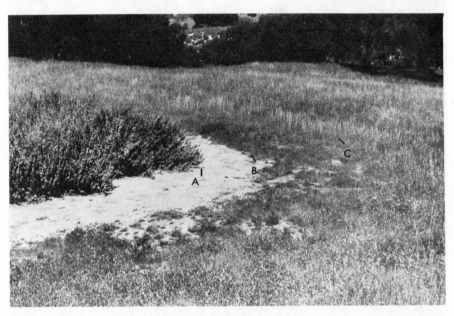

Fig. 22. *Salvia leucophylla* producing differential composition in annual grassland:
(1) to left of A, *Salvia* shrubs 1–2 m tall; (2) between A and B, zone 2 m wide bare of all
herbs except a few tiny seedlings of same age as the large herbs to the right; (3) between
B and C, zone of inhibited grassland consisting of several grass species but lacking
Bromus rigidus and *Avena fatua;* (4) to right of C, uninhibited grassland with large
plants of numerous grass species including *Bromus rigidus* and *Avena fatua.* (From
Muller, 1966.)

from addition of cattle droppings reinforced the conclusion that mineral deficiencies were not involved. There was no response to the manure in the bare zone; a slight increase in vigor resulted in the inhibited zone, and a great increase in growth and vigor resulted in the uninhibited zone. Observations and measurements during periods of very favorable moisture indicated that the differential growth was maintained and thus eliminated moisture as the determining factor in initiating and maintaining the observed zones.

The possibility of predation damage was investigated, and it was found that there was some damge to seedlings during the first few days of growth, especially by the golden-crowned sparrow, *Zonotrichia atricapilla,* and more near the shrubs than away from them (Muller, 1966). When individual seedlings were marked along permanent transects, it was found that few seedlings were totally lost to grazing, that many seedlings remained stunted even if they were protected from grazing damage, and that some inhibition zones showed no grazing damage at all. It was concluded that grazing by small animals may augment the effect of inhibition, but it cannot initiate or maintain the zones of inhibition.

The evidence suggested that chemical inhibitors might be responsible for the zones, so investigations were made to check this possibility. It was noted that inhibition zones on the uphill side of *Salvia* thickets were about equal to those on the downhill side. This indicated that water-soluble inhibitors could not account for the bare or retarded zones, and suggested the possiblity of volatile inhibitors being involved.

An assay technique was developed in which assay seeds were placed between sheets of filter paper on a moist sponge on the floor of a storage dish of 500 ml capacity. Two beakers, each containing 1 gm of the plant material to be assayed, were placed in the storage dish beside the sponge. The dish was covered with parafilm and incubated at 25°–28°C for 48–96 hours, depending on the assay seeds. Results with cucumber, *Cucumis sativus,* were always recorded as the average length of radicles produced by the germinating seeds in 48 hours (Muller, 1966). Initial experiments indicated that leaves of *Salvia leucophylla, S. apiana,* and *Artemisia californica* produced volatile inhibitors of root growth of cucumber and *Avena fatua* seedlings (Muller *et al.,* 1964). Roots of *Salvia leucophylla* failed to inhibit the growth of cucumber seedlings even when the filter paper on which the cucumber seedlings were growing was in contact with the roots. Muller and Muller (1964) identified six terpenes in ether extracts of leaves of each of three species of *Salvia, S. leucophylla, S. apiana,* and

S. *mellifera,* using gas chromatography. The identified terpenes were α-pinene, β-pinene camphene, camphor, cineole, and dipentene. The same compounds were identified also from the atmosphere in dishes in which leaves of the species were sealed.

The identified terpenes were tested for inhibitory activity against root growth of cucumber seedlings. A measured amount of each was placed separately on filter-paper disks, and each disk containing a terpene was placed in a beaker inside a container with a moist sponge and filter paper on which were placed soaked cucumber seeds as previously described. The containers were sealed, and after 48 hours at 28°C the lengths of the radicles were measured. Muller and Muller (1964) found that all the terpenes were toxic, with camphor being most toxic and the two pinenes the least toxic. When equal amounts of leaves of the three *Salvia* species were placed separately in sealed containers of the same size, the order based on decreasing inhibitory activity was S. *mellifera,* S. *leucophylla,* and S. *apiana.* This was the same order as that based on decreasing amounts of terpenes emanating from the leaves. They concluded, therefore, that inhibition of growth of annual grassland species in and around *Salvia* thickets is due to the production of volatile terpenes.

C. H. Muller (1965) collected air samples from among leafy branches of *Salvia leucophylla* and S. *mellifera* in the field and identified cineole and camphor from these samples. The same two compounds were identified consistently from air around S. *leucophylla* in the greenhouse and from the liquid collected in a dry ice-cold trap in the field when air was forced through the trap near *Salvia* patches.

Muller *et al.* (1964) suggested that the method of deposition of the terpenes on inhibited plants might be in dew; they collected artificial dew from cooling coils near a group of *Salvia* plants in the greenhouse and found that the artificial dew was slightly toxic in some tests to the growth of roots of cucumber seedlings. Later, C. H. Muller (1965) decided that perhaps the terpenes might accumulate in the seedling cuticle because oils and waxes are efficient solvents for volatile terpenes. He proceeded to test this possibility by injecting air from a flask containing *Salvia leucophylla* leaves into sealed flasks containing unbroken ampoules of granulated paraffin. Immediately after this air was injected, a 1 ml sample was withdrawn to determine the original concentration and the jars were shaken to break the ampoules in order to release the paraffin. Aliquots of 1 ml were withdrawn subsequently at 5 and 45 minutes after the original injection of terpene containing air into the flasks. The results indicated that there was a rapid uptake of the terpenes by the paraffin (Fig. 23).

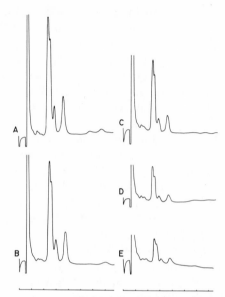

Fig. 23. Extraction of vapors of *Salvia leucophylla* terpenes from atmosphere by paraffin: (A) control at beginning of experiment; (B) control at end of experiment; (C) treatment at beginning of experiment; (D) treatment after 5 minutes' exposure to paraffin; (E) treatment after 45 minutes' exposure to paraffin. (From C. H. Muller, 1965.)

C. H. Muller (1965) suggested from the evidence just presented that the volatile terpenes may dissolve in the cuticular layer of the epidermis or mesophyll cells (Scott *et al.*, 1948) and then pass through the plasmodesmata into the insides of the cells. He suggested further that in young leaves where formation of the cuticle is still in progress, the terpenes may dissolve in fatty acids and lipids present on the exposed cell wall surfaces, in the adjacent plasma membranes, and in the cytoplasm.

Muller and del Moral (1966) suggested a third possible method by which the volatile terpenes may be absorbed or adsorbed and brought in contact with the affected plants. Dr. Muller had noted from the beginning of his work on the zonation around certain shrubs in the chaparral that the patterns were most pronounced in fine-textured soil and particularly on heavy Zaca clay soils, which are widely distributed in the Santa Ynez Valley where he did most of his research. He and del Moral hypothesized, therefore, that perhaps the volatile terpenes may be adsorbed on colloidal material in soil and come into contact in this way with roots of affected plants. They obtained Zaca clay from gopher mounds in grassland portions of the patterned area and placed aliquots of this soil in vacuum flasks. The side arms of the flasks were stoppered with rubber serum caps, and the mouths were sealed with rubber stoppers wrapped in cellophane to reduce solution of atmospheric terpenes in the rubber. The soil was kept air dried in some flasks, moist to field capacity in others, and still others had layers of 5-mm glass beads to serve as controls. A measured amount of air obtained from a flask containing fresh *Salvia leucophylla* leaves was injected into each of the test flasks. A 1 ml sample was taken from each flask immediately to determine the initial concentrations, and other 1 ml samples were analyzed at 10 minutes and 1 hour after the original injection of air containing terpenes. The results clearly indicated that the terpenes were adsorbed by the soil and a greater amount was adsorbed by dry soil than by moist soil (Fig. 24).

Subsequently, Zaca clay soil was dried, some was exposed to *Salvia* volatiles for 18 hours (heavily charged), and some for 1 hour (lightly charged). The soil was moistened to field capacity, and *Bromus rigidus* seeds were planted in aliquots of the charged soils and sealed in containers. Controls consisted of flasks of similar soil not exposed to *Salvia* terpenes. All the flasks were kept in darkness for 48 hours at 25°C, after which the germination percentage and root growth were determined. No germination occurred in the heavily charged soil when assayed immediately. Therefore, open containers of the heavily charged soil were kept in a growth chamber for 2 months and assayed again. Germination reached 43% this time and growth of roots averaged only 7% of that of the controls. The lightly charged soil was very inhibitory to radicle growth of *Bromus rigidus* seedlings when assayed immediately and was still inhibitory 4 months later when root growth of seedlings in test soil was only 60% of control growth (Fig.

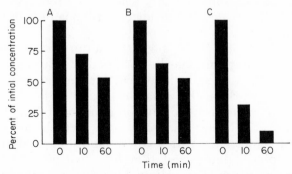

Fig. 24. Rate of terpene adsorption by soils: (A) control, 5 mm glass beads; (B) moist soil; (C) dry soil. Each sampled initially and at 10 and 60 minutes. Each quantity is expressed as percent of initial concentration. (From Muller and del Moral, 1966.)

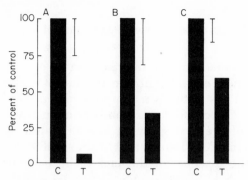

Fig. 25. Bioassay of lightly charged soils: (A) and (B), results of two typical preparations, assayed immediately; (C) assay of soil from B after four months' storage. The
quantity of growth under each treatment is expressed as percent of a simultaneous
control. Least significant difference at 5% confidence interval is shown by vertical
lines. (From Muller and del Moral, 1966.)

25). It was clear from these experiments that the volatile terpenes
from *Salvia* which were adsorbed on soil remained in an active state
and that they migrated from the surfaces of soil particles to the sites of
inhibition within the plants.

Based on all investigations to this point in time, Muller and del
Moral summarized as follows their inferences as to the steps by which
Salvia and other volatile terpene-producing plants initiate and perpet-
uate the patterns of zonation. (1) Terpenes are evolved into the air at a
maximum rate during periods of high temperatures and are adsorbed
in greatest amounts at this time by the soil because the period of
highest temperatures corresponds to the period of driest soils. (2) The
terpenes are held on the soil at least until the early part of the following growing season. (3) Seeds and seedlings in contact with the ter-
pene-containing soils extract some of the terpenes by solution in cutin
which is in direct contact with the soil particles. (4) The terpenes are
transported into the cells by means of the phospholipids in the plasmodesmata.

Muller (1966) analyzed numerous species of plants from the chaparral for production of volatile terpenes and found that, in addition to
the species of *Salvia* and *Artemisia* previously discussed, the following species produce high amounts of terpenes: *Lepechinia calycina,
Heteromeles arbutifolia, Prunus ilicifolia, Prunus lyoni, Umbellularia californica,* and *Artemisia tridentata.* All of these species
proved to be toxic in the usual assay tests. Many of these are common
species in the chaparral as previously indicated.

B. Allelopathic Effects of *Adenostoma fasciculatum*

The most common dominant in the chaparral of southern California, *Adenostoma fasciculatum,* is not on the list of producers of volatile terpenes and still has virtually a complete absence of herbs in mature stands (Fig. 26). Of course, large numbers of such species come in at the beginning of the first growing season following a fire, as previously pointed out. McPherson and Muller (1969) decided, therefore, to investigate the reasons for the lack of herbaceous species in the

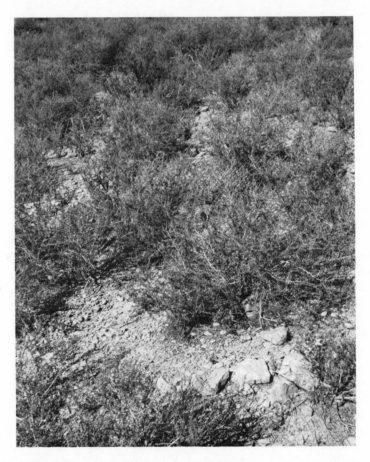

Fig. 26. Overview of relatively young (12 years since burning) open stand of *Adenostoma fasciculatum* showing bare ground between shrubs. (From McPherson and Muller, 1969.)

chamise stands. Initial experiments were designed to determine if the lack of herbs might be due to a deficiency of minerals. Excavations showed that the root system of chamise is directed downward and that there are very few roots in the upper part of the soil. Moreover, herbs grew readily on disturbed areas where the organic horizons were removed. Test plots were fertilized also at the rate of 33 lb of nitrogen, 55 lb of phosphoric acid, and 22 lb of potassium per acre plus traces of calcium, iron, manganese, sulfur, and zinc. Subsequent sampling in mid-January, when most herbs had germinated in the general study area, showed that there were no differences in the fertilizer plots and in the control areas. A second sampling about 1 month later indicated a decline in numbers of herbs per square meter in both areas, and there was no increase in size of herbs in treated or control areas since the January sampling time. Addition of ashes from burned chamise, in about the same amounts as result from fires, had no effect on numbers or growth of herbaceous plants.

Four clearings (6 × 6 m) were made in stands of chamise by cutting off the tops 5–10 cm above the soil in August. The tops were removed and the clearings were fenced to prevent small animals from entering the clearings. Comparable areas of undisturbed brush were fenced in the same way to serve as control areas. Sprouts formed from some chamise stumps in the areas soon after clearing. No herb growth occurred, however, until the first rain in early November. By the end of January large numbers of herbs were found in the cleared areas, but very few in the control areas. Twenty-nine herbaceous species were found in the cleared areas and only a few in the control areas (Table 24). An average of 40 seedlings/m² occurred under the shrubs, and they were stunted and visible only with careful searching. Herb populations on the clearings averaged over 1000/m², and these developed normally, reaching several times the sizes of the same species under the shrubs. The herb populations in the control plots reached a peak in mid-December, remained constant until late January, and then declined through the rest of the growing season. Herb numbers in the clearings continued to increase until late January and then remained almost constant (Fig. 27). There was no alteration in mineral supply in this experiment, furnishing more evidence that the lack of herbs in mature chamise stands is not due to mineral depletion by chamise.

Light did not appear to McPherson and Muller to be a critical factor because of the open nature of many chamise stands, but they investigated this factor anyway. They found a luxuriant ground cover of various herbaceous species in a grove of *Quercus agrifolia* and *Arbutus menziesii* near their study sites. They measured light intensity

TABLE 24

Species Occurring as Seedlings in the Clearing Experiment and Its Control Shrub Stands [a,b]

Species	A	B	C	D
Annual Herbs				
Allophyllum glutinosum			×	
Apiastrum angustifolium			×	×
Bromus rubens		×	×	×
Calandrinia ciliata	×		×	
Chorizanthe staticoides		×	×	
Conyza canadensis		×	×	
Cryptantha clevelandii		×	×	
Cryptantha micromeres		×	×	
Cynosurus echinatus		×	×	
Daucus pusillus			×	
Eucrypta chrysanthemifolia			×	
Festuca octoflora	×		×	×
Filago californica	×	×	×	×
Hemizonia ramosissima		×	×	
Lotus strigosus		×	×	
Oenothera micrantha			×	×
Phacelia grandiflora			×	
Silene multinervia		×	×	
Tillaea erecta	×		×	
Bulb-forming Herbs				
Brodiaea pulchella	×	×	×	×
Chlorogalum pomeridianum	×		×	×
Other perennial Herbs				
Convolvulus cyclostegius		×	×	
Eriophyllum confertiflorum		×	×	
Gnaphalium californicum		×	×	
Scutellaria tuberosa			×	×
Shrubs				
Adenostoma fasciculatum			×	
Helianthemum scoparium		×	×	
Lotus scoparius	×	×	×	×
Salvia mellifera			×	

[a] Modified from McPherson and Muller (1969).

[b] Species also found by Sweeney (1956) as fire response herbs in Lake County, California are indicated, At least five occurrences by a species are required for an entry under the presence heading, the only exception being disturbed site entries which were based on close observation: (A) in undisturbed *Adenostoma fasciculatum* stands; (B) in disturbed sites; (C) in experimental clearings; (D) on Sweeney's list.

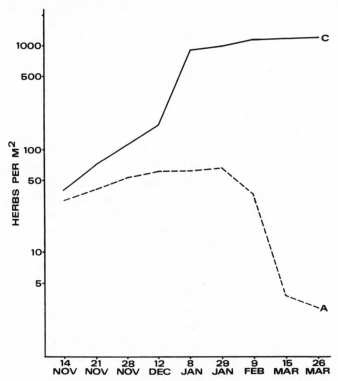

Fig. 27. Herb populations in experimental clearings and controls during the 1966–1967 growing season (C, in clearings; A, in adjacent, undisturbed *Adenostoma fasciculatum* stands). (From McPherson and Muller, 1969.)

at 1 dm above ground along a transect in the chamise chaparral and along a similar transect in the *Quercus–Arbutus* stand, except measurements were taken at 4 dm above ground to prevent shading of the light meter by the herbs. Light values were uniformly low along the transect in the *Quercus–Arbutus* stand with most values being less than 30% of full sunlight. Nevertheless, thriving plants of several herbaceous species were present along the entire transect. On the other hand, light values were relatively high on the average in the chamise stand with a mean approaching 65% of full sunlight. Actually, values equal to full sunlight were found to alternate with lower values. Virtually no herbaceous plants were found along the entire transect in spite of the relatively good light conditions.

Light requirements of fire-response species were checked further by placing artificial shading devices over parts of freshly cleared areas. Sampling of the shaded and unshaded cleared areas during the following growing season indicated no differences in size and numbers of herbs in the two areas. They concluded that light competition cannot account for the lack of herbs in chamise stands.

McPherson and Muller felt that competition for soil moisture was not an important factor in the exclusion of herbaceous species from the chamise stands because of the deep root systems of chamise and the fact that the rainfall pattern is such that annual plants suffer little from drought. Rainfall is generally confined to the winter months, and germination of most annuals outside the influence of shrubs occurs simultaneously within a few days after the season's first significant rain. They pointed out that during the germination period, soils are near field capacity throughout the region and thus differences in soil moisture could not account for the differential germination. Droughts of sufficient magnitudes to kill annuals are uncommon. In spite of logical evidence against soil moisture as a determining factor in the absence of herbs in chamise stands, McPherson and Muller investigated the possibility further. They measured soil moisture in chamise stands and in adjacent stands of herbaceous plants along roadsides throughout a growing season and found no appreciable differences. At no time did the soil moisture values in either type of stand get as low as the wilting ranges of the soils involved.

Counts of herbaceous seedlings in fenced and unfenced areas within the chamise chaparral indicated that small animals have a slight impact on numbers of herbs in such areas. However, when the number of herbs per square meter in the cleared area (over 1000) was compared with the number per square meter in the fenced uncleared area (70), it was obvious that the effect of the animals was slight compared with the effect of the shrub.

McPherson and Muller (1969) stated that several workers had demonstrated that seeds of many of the chaparral shrub species are stimulated to germinate by heating, but that seeds of fire-response herbs do not appear to be stimulated by heat. They decided to determine what effect heat would have on the soil–litter–seed system of chaparral in field and laboratory tests. According to these workers, Sweeney (1956) found that 70°C was near the middle of the temperature range encountered in chaparral soils at 1 cm depth during fires. Therefore, they heated the soil of several plots to 70°C and then allowed it to cool. The heating was done in August and seedling counts were made in late February. The seedling counts in the heated plots averaged 712 seedlings/m², whereas the control plots averaged only 70 seedlings/m². More species occurred in the heated plots also. A laboratory experiment was run also at temperatures of 40°, 60°, and 80°C, plus unheated controls. Seedlings were counted 66 days later and much larger numbers were found in the soil heated to 80°C. No significant differences were found between any other treatments. They inferred from the field and laboratory experiments that heat either stimulated germination of some of the herbaceous species or degraded some germination-inhibiting substance in the soil. Subsequent experiments agreed with results of others that heat does not stimulate germination of fire-response herbs. Thus, McPherson and Muller inferred that heating degraded some inhibitor or inhibitors in the soil. All the evidence to this point suggested an allelopathic mechanism of herb suppression. Tests were initiated, therefore, to determine if tops of chamise produce water-soluble toxic materials. Chamise does not produce volatile terpenes as was previously stated.

Aqueous extracts of the leaves of *Adenostoma fasciculatum* were found to inhibit growth of roots of seedlings of *Bromus rigidus* in the usual moist-sponge bioassay procedure, but similar extracts of roots had no effect. Aqueous extracts of stems of chamise, with and without a common lichen encrustation, had no effect on root growth of *Bromus rigidus*, but fresh leaves of chamise placed in direct contact with the seedbed in the bioassay did significantly inhibit *Bromus* roots.

A leachate of leafy branches of chamise obtained by means of artificial rain in the laboratory was very inhibitory to root growth of *Bromus rigidus*, after the leachate was evaporated to about one-ninth of its original volume in a flash evaporator. Leachates of chamise collected in the field from intact plants, both from artificial and natural rainfall, were inhibitory to *Bromus* in the assay. When leachate was applied to surface soil collected in one of the field sites and the soil was then used in the bioassay, it was found to be inhibitory to *Bromus* also.

Bromus rigidus is not of much importance in the fire cycle, so McPherson and Muller decided to try some true fire-response species in similar assays. By scarifying seeds, they were able to obtain satisfactory assays with *Calandrinia ciliata, Helianthemum scoparium*, and *Silene multinervia*. All were found to be inhibited in both seed germination and root growth by natural rainfall leachate of chamise tops. This was particularly striking because germination of *Bromus rigidus* was not affected in any of the tests. Moreover, root growth of seedlings of *Helianthemum* and *Silene* was much more markedly reduced by the leachate than was that of *Bromus rigidus*.

McPherson and Muller concluded from their experiments that (1) leaves of mature *Adenostoma fasciculatum* shrubs accumulate toxins on their surfaces during the dry summer season; (2) these toxins are washed off the leaves by the rains which initiate a new growing season; (3) the toxins are retained in the soil and possibly in the upper 1–3 cm; (4) additional increments of toxins are added with each rain; (5) most seeds in the soil of mature chamise stands are prevented from germinating by the toxins; (6) seeds of a few resistant species do germinate but the seedlings usually fail to mature and reproduce; (7) under natural circumstances, these conditions continue until a fire consumes the aerial parts of the shrubs; (8) natural degradation of the toxin has eliminated it before and during the fire; (9) seeds of the fire-response species, which have been present in the soil and inhibited from germinating, are able to germinate as soon as rain comes; (10) during the early phases of recovery from fire, the aerial parts of chamise are reduced in size and thus in toxin output; (11) herbs continue to flourish for a few years; and (12) toxin production increases with regrowth of leafy crowns on the chamise and the level of toxin is finally sufficient to provide the suppression of herbs which occurs in mature stands.

C. Allelopathic Effects of *Arctostaphylos*

Species of *Arctostaphylos* (manzanita) are other important shrubs in the California chaparral that do not produce volatile inhibitors (Muller *et al.*, 1968). These investigators found, however, that *Arctostaphylos glauca* and *A. glandulosa* inhibit herbs for a distance of 1–2 m from the edge of the drip lines of their canopies. This results in a virtually bare zone between the shrubs and adjacent grassland which is occupied only by a few species of perennial herbs. Sampling of transects at right angles to lines of contact demonstrated an inverse correlation between litter and density of seedlings of herbs (Table 25). Pure

TABLE 25

Relationship of Herb Seedling Populations to Litter Cover about the Margins of *Arctostaphylos glauca* Stands [a]

Distance from canopy edge (m)	0.0	0.5	1.0	2.0	4.0	8.0
Cover by litter (%)	55	22	18	3	8	1
Seedlings per m²	30	60	60	620	1210	2650

[a] From Muller *et al.* (1968).

stands of either of the species of *Arctostaphylos,* as well as mixed chaparral stands having significant amounts of *Arctostaphylos,* have the same dearth of herbs as chamise stands. Leaf litter of both species of *Arctostaphylos* was found to contain water-soluble inhibitors of seed germination and seedling growth. Leachate from uninjured foliar branches was found to be inhibitory also.

Based on results of the early experiments on species of *Arctostaphylos,* Chou and Muller (1972) decided to investigate more thoroughly the allelopathic effects of *A. glandulosa* var. *zacaensis.* This shrub occurs in extensive pure stands on Zaca Ridge in the San Rafael Mountains of California. The same type of zonation occurs around these stands as described above, and initial experiments were designed to determine if the zones could be due to differences in mineral levels or pH. The mineral elements sodium, copper, zinc, manganese, iron, nitrogen, phosphorus, and potassium were determined. In general, the mineral content in the shrub soil was higher than in herb zone soil except for sodium and manganese. There was no significant difference, however, in total exchangeable bases and the pH was virtually the same in both areas. There was a considerably higher organic matter content in the shrub soil (29%) than in the bare zone soil (9–18%) or the herb zone soil (5%).

Competition for light was evaluated next by Chou and Muller. They found no herbs under or between *Arctostaphylos* shrubs even when the canopies were very open (as little as 50% covered). Moreover, herbs remained absent in artificially cleared quadrats during the first growing season. Additionally, zones around *Arctostaphylos* often lacked any herbs even though some of these bare zones were observed several years earlier to have a dense cover of annual herbs. They concluded that light was not the limiting factor in herb growth.

They investigated the distribution of *Arctostaphylos* roots in the soil and found them to be distributed principally at depths between 20 and 70 cm. Only a few roots were found in the top 10 cm of soil where most of the herb roots are typically found. *Adenostoma* has a similar root distribution, and McPherson and Muller (1969) demonstrated that soil moisture was not important in the elimination of herbs from the chamise stands. Chou and Muller (1972) concluded from the evidence that soil moisture is not the deciding factor in the elimination of herbs from the manzanita stands or the bare zones around them, and that the overall similarity with the situation in chamise indicates a similar allelopathic role for manzanita.

Several plots, 10 × 15 m each, were marked in manzanita stands and the downhill half of each was cleared of shrubs in the summer.

The upper half of each was left as a control. The shrubs were cut off about 5 cm above the soil, and the tops were removed from the plots. Each plot was fenced to keep small animals out of both the control half and the cleared half. Stump sprouts were removed periodically from the cleared areas over the 3-year duration of the experiment.

Only four seedlings occurred in the total cleared area during the first year. There was one seedling of each of the following species: *Emmenanthe penduliflora, Avena fatua, Rhamnus californica,* and *Ceanothus oliganthus.* The density of seedlings in the cleared area the second year rose to 36/m², and fell again in the third growing season to about 15/m². These results strongly contrasted with the results from the clearing of *Adenostoma* because McPherson and Muller (1969) found a luxuriant growth of seedlings during the first growing season after clearing the chamise (1000 seedlings/m²). These differences suggested the presence of persistent phytotoxins in manzanita.

A zone 1.5–2 m broad in which no seed germination occurred developed adjacent to the control in each clearing during the third growing season. This zone contained many manzanita seedlings from the previous growing season, but no new seedlings appeared, in spite of the fact that they appeared abundantly elsewhere in the cleared areas during the third growing season. Clearing had thus caused favorable conditions for germination of *Arctostaphylos* seeds to occur for only 1 year in the zone next to mature *Arctostaphylos* plants, and the following year the toxin content of the soil had apparently already become too great for seeds of this species or any other to germinate. Chou and Muller concluded that waterborne toxins from the manzanita were probably responsible for the observed results.

They used seeds of *Bromus rigidus* and *Avena fatua* in their standard sponge or sand assay to determine whether aqueous extracts of various parts of *Arctostaphylos glandulosa* plants produce phytotoxins. They tested extracts of fresh fallen leaves, bark, roots, and pericarp, and they determined the osmotic concentration of each extract cryoscopically with an osmometer. Extracts of all parts were found to be inhibitory to some extent. Those of leaves and bark were most inhibitory, and the effects were not due to the osmotic concentrations. The osmotic concentrations of the pericarp extracts were so high, however, that Chou and Muller concluded that inhibition of *Bromus* and *Avena* in this case was probably due to the osmotic effect of the extracts.

Leachates of leafy branches of manzanita obtained by use of artificial rain were found to be inhibitory also, and this was not due to an osmotic effect.

Living leaves and leaf litter of different ages were collected in the field. The leaf litter was divided into three stages: the oldest was 2 years old and partially rotted, the youngest was less than 1 year old and partially intact, and the last was intermediate in age. Extracts of living leaves and youngest leaf litter inhibited root growth of test seedlings by 40% or more, extracts of leaf litter of intermediate age inhibited growth by 20%, and extracts of the oldest litter were only slightly inhibitory. Extracts of fresh leaf litter were tested against several important herbaceous species in the usual assay procedures, and all were greatly inhibited (Fig. 28).

Soil was collected from the shrub, bare, and herb zones in field plots; wetted to field capacity with distilled water; and used in assays with *Bromus rigidus*. The *Arctostaphylos* soil caused inhibitions in root growth of 15–20%, and the bare zone soil inhibited root growth by about 40%. Thus, Chou and Muller concluded that water-soluble toxins are leached out of the manzanita stands and accumulate in the bare zone soil downhill.

Numerous toxins were identified in leaves and leaf litter of manzanita, in the soil under manzanita, and in the bare zone. These will be discussed in Chapter 12 along with phytotoxins from many other

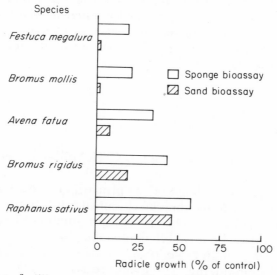

Fig. 28. Effect of a 5% aqueous extract of freshly fallen leaves on growth of various species in sand and sponge bioassays. Values are expressed as percent of distilled water controls. Tests are significantly different from control at 0.1% level. (From Chou and Muller, 1972.)

sources. One potent toxin identified in the leachate of leafy branches of *Arctostaphylos glandulosa* was hydroquinone. This was tested in the sand assay against *Avena fatua* and *Bromus rigidus,* and it inhibited root growth of both species in a concentration at least as low as 50 ppm, which was the lowest tested. Other identified inhibitors were tested against *Lactuca sativa* seedlings, and all were found to be inhibitory to root growth of that species.

Chou and Muller tested the effects of heat on the toxins in fresh leaf litter of *Arctostaphylos* by grinding the litter and exposing the ground material to various temperatures up to 240°C for 2 hours. The samples were subsequently extracted with distilled water (5 gm per 95 ml water), and the extracts were tested against *Bromus rigidus* in the sponge assay. Toxicity increased with heating up to 160°C, but rapidly declined after that and disappeared at 200°C. They concluded that the phytotoxins produced by *Arctostaphylos* can apparently be denatured under conditions of a severe fire, thus permitting the flush of herb growth which follows a fire in the chaparral.

Chou and Muller concluded from their many experiments that (1) the exclusion of herbaceous species from areas strongly influenced by *Arctostaphylos glandulosa* var. *zacaensis* clearly results from the allelopathic effects of this shrub; (2) the similarity of this mechanism to the mode of dominance exerted by *Adenostoma fasciculatum* is very close and establishes the proportionally equal involvement of these allelopathic mechanisms in the fire cycle in chaparral; and (3) the toxic effects of *Arctostaphylos* are somewhat greater and persist longer than those of *Adenostoma.*

III. CONCLUSIONS

I feel that the evidence obtained by C. H. Muller and his co-workers indicates overwhelmingly that allelopathic effects of numerous shrubs in the California chaparral are primarily responsible for the fire cycle. It seems clear to me that the chemical inhibition exerted by the mature shrubs is sufficient to prevent germination of seeds of most herbs, and that this chemical effect plus the competitive effects of the shrubs are great enough to keep any herbs which do germinate from maturing and reproducing. The evidence seems clear also that fires release the allelopathic effects of the shrubs by removing the sources of toxins and by destroying some of the toxins present in the soil and litter. Thus, a flush of herbs appears from seeds that have been dormant in the soil since the previous fire and which are no longer inhibited by toxins.

As the shrubs develop in prominence again after the fire, interference increases due to the increased addition of toxins and to competition that accentuates any inhibition caused by toxins.

7

Roles of Allelopathy in Patterning
of Vegetation and Creation
# of Bare Areas

I. CONCEPTS OF PATTERNING

The term patterning is used in a restricted sense by many ecologists to refer to a mathematical expression of the spatial distribution of organisms within a community. If the individuals of a species are regularly dispersed like plants in a corn field, the species is said to be hypodispersed or underdispersed; if the individuals of a species occur in clumps, the species is said to be hyperdispersed or aggregated; and finally, if the individuals of a species are so dispersed that mathematically each individual has an equal chance of occurring at any point within the area involved, the species is said to be randomly dispersed. I feel that this concept of patterning is very important, and I have used it often myself (Rice and Penfound, 1955). Obviously, in most instances one can determine the type of dispersion only by appropriate sampling procedures and mathematical treatment of the sampling data.

The term patterning has been widely used by ecologists also to refer to spatial arrangements of individuals which are visually apparent in the field, such as the zonation around *Artemisia absinthium* (Bode, 1940; Funke, 1943), *Helianthus annuus* (Wilson and Rice, 1968), *Salvia* spp., *Artemisia californica* (Muller *et al.*, 1964; Muller, 1966), and many other species. Naturally, the two concepts are interrelated because spatial distributions that result in visually obvious zones of distribution of individuals would be reflected in the type of mathematical expression of distribution based on appropriate sampling. In this chapter, I will use the term patterning to refer to the obvious zones of distribution of plants around individuals of selected species.

Since von Liebig (1843) stressed the importance of mineral nutrition in the growth of plants, most ecologists have attempted to explain the patterning of vegetation and the general distribution of plants largely on the basis of competition. Virtually none of the ecologists who have attributed specific patterns to competition have in any way eliminated the possibility of allelopathy as the primary cause. Of course, it is obviously easier to design experiments to eliminate competition than it is to eliminate allelopathy. It is interesting that most ecologists have assumed for many years that soil moisture and mineral levels are lower under trees than away from them, and the reverse has proved to be true for moisture in all our work in Oklahoma and often for minerals in the upper layers of soil where herbs root (Al-Naib and Rice, 1971; Lodhi and Rice, 1971). We have never found significantly lower amounts of minerals under trees than away from them, but the amounts are sometimes not significantly different in the two regions. Actually, it is logical that the moisture in the upper levels of soil under trees would remain higher than away from them, particularly in areas subject to water stress, because of the lower temperatures, higher humidities, and lower wind velocities under the trees and fewer roots generally in the upper levels of soil. It is illogical to assume that the virtually complete absence of herbs under many trees is due to shading also, because there are obviously many herbs that grow better in low light than in high light intensity. Thus, logic should cause one to infer that something other than competition is basically responsible for the absence of herbs in such cases. I should emphasize here again that competition probably plays a secondary role even if the basic cause of a particular patterning is allelopathy. The reinforcing effect of competition in retarding the growth of a plant once its germination and growth have been slowed by toxins should never be overlooked.

I will discuss in detail in this chapter several examples of patterning in which the primary cause has been fairly clearly demonstrated to be allelopathy. Certain other examples will be mentioned for historical reasons because the patterns were suggested to be due to allelopathy, even though insufficient evidence was available to support the statement.

Probably all allelopathic effects of any ecological significance would have some effect on the dispersion of plants in an area and thus on patterning, even though the effect might not be visually evident in the field. Lieth (1960) studied plant migration within a grassland community at Hohenheim, Germany by mapping the exact location of individuals over a period of a few years, and he found that individuals of all species migrate constantly. Thus, they do not stay in one spot even for a period of a year or two. This was true even of clones of bunch grasses. Lieth termed the phenomenon "internal crop rotation." Szczepańska (1971) compared this with the situation in agriculture where crops are rotated (by man) to prevent the soil sickness problem, which appears to be due to the contamination of the soil by toxins that are the products of metabolism and plant decomposition and not to the lack of nutrients. Szczepańska (1971) stated also that Nowinski (1961) believed that the type of internal rotation observed by Lieth is often due to autotoxins, especially in the case of perennials with clones expanding by vegetative growth in all directions. In some years, such clones divide on the outside into a number of separate individuals.

Selleck (1972) found in laboratory experiments that *Antennaria microphylla* and *Euphorbia esula* were inhibitory to seed germination and seedling growth of several species often associated with them in natural areas. Moreover, *A. microphylla* produced toxins inhibitory to the growth of *E. esula*. In field experiments also, the former was found to be very inhibitory to the latter. This was true also of soil formerly in contact with the roots of *A. microphylla*. He found that in natural stands of either of these species there is a paucity of growth of other forbs even when much bare gound is present. Selleck suggested, as a result of his research, that allelopathy is probably a significant influence in the interspatial relationships of species in most plant communities.

II. PATTERNING DUE TO ALLELOPATHIC EFFECTS OF HERBACEOUS SPECIES

A. *Helianthus rigidus*

Cooper and Stoesz (1931) observed the fairy-ring pattern of the prairie sunflower, *Helianthus rigidus* (= *H. scaberrimus*), which is due to a pronounced reduction in plant numbers, size, and inflorescences in the center of the clone. Curtis and Cottam (1950) observed the same phenomenon and became curious as to its cause. They located a group of plots within several of the fairy rings and manipulated them in different ways. Some had the soil removed and replaced without any other treatment, others had the soil removed and all roots and rhizomes taken out before the soil was replaced, a few plots were fertilized, and in several plots the soil was cleared away and replaced with soil taken from a spot in the prairie where there were no prairie sunflowers. They found that fertilizing or removing the soil and replacing it directly did not alter the growth of the sunflower. On the other hand, removal of roots and rhizomes of the prairie sunflower from the soil in the fairy rings or replacement with soil from outside the rings resulted in normal growth and flowering of the sunflower. They concluded that inhibition inside the clones resulted from autotoxins produced by decay of dead plant parts of the prairie sunflower.

B. Miscellaneous Species

Guyot *et al.* (1951) and Guyot (1957) investigated allelopathic effects of several important herbaceous species in old-field succession in southern France, and, based on these studies, they attributed the mosaiclike dominance patches of different species in successional communities to allelopathic influences of the dominant species in each patch.

C. *Helianthus annuus*

Wilson and Rice (1968) observed striking patterns of distribution of herbaceous species around individuals of the annual sunflower, *Helianthus annuus,* in the pioneer weed stage of old-field succession in Oklahoma as I discussed in Chapter 4 (Fig. 29 and Table 5). Field sampling through two growing seasons indicated that *Erigeron canadensis* and *Rudbeckia hirta* were significantly inhibited near *Helianthus annuus. Haplopappus ciliatus* and *Bromus japonicus* were slightly inhibited, but the effect was small and variable so it was not statistically significant. *Croton glandulosus* was stimulated in growth near sunflower plants, but the variability was such that the effect over the 2 year period was not statistically significant.

The patterns around annual sunflower plants could not have been due to light competition because they were the same on all sides of the sunflower plants, and these plants do not cast a very pronounced shadow anyway when growing alone. Analyses of pH and mineral elements reported to be most likely deficient in the soils involved

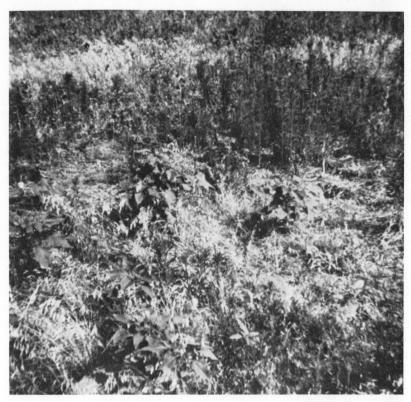

Fig. 29. Zonation of species around *Helianthus annuus* in field plots near Norman, Oklahoma. (Photographed by Dr. Roger Wilson, Miami University, Oxford, Ohio.) *Bromus japonicus* near sunflower; *Erigeron canadensis, Rudbeckia hirta,* and *Haplopappus ciliatus* in zone away from sunflower.

suggested that the zonation was not likely due to competition for minerals or pH.

Nevertheless, soil obtained near sunflower plants in the field was found to inhibit seed germination and growth of *Erigeron canadensis* and *Rudbeckia hirta* when compared with results in soil taken at least 1 m from sunflower plants, whether the soil was obtained in July or October from the field (Table 6). The soil collected in October after leaf fall was found to be inhibitory also to *Haplopappus ciliatus* and *Bromus japonicus*, but not to *Croton glandulosus* (Table 6). Results with soil taken near sunflower plants correlated well with the patterns around sunflower plants, even though no competition with sunflower was present. This suggested that some compounds must have been added to the soil by the sunflower while it was present, or, in other words, that the patterning might be due to allelopathy. Subsequent experiments indicated that small amounts of decaying sunflower leaves in soil were inhibitory to germination and growth of *Erigeron canadensis* and *Haplopappus ciliatus* and were inhibitory to growth of *Rudbeckia hirta* and *Bromus japonicus* (Table 7, Chapter 4). Root exudate of sunflower was inhibitory to growth of *Erigeron canadensis* and *Rudbeckia hirta,* but not to the other three species under consideration here (Table 8, Chapter 4). Leachate of sunflower leaves was inhibitory to growth in soil of *Erigeron canadensis, Rudbeckia hirta,* and *Haplopappus ciliatus,* but not to *Bromus japonicus* and *Croton glandulosus* (Table 9, Chapter 4).

Croton glandulosus was not inhibited by any of the three sources of toxins from sunflower, and it grows better in the field close to the sunflower than it does a meter or so away. *Erigeron canadensis* and *Rudbeckia hirta* were inhibited in all tests and were found to be significantly inhibited near sunflower plants in the field. *Bromus japonicus* was inhibited by only one source of toxin, and *Haplopappus ciliatus* was inhibited by only two sources of toxin; these two species were found to be inhibited somewhat in the field, but not significantly so over the 2-year sampling period. Thus, field results were well correlated with results of laboratory tests of allelopathic effects of sunflower. *Rudbeckia hirta, Erigeron canadensis,* and *Bromus japonicus* occur as winter annuals in revegetating old fields, and thus the patterns are obvious around dead sunflower stalks during the late winter months also.

The chief phytotoxins identified were chlorogenic and isochlorogenic acids in aqueous extracts of all organs of the sunflower plant and scopolin and a suspected α-naphthol derivative in leaf leachate (Wilson and Rice, 1968).

D. *Brassica nigra*

Muller (1969) reported that mustard, *Brassica nigra*, forms pure stands that have invaded slopes in the annual grasslands of coastal southern California. All the species involved are annual plants that pass the dry summer and early fall as seeds, and the supply of grass seed is plentiful both inside and outside the mustard stand. There is a clear-cut time of seed germination, and it occurs at the time of the first significant winter rain. It is usually completed within a 2–3 day period while the rain is still falling and the ground is saturated. There is no competition during this period in the grass or mustard area because only the dead parts of the plants of the previous growing season are present. Nevertheless, Muller repeatedly observed during many years that the grass seeds germinated in great density in the grassed areas, but not at all in immediately adjacent areas within the mustard stand, despite plentiful supplies of grass seeds and moisture. Mustard seeds germinated well in the mustard stand.

Bell and Muller (1973) investigated the causes for the failure of grasses to invade the mustard stands, and initial tests indicated that soil factors were not responsible. There were no significant differences in texture, pH, temperature, minerals, or moisture, and as Muller previously pointed out, the pattern is established at the time of germination when no competition is present anyway. Foraging studies indicated that seeds of *Avena fatua* could be markedly reduced in the mustard stands by animals, but none of the other species was appreciably affected. It was concluded, therefore, that the almost total lack of grass seedlings in the mustard zone could not be due solely to foraging activities. Light measurements and the use of artificial shading screens demonstrated that light was not a factor in the patterning. Thus, they concluded that some sort of allelopathic mechanism must be involved and proceeded to test this hypothesis.

Their early tests for the presence of inhibitors were concerned with the possible role of volatile toxins because several persons had previously reported that certain volatile compounds resulting from the hydrolysis of mustard oil glycosides are toxic to some microorganisms. Using gas chromatography, they found that large quantities of allyl isothiocyanate are produced when living vegetative parts of *B. nigra* are crushed. Tests of the volatile materials from macerated tissue and of the pure compound using the sponge bioassay method of Muller *et al.* (1964) showed that both are very inhibitory to radicle growth of *Bromus rigidus*. It was found also that the compound is adsorbed on soil to the extent that the soil is very inhibitory to radicle growth of *B. rigidus*. Tests made periodically after the soil was allowed to stand indicated that all inhibitory activity was gone after 9 weeks. They found that seeds exposed to the vapors are retarded in germination and root growth initially; however after open-air storage for 6 weeks, very little inhibitory activity remains. They concluded, therefore, that the volatile inhibitors are not responsible for patterning.

Experiments were run next to determine if germinating mustard seeds are inhibitory to seed germination of some of the grasses involved. No effects were found.

Bell and Muller observed that the invasion of grassland by mustard was more marked on the downhill side, which made them suspect that water-soluble toxins are involved. Water extracts of the tops of living seedlings, dead roots, dead stems, and dead leaves were tested against root growth of three grass seedlings in the sponge bioassay, and the extracts of the dead stems and leaves were found to be very inhibitory. Extracts of living tops and of dead roots had no effects. Leachates of dead stems were collected in the field during rains and were found to be inhibitory to root growth of grass seedlings also. Subsequent studies indicated that all the toxins were washed out by the first rain of the season. Thus the introduction of toxic leachates into the soil coincides with the time during which the vegetational pattern is established.

The incorporation of macerated dead leaves into the soil markedly inhibited root growth of test seedlings when added in amounts even lower than calculated amounts in the field.

Field plots were established in mustard stands in which some were cleared of all debris; a few had the dead stalks cut, broken into pieces, and replaced, and others were left as controls. Other plots were established in the neighboring grassland. Density of seedlings of each species in each plot was determined following the first rainfall. The resulting seedling density of the various grass species was virtually the same in the plots cleared of mustard stalks as in the undisturbed grassland. Plots with broken-up pieces of mustard stalks had significant reductions in numbers of seedlings of both grasses and mustard, however.

The overall conclusion of Bell and Muller (1973) was that the establishment and maintenance of *Brassica nigra* in virtually pure stands is the result of toxins in the rainwater leachates from dead stalks and leaves of the *Brassica* crop of the previous year.

Chou and Muller (1972) stated, "Pure stands of any long-lived species are highly suggestive of chemical dominance." I suspect that pure stands of any species, long-lived or annual, suggest chemical dominance if maintained for several years in a given area.

E. *Sporobolus pyramidatus*

A few years back, I observed that *Sporobolus pyramidatus* often expanded the size of its stands in the University of Oklahoma Golf Course from a few plants to rather large areas in a short time, in spite of the heavy stand of Bermuda grass, *Cynodon dactylon,* on the course. As the *Sporobolus* spread, it almost completely eliminated the Bermuda grass and occurred in virtually pure stands itself. As the

Sporobolus stands spread, however, the *Sporobolus* died out partially in the center of the stand and appeared to be less vigorous in vegetative growth and inflorescence production than around the margin (Fig. 30). Thus, very striking patterns were created, and similar patterns were found in the Wichita Mountains Wildlife Refuge in southwestern Oklahoma in natural buffalo grass, *Buchloe dactyloides*, areas (Rasmussen and Rice, 1971).

   Sporobolus pyramidatus is a small grass, usually attaining a height in our area of no more than 1 dm or so even in flower. Thus, it does very little shading of other plants. Because of its small size, the pure stands in which it occurs, its edge effect, and its rapid invasion of other vegetation, Rasmussen and I suspected allelopathy and proceeded to investigate this possibility (Rasmussen and Rice, 1971). Quantitative sampling of the *Sporobolus* stands and the areas surrounding them in the golf course site demonstrated that moderate amounts of three species other than *Sporobolus* occurred in the stands in the early part of the growing season. A little *Cynodon* occurred plus two winter annuals, *Bromus catharticus* and *Hordeum pusillum*. These last two were not present in the August sampling. Outside the

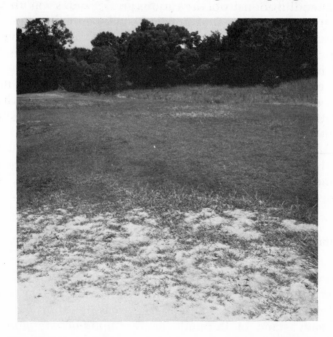

Fig. 30.   *Sporobolus pyramidatus* stand associated with *Cynodon dactylon* showing edge effect; *S. pyramidatus* in foreground. (From Rasmussen and Rice, 1971.)

Sporobolus stand, *Cynodon dactylon* was the only species of con-sequence. In the Wichita Mountains Wildlife Refuge, the only species that occurred in the *Sporobolus* stands was buffalo grass, and it was present only in minute amounts. Outside the *Sporobolus* stands, *Buch-loe dactyloides* was the only species of any consequence present.

The species chosen to be tested for possible allelopathic reaction to *Sporobolus pyramidatus* were *Cynodon dactylon, Buchloe dacty-loides, S. pyramidatus, Bromus japonicus, Amaranthus retroflexus, Hordeum pusillum,* and *Aristida purpurea. Cyndon dactylon, Buch-loe dactyloides, S. pyramidatus,* and *Hordeum pusillum* were obvious choices. *Bromus japonicus* and *Amaranthus retroflexus* were chosen because they are commonly used indicator species of allelopathy in our area. Also, good seed sources of both species are available. Al-though *Aristida purpurea* was not sampled, its seeds were found in great quantity in the *Sporobolus* stands at the Wichita Mountains Wildlife Refuge site, and plants grew profusely in the areas surround-ing buffalo grass.

Initial experiments were designed to determine if *Sporobolus* was causing marked changes in selected physical and mineral factors in the soil to a depth of 30 cm, which would certainly include most of the roots of the species involved. No differences were found in pH, or-ganic matter, total nitrogen, total phosphorus, or soil moisture. Soil moisture was measured in August also when it is most likely to be deficient in central Oklahoma. Obviously the analyses were not in-clusive enough to exclude all soil factors as possible causes of the virtual exclusion of *Cynodon* from the *Sporobolus* stand, but they did indicate no obvious changes.

In order to eliminate competition from *Sporobolus* and to deter-mine if inhibitors were present in soil in the *Sporobolus* stands, soil minus litter was taken from within such stands and outside them in the golf course site in July and in January, and each collection was used as a separate experiment. Thirty seeds of all test species except *Sporobolus* were planted in their respective pots. Germination was counted on the second day after it began and again 2 weeks after planting. The earliest determination of germination was done to see the initial effects on seed germination, which may be of great con-sequence to plants exposed to the competitive mechanisms of their natural environment. Two weeks after planting, the plants were thinned to the five largest per pot and allowed to grow an additional 2 weeks. *Sporobolus* did not germinate well in soil even after pre-treatment, so it was allowed to germinate and grow in sand for 1 week and then transplanted to the soil, where it was allowed to grow an additional 3 weeks. All species were compared on an oven-dried weight basis. All experiments on *Sporobolus* were run in a growth chamber on a 16-hour photoperiod at 28°C and a night temperature of 21°C.

The July soils collected within *Sporobolus* stands significantly reduced the oven-dried weights of *Hordeum pusillum, Bromus japonicus,* and *Aristida purpurea,* but stimulated growth of *Cynodon dactylon* (Table 26). *Sporobolus pyramidatus* and *Buchloe dactyloides* were also stimulated, but not to a statistically significant level. Germination was appreciably reduced in all species at the second day, but recovered considerably in some after 2 weeks. The stimulation of Bermuda grass and buffalo grass growth demonstrated that there was no deficiency of minerals in the soil in *Sporobolus* stands.

Soils collected in January from *Sporobolus* stands significantly inhibited all test species except *S. pyramidatus* itself, and germination of all tested species was markedly affected (Table 26). Dry weight of *Sporobolus* was reduced in the test, but not significantly. These re-

TABLE 26

Effects of Field Soils Previously in Contact with *Sporobolus* on Germination and Growth of Test Species [a]

		Mean dry weight and S.E.(mg)		Germination (% of control)	
Species	Date soil taken	Control	Test	Second day	Two weeks
Cynodon	July	34 ± 4.3	73 ± 7.4 [b]	10	46
dactylon	Jan.	21 ± 2.8	9 ± 0.1 [b]	17	29
Hordeum	July	62 ± 3.5	46 ± 2.6 [b]	16	77
pusillum	Jan.	21 ± 1.1	14 ± 1.8 [b]	3	12
Bromus	July	189 ± 10.0	114 ± 8.0 [b]	53	92
japonicus	Jan.	55 ± 2.7	27 ± 2.7 [b]	8	13
Amaranthus	July	216 ± 29.3	161 ± 15.8	62	88
retroflexus	Jan.	141 ± 12.8	90 ± 15.7 [b]	15	26
Sporobolus	July	61 ± 9.6	84 ± 6.8	—	—
pyramidatus	Jan.	42 ± 3.2	37 ± 3.0	—	—
Buchloe	July	31 ± 3.4	40 ± 3.4	70	90
dactyloides	Jan.	33 ± 1.6	24 ± 2.0 [b]	65	60
Aristida	July	41 ± 3.4	14 ± 1.9 [b]	10	50
purpurea	Jan.	14 ± 0.1	6 ± 0.5 [b]	40	32

[a] From Rasmussen and Rice (1971).
[b] Dry weight significantly different from control at 0.05 level or better.

sults indicate a phytotoxic effect of the soils closely associated with *Sporobolus* and eliminate any competitive mechanism associated with the presence of the *Sporobolus* plant.

Studies were undertaken next to determine the sources of the toxins in the soil of the *Sporobolus* plots. In one type of experiment, leachate collected from shoots of *Sporobolus* by use of artifical rain was used to water the test species in soil. Control pots were watered with water that had not passed over shoots of *Sporobolus*. All experiments were repeated.

The leachate was not inhibitory generally to most test species. Only *Bromus japonicus* was inhibited in one experiment, and *Bromus, Amaranthus retroflexus,* and *Sporobolus* itself in the second experiment.

It was noted from field observations that even in early June, *Sporobolus* leaves begin to die and are associated in large quantities with the living plant. As much as 8–10 gm of dead material could be found on a single plant. To determine the effect of decaying *Sporobolus* shoots on the test species, 1 gm of shoots (air-dried 3 weeks) was added to each 454 gm of soil. A control series was run with 1 gm of extra peat moss added per 454 gm of soil. The test and control series were watered equally with distilled water. Thirty seeds were planted in each pot, and germination was determined 2 days after it had begun and at 2 weeks.

The dry weights of all test species except *Aristida purpurea* were significantly decreased by decaying *Sporobolus* shoot material (Table 27). *Cynodon dactylon* and *Amaranthus retroflexus* were greatly reduced in dry weight in the second test, and the latter never attained growth past the cotyledon stage in the month that it grew. Seed germination was appreciably reduced in all species at both check periods.

A similar type of experiment was run using decaying root material of *Sporobolus* rather than shoot material. *Cynodon dactylon* was significantly inhibited in both germination and growth, but no other species was inhibited.

An experiment was designed next to determine if exudates from *Sporobolus* roots were inhibitory to the test species. The experimental design was modified from Parenti and Rice (1969) in that the staircase structure was used only as a method for collecting exudate each day of the experiment. The water that had passed over *Sporobolus* roots was used to water a set of pots containing soil. A control series of pots was watered with distilled water that had not passed over *Sporobolus* roots.

TABLE 27

Effects of Decaying *Sporobolus* **Shoots (Air-Dried 3 Weeks) on Seed Germination and Seedling Growth** [a]

Species	Experiment No.	Mean dry weight and S.E. (mg)		Germination (% of control)	
		Control	Test	Second day	Two weeks
Cynodon	1	6 ± 0.4	4 ± 0.3 [b]	22	43
dactylon	2	7 ± 0.4	1 ± 0.1 [b]	20	47
Hordeum	1	13 ± 0.8	11 ± 0.7 [b]	40	60
pusillum	2	14 ± 0.8	12 ± 0.5 [b]	53	49
Bromus	1	26 ± 1.3	13 ± 1.0 [b]	54	80
japonicus	2	25 ± 1.4	10 ± 0.4 [b]	68	78
Amaranthus	1	75 ± 5.7	37 ± 4.7 [b]	56	65
retroflexus	2	21 ± 2.1	1 ± 0.1 [b]	40	62
Sporobolus	1	19 ± 2.1	13 ± 1.2 [b]	—	—
pyramidatus	2	20 ± 2.5	13 ± 1.3 [b]	—	—
Buchloe	1	26 ± 1.1	21 ± 1.0 [b]	41	78
dactyloides	2	27 ± 1.0	18 ± 1.0 [b]	55	70
Aristida	1	8 ± 0.3	7 ± 0.4	40	55
purpurea	2	8 ± 0.4	7 ± 0.4	42	51

[a] From Rasmussen and Rice (1971).
[b] Dry weight significantly different from control at 0.05 level or better.

Root exudates significantly reduced the dry weight of *Cynodon dactylon* in both tests and markedly reduced its germination (Table 28). The dry weights of *Hordeum pusillum, Bromus japonicus, Sporobolus pyramidatus,* and *Aristida purpurea* were significantly reduced in one test. *Buchloe dactyloides* was not inhibited in either experiment, but its seed germination was reduced in one test.

Five *Sporobolus* stands on the University of Oklahoma Golf Course were measured and stakes were placed around the perimeter of each stand in July of 1969 to determine the rate of spread. In June, 1970, measurements were taken and results showed a very rapid spread of *Sporobolus*. The stands increased in diameter by 1–4 m, and this rate of spread occurred even though a heavy Bermuda grass sod completely surrounded each stand of *Sporobolus*.

The evidence seems clear that *Sporobolus pyramidatus* is able to spread rapidly into heavy sods of *Cyndon dactylon* or *Buchloe dactyloides* because it produces toxins that are exuded from living roots or diffuse from decaying roots or shoots and inhibit seed germination and growth. Bermuda grass and buffalo grass are both perennials, of course, and both generally spread rapidly vegetatively—Bermuda grass by rhizomes and buffalo grass by runners. It might appear, therefore, that inhibition of seed germination of these species is not important in the patterning. As previously pointed out, however, the *Sporobolus* stands are very open, especially at the center, and could be reseeded even though encroachment by rhizomes or runners is eliminated.

Pioneer weed species are apparently prevented from invading the bare centers of the *Sporobolus* stands because of the demonstrated toxic effects of leachates, root exudates, and decaying material of *Sporobolus* on seed germination and growth of representative species. *Hordeum pusillum,* which was found in small amounts in the *Sporobolus* stands in late winter and spring, was adversely affected by root exudate and decaying material of *Sporobolus*. It grows to maturity and flowers, however, at a time when inhibitors produced by *Sporobolus* are at their lowest concentration in the soil.

To be able to survive the allelopathic effects on itself, *Sporobolus* must be able to move constantly into new areas. To do this it must be less inhibitory to itself than to the surrounding vegetation, which is

TABLE 28

Effects of *Sporobolus* Root Exudate on Seed Germination and Seedling Growth [a]

Species	Experiment No.	Mean dry weight and S.E. (mg)		Germination (% of control)	
		Control	Test	Second day	Two weeks
Cynodon	1	9 ± 0.6	4 ± 0.4 [b]	28	40
dactylon	2	14 ± 0.7	10 ± 0.7 [b]	42	54
Hordeum	1	13 ± 0.7	13 ± 0.7	59	87
pusillum	2	20 ± 1.1	18 ± 0.8 [b]	63	79
Bromus	1	29 ± 1.8	24 ± 1.2 [b]	98	95
japonicus	2	47 ± 1.8	44 ± 1.8	96	95
Amaranthus	1	18 ± 1.6	31 ± 2.7 [b]	150	111
retroflexus	2	41 ± 4.8	55 ± 4.6	260	132
Sporobolus	1	18 ± 2.2	19 ± 2.0	—	—
pyramidatus	2	42 ± 2.3	35 ± 2.2 [b]	—	—
Buchloe	1	25 ± 1.3	24 ± 1.0	116	123
dactyloides	2	42 ± 1.2	48 ± 1.9 [b]	50	69
Aristida	1	9 ± 0.4	7 ± 0.3 [b]	70	105
purpurea	2	10 ± 0.9	11 ± 1.0	122	90

[a] From Rasmussen and Rice (1971).
[b] Dry weight significantly different from control at 0.05 level or better.

apparently the case because field soils did not affect *Sporobolus* at either collection date. This probably means that the effective concentrations inhibitory to *Sporobolus* can be maintained only by continued association with its own decay material.

Aristida purpurea is probably prevented from germinating and growing in the *Sporobolus* stands in the buffalo grass areas of southwestern Oklahoma by a combination of unfavorable soil factors and allelopathic effects of *Sporobolus*.

The initial entry of *Sporobolus pyramidatus* into dense Bermuda grass or buffalo grass sod apparently requires some disturbance. *Sporobolus* seeds have a light requirement for germination and the *Sporobolus* stands start, therefore, in tiny disturbed areas created by divots in the golf course or cattle tracks in the buffalo grass areas.

p-Coumaric acid and ferulic acid were extracted from shoot residue in large quantities, and both compounds were very inhibitory to germination of *Amaranthus palmeri* seeds.

F. *Ambrosia psilostachya*

Neill and Rice (1971) observed in an old field near Norman, Oklahoma abandoned for 25 years that the composition of vegetation adjacent to western ragweed, *Ambrosia psilostachya,* was different from that apart from it. These observations were quantified using $0.25m^2$ quadrats. Clippings were made in quadrats with western ragweed, in quadrats 1 m removed from the first quadrat and in an area that included no *A. psilostachya.* The second quadrat was always located in the same direction from the first unless the above conditions were not met in that location. The clippings were separated as to species and dry weights were taken. Five sets of quadrats were clipped every 2 weeks from June through October.

The mean oven-dried weights of the forbs were not statistically different in the quadrats with *A. psilostachya* as compared with those 1 m away (Table 29). On the other hand, *Andropogon ternarius* had a significantly lower mean oven-dried weight near *Ambrosia psilostachya,* and *Leptoloma cognatum* had a significantly greater mean dry weight near western ragweed than 1 m away. *Tridens flavus* also had a higher mean dry weight near western ragweed, but not at the 0.05 level of significance.

Several chemical and physical soil factors were measured to a depth of 30 cm and found to be no different near the western ragweed plants than at least 1 m away. Soil moisture measured in July after a lengthy

TABLE 29

Results of Field Clippings of Species Associated with *Ambrosia psilostachya* [a]

Species	Mean oven-dried weight in gm/0.25 m² with S.E.	
	Quadrat A [b]	Quadrat B [b]
Andropogon ternarius	0.97 ± 0.31	6.37 ± 1.19 [c]
Aristida oligantha	2.14 ± 0.63	2.89 ± 0.64
Bromus japonicus	1.22 ± 0.50	2.48 ± 0.97
Erigeron canadensis	0.66 ± 0.36	0.55 ± 0.43
Haplopappus ciliatus	0.47 ± 0.27	0.59 ± 0.42
Leptoloma cognatum	1.26 ± 0.35	0.43 ± 0.12 [c]
Rudbeckia hirta	0.32 ± 0.11	0.26 ± 0.09
Tridens flavus	1.03 ± 0.34	0.56 ± 0.30

[a] From Neill and Rice (1971).
[b] Quadrat A includes the *A. psilostachya* plants; quadrat B starts 1 m from quadrat A.
[c] Significant difference among quadrats.

period without rain indicated no significant difference near the ragweed plants and 1 m away.

It was decided, therefore, to determine whether the differential growth patterns observed and confirmed by sampling would occur in soil obtained near ragweed plants without the presence of competition from the ragweeds. In July and again in January, a series of eight soil samples, minus litter, was taken within 0.25 m of several *A. psilostachya* plants, and another series of eight was taken over 1 m away from the same plants to be used for controls. The samples were collected with a sharp-nosed shovel and placed in plastic pots. The soil collections from the two dates were treated as separate experiments. Seeds of test species collected from abandoned fields near Norman were planted in their respective pots and grown in the greenhouse immediately after the soil was collected each time. Germination was recorded at the end of 2 weeks, after which the plants were thinned to the five largest plants per pot. They were allowed to grow for 3 more weeks, and dry weights were then determined. Field soil taken in July from near the *A. psilostachya* plants proved to be significantly stimulatory to *Andropogon ternarius, Bromus japonicus, Leptoloma cognatum, Rudbeckia hirta,* and *Tridens flavus* (Table 30). However, soil collected in January prior to the onset of germination in the field and after accumulation of *A. psilostachya* leaves stimulated only *Leptoloma cognatum* and *Tridens flavus* and not at the 0.05 level

TABLE 30

**Effects of Field Soils Previously in Contact with _Ambrosia psilostachya_
Roots on Germination and Growth of Test Species** [a]

Species	Date soil taken	Mean dry weight (mg) with S.E.		Germination (% of control)
		Control	Test	
Andropogon	July	25 ± 1.4	33 ± 2.1 [b]	80
ternarius	Jan.	10 ± 0.6	10 ± 0.5	66
Aristida	July	31 ± 1.8	26 ± 1.7	100
oligantha	Jan.	11 ± 0.5	11 ± 0.5	105
Bromus	July	22 ± 1.1	46 ± 3.3 [b]	112
japonicus	Jan.	17 ± 1.0	14 ± 0.6	97
Erigeron	July	13 ± 1.0	13 ± 0.8	92
canadensis	Jan.	8 ± 0.6	7 ± 0.6	85
Haplopappus	July	18 ± 1.2	20 ± 1.9	77
ciliatus	Jan.	10 ± 0.5	7 ± 0.5 [b]	83
Leptoloma	July	20 ± 1.9	36 ± 1.8 [b]	90
cognatum	Jan.	13 ± 1.0	15 ± 1.1	114
Rudbeckia	July	16 ± 0.8	25 ± 1.6 [b]	83
hirta	Jan.	8 ± 0.7	6 ± 0.4 [b]	130
Tridens	July	27 ± 1.6	43 ± 3.2 [b]	102
flavus	Jan.	6 ± 0.8	8 ± 1.4	100

[a] Modified from Neill and Rice (1971).
[b] Dry weight significantly different from control at 0.05 level or better.

of significance. The January soil significantly inhibited growth of _Rudbeckia hirta_.

There were some interesting correlations with field patterns. _Leptoloma cognatum_ and _Tridens flavus_, which grew better near _A. psilostachya_ in the field, were stimulated by soil collected near _A. psilostachya_ during both sampling periods. The results to this point suggested that the _A. psilostachya_ plants were producing organic compounds that stimulated some plants and inhibited others. Experiments were designed to investigate this possibility.

Initial experiments concerned effects of decaying air-dried fresh leaves of western ragweed. Seeds of test species often associated with _A. psilostachya_ were germinated in pots containing soil mixed with 1 gm air-dried powdered leaf material per 454 gm of soil, or 1 gm of air-dried peat moss in control pots. Rice (1968) determined that mature stands of _A. psilostachya_ produced more than 1 gm of air-dried weight of leaves per 454 gm of soil to the depth of plowing, the top 17 cm. Percentage germination of the greenhouse grown plants was determined after 14 days, the plants were thinned to the five largest per pot, and the oven-dried weights of the seedlings were taken after 3 more weeks growth.

The air-dried leaves inhibited growth of *Andropogon ternarius* seedlings, but signficantly stimulated *Aristida oligantha, Bromus japonicus, Haplopappus ciliatus,* and *Rudbeckia hirta* (Table 31). All other species were stimulated to some degree. *Leptoloma* and *Tridens* were slightly stimulated also, but the differences were not statistically significant.

This experiment was repeated using old leaves that had aged on the *A. psilostachya* plants and were starting to drop. These leaves produced contrasting results, with significant inhibition in dry weights occurring in four of the test species (Table 32). The percentage germination of *Haplopappus ciliatus* was reduced appreciably.

Leachates of the tops of western ragweed obtained by use of artificial rain were used to water the same test species growing in soil and were found to significantly stimulate growth of *Aristida oligantha, Leptoloma cognatum,* and *Tridens flavus.* Leachates inhibited growth of *Bromus japonicus* and *Haplopappus ciliatus.*

TABLE 31

Effects of Decaying *Ambrosia psilostachya* (Air-Dried Fresh Leaves) on Seedling Growth [a]

Species	Experiment No.	Mean dry weight of seedlings (mg)		Germination (% of control)
		Control	Test	
Andropogon	1	51.7 ± 4.3	12.1 ± 1.6 [b]	110
ternarius	2	35.2 ± 2.4	21.4 ± 1.9 [b]	92
Aristida	1	55.7 ± 3.3	105.2 ± 5.2 [b]	84
oligantha	2	75.9 ± 7.8	105.5 ± 5.9 [b]	86
Bromus	1	43.8 ± 3.1	102.8 ± 9.8 [b]	98
japonicus	2	121.3 ± 6.1	143.4 ± 6.9 [b]	100
Erigeron	1	13.7 ± 1.3	14.2 ± 1.2	70
canadensis	2	12.3 ± 0.9	13.2 ± 0.9	70
Haplopappus	1	19.7 ± 1.7	57.1 ± 5.9 [b]	136
ciliatus	2	25.9 ± 3.2	29.7 ± 3.3	100
Leptoloma	1	94.0 ± 6.3	114.1 ± 8.6	127
cognatum	2	106.1 ± 9.0	114.7 ± 7.7	97
Rudbeckia	1	30.0 ± 2.9	92.8 ± 8.2 [b]	193
hirta	2	43.9 ± 4.3	68.1 ± 6.2 [b]	77
Tridens	1	375.9 ± 24.5	386.0 ± 27.2	137
flavus	2	376.0 ± 35.3	387.6 ± 24.8	78

[a] Modified from Neill and Rice (1971).
[b] Dry weight significantly different from control at 0.05 level or better.

TABLE 32

Effects of Decaying *Ambrosia psilostachya* Leaves (Overwintered on Plant) on Seedling Growth and Germination [a]

Species	Experiment No.	Mean dry weight (mg) with S.E.		Germination (% of control)
		Control	Test	
Andropogon	1	14 ± 0.9	12 ± 0.8	100
ternarius	2	15 ± 1.4	12 ± 0.9	91
Aristida	1	32 ± 0.5	25 ± 1.4 [b]	87
oligantha	2	90 ± 6.2	67 ± 5.2 [b]	80
Bromus	1	69 ± 4.6	53 ± 3.4 [b]	92
japonicus	2	78 ± 4.7	69 ± 4.6	99
Erigeron	1	24 ± 1.8	12 ± 1.1 [b]	98
canadensis	2	9 ± 0.9	4 ± 0.4 [b]	92
Haplopappus	1	39 ± 6.3	26 ± 5.0	55
ciliatus	2	36 ± 5.6	26 ± 4.5	80
Leptoloma	1	156 ± 15.2	84 ± 7.9 [b]	91
cognatum	2	20 ± 2.1	11 ± 0.8 [b]	87
Rudbeckia	1	9 ± 0.9	12 ± 1.4 [b]	87
hirta	2	11 ± 0.8	13 ± 1.0	80
Tridens	1	104 ± 17.1	84 ± 18.3	98
flavus	2	62 ± 5.7	52 ± 4.0	107

[a] Modified from Neill and Rice (1971).
[b] Dry weight significantly different from control at 0.05 level or better.

Root exudates obtained as described for *Helianthus annuus* (Chapter 4) were significantly inhibitory to the growth of *Andropogon ternarius, Bromus japonicus, Erigeron canadensis,* and *Rudbeckia hirta. Aristida oligantha* was significantly stimulated in one experiment and *Tridens flavus* was significantly stimulated in both.

The correlations between field patterns of associated species and results of the various experiments were generally good. *Andropogon ternarius,* which was significantly inhibited near ragweed in the field was significantly inhibited by root exudate and decaying material of western ragweed. *Leptoloma cognatum* was stimulated by soil obtained near western ragweed and by leaf leachate of ragweed, and it grew slightly better near ragweed in the field. *Tridens flavus* grew better near ragweed in the field, and it was stimulated by field soil, leaf leachate, and root exudate. *Bromus japonicus* was inhibited by decaying overwintered leaves, leachate, and root exudate and did not grow quite as well near western ragweed in the field as 1 m or more away. *Aristida oligantha* was inhibited in some tests and stimulated in an equal number of tests and it grew about as well in the field near ragweed as 1 m or more away.

Based on the results of the experimentation, Neill and Rice (1971) concluded that the vegetational patterns around *Ambrosia psilostachya* in revegetating old fields are probably due primarily to organic compounds produced by western ragweed, which stimulate growth of some associated species and inhibit others.

G. *Avena fatua*

Tinnin and Muller (1971) reported that the annual grasslands of California (see Chapter 6) are best developed on deep clay soils, whereas the hard chaparral dominated by deep-rooted evergreen shrubs, such as *Adenostoma fasciculatum* (chamise), occurs generally on better-drained and shallower soils. Contacts between the hard chaparral and grassland are generally occupied by soft chaparral dominated by such species as *Salvia californica* and *Artemisia californica*. Tinnin and Muller found one area in the foothills of the San Rafael Mountains near Santa Barbara, California where direct contact occurred between hard chaparral dominated by chamise and the annual grassland. In that area clay soils were present over Careaga sandstone at an elevation of 560 m. Herbaceous species in the contact area were separated into three zones, with one group occupying chiefly the shrub zone, another group chiefly the normal grassland, and a third group chiefly the border zone between the other two zones (Fig. 31). This third zone was about 1 m wide and extended completely around the margin of the shrub stand. The grassland zone adjacent to the border zone consisted almost exclusively of *Avena fatua*. This fact, together with the fact that *A. fatua* dominates vast areas of annual grassland, where it sometimes represents virtually the entire complement of vascular plants in sizable areas, caused Tinnin and Muller to suspect that interference from *A. fatua* might be involved in the pattern of zonation around chamise in the study area.

The three herb zones were sampled separately by permanently located quadrats, and it was found that, of a total of 28 annual species, eight occurred only in the grassland zone, three only in the border zone, and three only in the shrub zone. In addition, three other annual herbs occurred only in the grassland and border zones, and one species only in the border and shrub zones. This demonstrated that there was a clear-cut pattern of species distribution and not just of growth.

After the first rainstorm of the growing season, seedlings were iden-

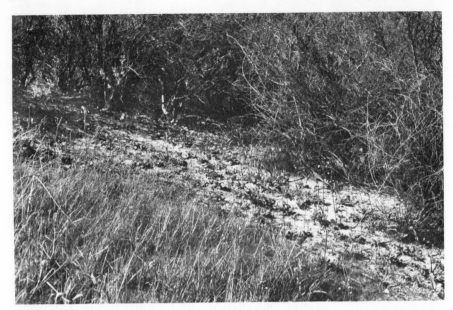

Fig. 31. The three herb zones, as viewed from grass zone, showing *Adenostoma fasciculatum* in background (shrub zone), the adjacent conspicuous *Dodecatheon clevelandii* in the border zone, and primarily *Avena fatua* in the foreground (grass zone). (From Tinnin and Muller, 1971.)

tified and counted in all the marked quadrats and were followed throughout the growing season. Seed germination occurred within a 3-day period after the first rain, and no differential mortality occurred during the growing season. The pattern of distribution of seedlings was found to be the same as the pattern identified by previous sampling. Tinnin and Muller concluded, therefore, that the pattern was established at the time of seed germination.

Investigations were carried out to determine the reasons for the pattern of germination, particularly for the failure of annual herbs from the shrub and border zone to occur in the grassland. It was previously shown by McPherson and Muller (1969) that chamise produces toxins that inhibit germination and growth of annual herbs from the grassland. Initially, a study was made of the possible role of small animals because there was evidence of light grazing in all zones. Of the seedlings that were marked, however, one occasionally had a leaf clipped, but seedling density was never influenced greatly. There was additional evidence that animals did not significantly influence the density of seeds.

Soil analyses were made of texture, moisture, pH, electrical conductivity, cation exchange capacity, available phosphorus, nitrate, and total nitrogen in the top 6 cm. No differences were found that could account for the pattern of herbs. Soil moisture was consistently higher in the grassland, although the difference from the other zones was small.

Light intensities at the soil surface averaged approximately 1880 ft-c in the grass zone, 1130 ft-c in the shaded portions of the border zone, and 790 ft-c in the shrub zone. Openings were present in all zones which allowed 100% of full sunlight to reach the soil surface. Light competition was obviously not responsible for the failure of shrub and border zone seeds to germinate in the grass zone, even if they had light requirements for germination.

Soil temperatures in the top 2 cm were found to be similar in the shrub and grass zones even on sunny days, and this was true in all zones on the cloudy and rainy days when germination occurred and the herb pattern was established.

Tinnin and Muller (1971) decided, therefore, that an allelopathic mechanism must be involved in the failure of shrub and border zone herbs to grow in the grass zone. They designed experiments to test this hypothesis. Field plots were established in the grass zone and part of the plots were clipped to remove dead growth of the previous growing season. The clipped material consisted primarily of *Avena fatua*. The clipping was done in early summer in each year of study. Abundant supplies of one of the shrub border zone species, *Centaurea melitensis,* were introduced into clipped and unclipped grass zone plots by hand. Germination and survival of herb species were observed throughout the winter growing season, and it was found that *C. melitensis* germinated in clipped and unclipped plots. A density of only 200 individuals/m² occurred in the unclipped plots, whereas 1200 individuals/m² occurred in the clipped plots. These investigators concluded, therefore, that the results supported the hypothesis of an allelopathic control of germination because success of germination was directly correlated with the absence of dead grass straw, primarily of *Avena fatua*. Late in the growing season, the *Centaurea* plants in the border zone were 0.5 m tall and had many floral heads per plant; those in the unclipped grass zone which survived were less than 1 dm tall bearing zero to three poorly developed floral heads; and in the clipped grass zone plots the plants were about 2 dm in height with one to ten poorly developed heads. Plants in the clipped area were obviously doing better than in the unclipped area, but were definitely inhibited in comparison with those in the border zone. Those in the clipped plots were growing with living *Avena fatua* plants, of course, which indicated interference from the living *Avena* plants.

In other experiments, Tinnin and Muller (1971) found that the dry straw of *Avena fatua* from the previous growing season contains water-soluble toxins that are leached into the soil by the first rains of the growing season and selectively inhibit germination.

Results of previous studies by McPherson and Muller (1969), plus results just described, caused Tinnin and Muller (1971) to conclude the following concerning the three herb zones at the study site. (1) Several grass zone plants were excluded from the shrub and border zones by toxins produced by chamise; (2) the herbs that occur in the shrub and border zones do so only because of their tolerance for the toxins produced by chamise; (3) some of the shrub and border zone herbs are excluded from the grass zone by toxins present primarily in dry straw of *Avena fatua*; (4) after the toxic materials have washed out of the dead straw, the living grass zone seedlings help maintain the herb pattern through mechanisms of allelopathy and competition; (5) because of the differential susceptibility of the herbs to the inhibitors, the herbs are sorted initially into the three zones; (6) seeds of each species are deposited mainly near the parent plants and fall mainly in the same herb zones as the plants that produce them; (7) some seeds do reach other zones but germination is partially inhibited; (8) of those which do germinate, only a small percentage reaches maturity due to competition and inhibition by chemicals; and (9) the pattern is thus maintained.

H. Emergent Aquatic Plants

Szczepańska (1971) pointed out that beds of emergent aquatics are usually monospecific, and I am sure that most ecologists who have investigated the ecology of such plants have been impressed with this same fact. As I pointed out previously, this sort of situation is always at least suggestive of an allelopathic mechanism. Nevertheless, very little research has been done concerning allelopathic effects of emergent aquatics, and the results are not conclusive. I feel a brief discussion is worthwhile anyway to accentuate the need and potentialities for further research.

McNaughton (1968) studied the autotoxic effects of cattail, *Typha latifolia*, and found that aqueous extracts of its leaves completely inhibited germination of cattail seeds. In addition, he found that water from a cattail marsh slightly inhibited seedling growth of this species, and water squeezed from soil in which cattail was growing was highly inhibitory to its seedling growth. Seed germination was only partially inhibited when the water extract of the cattail leaves was treated with Polyclar AT (a polyamide) to remove phenolic compounds.

McNaughton did not investigate the allelopathic effects of cattail on other neighboring species; thus, the reason for the common occurrence of monospecific stands of cattail was not clarified. In most instances where an allelopathic mechanism has been found to be operative, however, toxins produced by a given species have generally been found to be much more toxic to numerous other species than to the one that produces them. This is perfectly logical, of course, from an evolutionary standpoint. It is certainly possible, therefore, that *Typha latifolia* is allelopathic to other emergent aquatics and that this is primarily responsible for its virtually pure stands, accentuated, of course, by competition.

Szczepańska (1971) investigated growth of *Phragmites communis, Typha latifolia, Equisetum limosum,* and *Schoenoplectus lacustris* in pure cultures and in various two-species combinations in several types of natural substrates. He found pronounced interference on the part of some species and pronounced stimulation on the part of others. These experiments did not elucidate the mechanism of interference.

Additional experiments were run, however, on effects of decaying aerial parts of *Typha latifolia, T. angustifolia, Heleocharis palustris, Glyceria aquatica, Schoenoplectus lacustris,* and *Acorus calamus* on growth of *Phragmites communis* seedlings in lake mud. Ten grams of plant material per 300 ml of mud killed the seedlings regardless of which species was used for the plant material. Even 3 gm of plant material of each test species per 500 ml of mud killed most of the *Phragmites* seedlings, and those that survived were very stunted and had necrotic areas. Szczepańska concluded that the interference against *Phragmites* when growing with other emergent aquatic species was due primarily to allelopathy on the part of the interfering species.

Szczepański (1971), a colleague of Szczepańska, stated that *Glyceria aquatica* seems to have the strongest allelopathic effects of any of the species studied in his laboratory. Substances that leach out of dead leaves of this species are very inhibitory to seed germination of other species. These substances become most toxic on the ninth day after the leaching begins, which suggests that they may be a product of microbial decomposition. One part of the leachate per 10,000 parts water causes inhibition of seed germination, so Szczepański estimated that inhibition starts at 1 ppm or lower owing to the fact that much of the leachate is material other than the toxin. He pointed out that this makes the activity at least as great as that of some well-known herbicides, such as trichloracetate (TCA).

III. PATTERNING DUE TO ALLELOPATHIC EFFECTS OF WOODY SPECIES

A. Summary of Earlier Investigations

Vegetational patterns associated with trees and shrubs are generally more striking than those associated with herbaceous species, regardless of the type of interference responsible. It was probably for this reason that more accounts occur in the early literature on allelopathy, suggesting that several observed patterns were due to chemical inhibition by certain woody species. Several were discussed in Chapter 2, but I will discuss them briefly again at this point to set the stage for more recent investigations. Unfortunately, some of the earliest suggestions were not supported with any experimental evidence, and most investigations prior to the present decade failed to eliminate adequately possible mechanisms other than allelopathy as primary causes of the observed results.

Stickney and Hoy (1881) suggested that the failure of most herbs to grow under black walnut, *Juglans nigra,* is due to toxins produced by the walnut tree. These observations were supported by Cook (1921), Massey (1925), and Davis (1928). Massey and Davis presented good evidence that the failure of herbs to grow under walnut trees is due to a toxin produced by the walnut trees.

Waks (1936) observed that parks of black locust, *Robinia pseudoacacia,* are nearly void of all other vegetation, and he found that the bark and wood of black locust contain toxins that inhibit the growth of barley *(Hordeum).* His results suggested, therefore, that the failure of herbs to grow under the black locust trees was due to allelopathy.

Bode (1940) obtained evidence that many herbaceous species fail to grow near hedges of *Artemisia absinthium* because of a toxin produced by the shrub. Bode's results were supported by the investigations of Funke (1943).

Went (1942) did a very careful study of the association between annual plants and shrubs in southern California deserts. He found, among other results, that annual plants were never associated with some shrubs unless the shrubs were dead. One of the shrubs that fits this category was *Encelia farinosa*, and Went suggested that this shrub might produce toxins that inhibit growth of annuals. He did not have any experimental evidence to support his suggestion, but Gray and Bonner (1948a,b) did obtain such evidence, and they isolated and identified a toxin from the leaves of *Encelia*.

Deleuil (1950, 1951a,b) observed that annual plants rarely occurred in the Rosmarino–Ericion association in France even where light was obviously adequate. He subsequently found that field soil from this shrub association contained potent toxins that could be leached out with water and would inhibit growth of numerous annuals when added to soil in which the annuals were growing.

Mergen (1959) reported that *Ailanthus altissima* remains in virtually pure stands for long periods of time, and he found that extracts of the rachis, leaflets, and stem of *Ailanthus* caused rapid wilting in 45 of 46 seed plant species when applied to the cut surface of the stems of the test species. The virtually pure stands may be due to allelopathic effects of *Ailanthus*, therefore, but numerous additional types of experiments should be run before such an inference is drawn.

B. *Juniperus* spp. and *Pinus edulis*

Arnold (1964) demonstrated definite zones of herb growth around one-seeded juniper, *Juniperus monosperma*, in Arizona. He suggested that the zonation was probably due to competition for light, moisture, and minerals. He did state, in addition, that the zonation warranted more detailed ecological studies. Jameson (1961) stated that junipers appear to have inhibitor effects in the field, and he demonstrated that water extracts of leaves of three species of *Juniperus*— *J. osteosperma, J. deppeana,* and *J. monosperma*—strongly inhibited growth of wheat radicles. He demonstrated that extracts of pinyon pine, *Pinus edulis*, were inhibitory also. Later, he reported that aqueous extracts of *J. osteosperma* and *Pinus edulis* were very inhibitory to root growth of seedlings of several native plants associated with *Pinus* and *Juniperus* (Jameson, 1963). One of these was *Bouteloua gracilis*, blue grama, which Arnold reported to show a strong zonation response around *Juniperus monosperma*. Jameson (1966) did multiple regression analyses of data from plots in Arizona in which the vegetation consisted chiefly of *Pinus edulis, Juniperus* spp., and blue grama grass. He found that tree litter was the major factor associated with reduction of blue grama. Tree cover either did not influence blue grama or in some cases appeared to be beneficial. He did not study root competition, but pointed out other studies indicating that root competition of *Pinus* spp. and *Juniperus* spp. against blue grama is probably slight. His overall results indicate that allelopathy has a strong influence on the zonation of herbaceous plants under pinyon pine and juniper trees.

C. *Pinus densiflora*

Lee and Monsi (1963) reported the results of a very comprehensive study on red pine, *Pinus densiflora*, forests in Korea and Japan. These are extremely widespread in Japan and cover 60–70% of forest land in South Korea. They found that vegetation under the trees was very sparse, and they noted that this had been pointed out by many researchers. According to Lee and Monsi, the interior of red pine forests is one of the brightest among forests. They presented data showing that of ten types of forests in which they measured light intensity, the intensity was highest in red pine forests. Moreover, many of the other forests have dense undergrowths of herbaceous plants.

Lee and Monsi rated understory plants in the many red pine stands for vitality using a scale of four classes, with class 1 representing highest vitality and class 4 representing the lowest. They found a very small number of annual and biennial herbs with a rating of 1 or 2 and a relatively small number of perennial herbs with high ratings. A great many herbs that were found growing profusely in cultivated fields or other areas adjacent to red pine trees or stands were not found under the red pine trees, or, if they were present, they had low vitality and did not reproduce.

Lee and Monsi (1963) suspected that the failure of many species of plants to grow in the red pine forests, or to reproduce if present, was due to allelopathic effects of red pine. In fact, in a study of some ancient documents of Japan, they found a report by Banzan Kumazawa, some 300 years old, that the rain or dew washing the leaves of red pine is harmful to crops growing under the pine. Lee and Monsi selected 15 test species, with five representing species characteristic of red pine forests and ten representing species not characteristic of red pine forests and of low vitality if present. Characteristic species used were *Miscanthus sinensis, Paederia chinensis, Platycodon grandiflorum, Atractylis ovata,* and *Pinus densiflora;* noncharacteristic species were *Setaria viridis, Amaranthus patulus, Achyranthes japonica, Chenopodium album, Polygonum blumei, Phytolacca ameri-*

cana, Desmodium fallax, Galinsoga ciliata, Aster scaber, and *In-digofera gerardiana.*

Initially, hot and cold water extracts of fresh and fallen leaves and of roots were tested against germination of seeds of four test species in petri dishes. Germination of red pine seeds was not affected by any dilutions of any of the extracts, but germination of seeds of three noncharacteristic species, *Achyranthes japonica, Amaranthus pa-tulus,* and *Indigofera gerardiana,* was markedly inhibited in all tests.

Numerous experiments were run to determine effects of soils taken from various red pine forests on germination of seeds and growth of several characteristic and noncharacteristic species. Controls were run with soils taken from experiment stations. Results indicated that no marked differences in germination occurred, although red pine seeds regularly germinated somewhat earlier in red pine soils than in control soils. The red pine soils markedly inhibited growth of non-characteristic species, whereas growth of characteristic species was virtually the same in red pine and control soils (Fig. 32). The results shown in Fig. 32 are representative of their overall results, and mea-

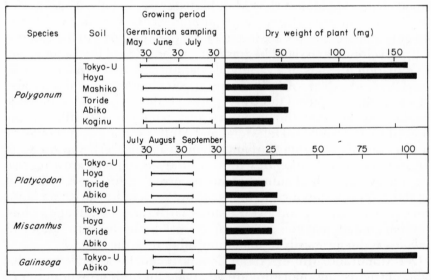

Fig. 32. Germination and growth in dry weight on various soils: farm soils, Tokyo University campus and Hoya Experimental Field; red-pine-forest soils, Mashiko, To-ride, Abiko, and Koginu; *Polygonum blumei,* sown on May 23, 1963; *Platycodon grandiflorum* and *Galinsoga ciliata,* sown on Aug. 5, 1963; *Miscanthus sinensis,* sown on July 20, 1963. (From Lee and Monsi, 1963.)

surements of physical and chemical factors of the soils used demonstrated no striking or consistent differences between control and the
various red pine test soils used.

Lee and Monsi (1963) concluded from their results that extracts of
various parts of *Pinus densiflora* and soils under this species contain
substances toxic to species which rarely occur in red pine forests.
They identified a tannin and *p*-coumaric acid in the extracts and in soil
from a red pine forest.

D. *Eucalyptus globulus*

Baker (1966) reported that *Eucalyptus globulus* produces volatile
materials that inhibit root growth of cucumber seedlings and also the
growth of hypocotyls, but not the roots of *Eucalyptus* seedlings.

Later, del Moral and Muller (1969) reported the abundance of this
species in parts of California, both as a planted and naturalized species. Moreover, they described the bare areas that regularly occur
under trees of this species and pointed out that most mature, undisturbed stands are almost devoid of herbaceous annuals. This species
often occurs in annual grasslands around Santa Barbara, California
and only stunted grasses are found under the outer part of the canopy.
Fully developed grassland begins right at the edge of the canopy, and
this situation prevails in a variety of edaphic and microclimatic conditions. A similar lack of herbaceous species under *E. globulus* also
occurs on the campus of the University of California at Santa Barbara,
despite the fact that the trees are kept trimmed and litter is not
allowed to accumulate. Del Moral and Muller reported an incidence
on the campus at Santa Barbara when heaps of fresh topsoil were
placed under two *E. globulus* trees. In the subsequent growing season, a heavy growth of annual plants occurred on the fresh soil. During the 2 years following the first growing season, however, no herbs
grew on the piles of soil even though no litter accumulated. Thus,
they concluded that the failure of annual herbs to grow under *E.
globulus* is due primarily to something other than the litter.

Del Moral and Muller (1969) demonstrated in several ways that
light, nutrients, and moisture are adequate for herb growth under *E.
globulus* and that small animals do not inhabit or visit *Eucalyptus*
stands frequently enough to influence the herbaceous vegetation. At
one time after a period of drought, the average soil moisture content in
one stand was 12.5%, whereas it was only 8.4% at a distance of 6 m
from the canopy in the grassland. One very large tree of *E. globulus* on

the Santa Barbara campus has its first branches 4–5 m above the ground so that full sunlight penetrates diagonally to the trunk. A new lawn was seeded, fertilized, and regularly watered under and to the southwest of the tree. The lawn developed rapidly except under the canopy where no germination occurred in spite of adequate light, water, and minerals.

Fog is very common in the area studied by del Moral and Muller, and large amounts of fog drip are common under trees. They hypothesized, therefore, that the fog drip might be primarily responsible for the lack of herb growth under the canopy of *E. globulus*. They collected fog drip under trees of this species on the Santa Barbara campus, filtered it to remove debris, and tested it against *Bromus rigidus* in the sponge assay procedure described in Chapter 6. Distilled water was used for controls. The fog drip was found to be very inhibitory to the growth of radicles of *Bromus* seedlings in six separate trials over a 6-month period.

Subsequent sponge assays were run using drip obtained by spraying a fine mist of distilled water over freshly collected leafy branches of *E. globulus*, and six test species found in annual grasslands adjacent to *Eucalyptus* groves, plus *E. globulus* itself. Significant reductions in radicle growth resulted in all test species due to the action of the artificial drip. This, of course, included *Eucalyptus globulus*.

Natural and artificial fog drip from *E. globulus* was tested against *Bromus rigidus* using the soil bioassay technique described in Chapter 6. Milpitas loam soil was substituted for sponges as the bed for germination, and both types of fog drip were inhibitory to root growth of *Bromus* in the assays. This demonstrated that the toxicity of fog drip is not lost in soil and supported the hypothesis that fog drip is responsible for the lack of annual herbs under *E. globulus*.

No terpenes were found in the fog drip from *E. globulus*, but numerous phenols were found including ellagic, chlorogenic, *p*-coumarylquinic, gentisic and gallic acids, and tannins. Del Moral and Muller stated that ellagic acid is a nontoxin, but work in my laboratory indicates it is toxic to nitrifying bacteria (Rice and Pancholy, 1973).

E. *Eucalyptus camaldulensis*

Del Moral and Muller (1970) observed characteristic zonations of herbaceous plants around groves of *Eucalyptus camaldulensis* and a virtual absence of herbs in the groves in Santa Barbara County,

California. These groves occur in annual grasslands in which the most important species are *Avena fatua, Bromus mollis, Bromus rigidus, Erodium cicutarium, Lolium multiflorum, Medicago hispida,* and *Trifolium hirtum. Festuca megalura* and *Hemizonia ramosissima* are sometimes important also.

The pattern associated with *E. camaldulensis* groves consists of (1) a litter zone covered by a moderately thick layer of leaves, bark, branches, and capsules which extended throughout the stand and to about the edge of the canopy; (2) a "bare" zone 2–5 m broad, devoid of litter and located between the edge of the litter zone and the edge of the grassland; and (3) the normal grassland (Fig. 33). Del Moral and Muller (1970) pointed out that virtually no annual herbs occur in the litter zone, but of those sporadic ones which occur, *Bromus mollis* and *Festuca megalura* are the most common. Occasionally a few seedlings of *Bromus rigidus, Trifolium hirtum,* and *Avena fatua* may appear. Seedlings of *Eucalyptus* itself are common but do not survive beyond the first season.

The "bare" zone appears bare but actually has herb densities higher than the litter zone. The densities are still low, and the plants are very stunted. *Bromus mollis* and *Festuca megalura* are most important

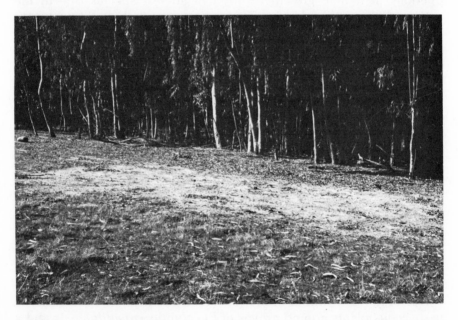

Fig. 33. Pattern of inhibition surrounding stand of *Eucalyptus camaldulensis.* (From del Moral and Muller, 1970.)

here also, just as in the litter zone. *Trifolium* seedlings are common but usually do not survive to maturity. *Avena fatua* and *Bromus rigidus* are uncommon in this zone. The grassland adjacent to the bare zone is dominated by *Bromus mollis, Festuca megalura, Trifolium hirtum,* and *Erodium,* and this dominance slowly shifts to *Avena fatua* and *Bromus rigidus.* This pattern is reestablished each year with the advent of winter rains and the germination of seeds of all the annual species within a period of a few days.

Del Moral and Muller (1970) decided to determine what phases of interference are responsible for the pattern of herbs associated with *E. camaldulensis.* Their initial thrust was aimed at the role of competition for minerals. They determined the levels of potassium, calcium, manganese, sodium, iron, magnesium, zinc, copper, nitrogen, phosphorus, and sulfur in each of the three zones described. No statistically significant differences in levels of any of the elements were found between zones. To test the possible role of competition for minerals still further, fertilizer containing most of the elements for which analyses were made was applied in bands 1.2 m broad across all zones. Herb growth was increased in all zones by the fertilizer, but the difference in growth between the litter zone and the grassland was even greater than in the untreated bands. Moreover, growth in the fertilized litter zone did not approach that even in the unfertilized grassland. They concluded, therefore, that nutrient limitations were not responsible for the pattern of herb growth inhibition.

Competition for light was investigated next by comparing light intensity in several stands of *E. camaldulensis* with that under *Quercus agrifolia* where herbaceous growth was good. The mean intensity under the *Quercus* trees was 45% of full sunlight, whereas it was 64% of full sunlight in *Eucalyptus* stands. It was thus concluded that competition for light is not likely to be an important mechanism of inhibition of herb growth.

Soil moisture measurements through two growing seasons indicated that the moisture content in the bare zone was consistently lower than in the grassland, whereas it was similar in the litter and grassland zones. Despite these facts, the density and vigor of the litter zone plants is less than for the bare zone plants. Thus, moisture differences could not explain the lack of herbs in the litter. Growth measurements were made of herbs in the litter zone and of similar species in the grassland zone early in the growing season when rains were common and soil moisture conditions were optimum in all zones. The litter zone plants were found to be markedly inhibited in growth even under the favorable moisture conditions existing at the time.

In another investigation of the soil moisture factor, del Moral and
Muller dug a trench around a plot in the litter zone to sever all roots of
Eucalyptus to a depth of 0.5 m, which was the depth of the hard pan.
Heavy plastic was placed in the trench before refilling to prevent
subsequent growth of roots into the plot. The results during a growing
season with normal rainfall indicated virtually no difference in herb
density and growth in the plot without root competition from *Eucalyptus* and the area in the litter zone with root competition. However, there was a marked increase in density and growth of species in
the plot without competition from *Eucalyptus* in an unusually wet
year (160% of normal rainfall). Del Moral and Muller concluded that
competition for water is not a sufficient mechanism alone to account
for the establishment of the inhibition pattern, but it could be important in the intensification and extension of the pattern.

Elimination of competition for light, water, and minerals as the
basic cause of the pattern of inhibition in and around *E. camaldulensis*
groves left only one aspect of interference to be investigated, allelopathy.

Much previous work indicated that various species of *Eucalyptus*
produce several terpenes. Therefore, del Moral and Muller (1970)
tested leaves for the presence of volatile inhibitors by use of the
sponge bioassay procedure with *Bromus rigidus* as the test species.
They found that leaves of *E. camaldulensis* produce strong volatile
toxins, and subsequently identified the major volatiles as α-pinene, β-
pinene, α-phellandrene, and cineole. Milpitas loam soil taken from
the field site was found to adsorb the volatile terpenes and to become
toxic to radicle growth of *Bromus rigidus*.

Del Moral and Muller obtained soil from the three zones in a *Eucalyptus* stand and heated it to drive off terpenes, if present, into
sealed flasks. The atmospheres of the flasks were subsequently analyzed by liquid-gas chromatography for terpenes, and large quantities
of α-pinene and cineole were obtained from litter zone soil. The same
terpenes were found in bare zone soil, but in lower concentrations,
and no terpenes were detected in the grassland soil. The concentrations of terpenes in litter zone soil were found to be great enough to
completely stop germination of the herb species involved, based on
previous tests. Subsequent tests confirmed a trend of decreasing terpene concentration from the litter zone to the grassland zone, and a
decrease in concentrations in all zones as the growing season progressed. They concluded that leaves of *E. camaldulensis* produce and
volatilize large quantities of terpenes during the hot, dry summer and
that these are adsorbed on dry soil in large amounts. Thus, the concen-

trations of terpenes in the soil would be at a peak at the beginning of the rainy season when seed germination occurs.

Experiments were carried out next to determine if various plant parts of *Eucalyptus* and litter in the groves contain water-soluble toxins. Aqueous extracts of green leaves, red leaf litter, brown leaf litter, bark, fresh roots, and partially decomposed roots were tested against *Bromus rigidus* in the sponge assay. The brown leaf litter was older than the red leaf litter. Both types of litter and bark were found to be very toxic to *Bromus* prior to the rainy season, but the toxicity of the leaf litter decreased markedly subsequent to the advent of the rains. They concluded that leaching by rain is an important mechanism for transfer of toxins from the litter into the soil.

Another test of the toxicity of litter was run by placing four or five layers of leaves from litter in a *Eucalyptus* grove on the surface of trays of soil in which four test species were planted. Half the trays of each species were irrigated by spraying from above so that the water would have to pass over the litter. The other trays were subirrigated so that the litter remained dry and was not leached (control). All test species were significantly inhibited in growth by the leachate from the litter (Table 33).

The effect of litter in the field was investigated by establishing two adjacent plots in a grove of *E. camaldulensis*. The litter was removed from one plot and allowed to remain on the other. One hundred seeds each of *Avena fatua* and *Festuca megalura* were carefully sown in each plot to ensure that all seeds fell in favorable spots for germination. Growth and survival were observed through a growing season,

TABLE 33

Height and Dry Weight of Herbs Growing under Greenhouse Conditions upon Treatment with Naturally Produced Litter Leachate [a]

Species	Control		Test	
	Height (mm)	Dry weight per pan (mg)	Height (mm)	Dry weight per pan (mg)
Avena fatua (20) [b]	113 ± 17	254	82 ± 13 [c]	134 [c]
Bromus rigidus (20)	114 ± 15	234	91 ± 17 [c]	177 [c]
Bromus mollis (30)	52 ± 8	13	30 ± 10 [c]	9 [c]
Festuca megalura (30)	50 ± 14	12	31 ± 12 [c]	7 [c]

[a] Modified from del Moral and Muller (1970).
[b] Number of plants per pan.
[c] Difference significant at the 5% level or better.

and it was found that survival and growth of both species were significantly reduced in the plot with litter. This was especially significant because the soil of the plot without litter was perceptibly drier.

Ten toxins were found in the aqueous extracts of leaf litter, five of which were identified. The five identified were the phenolics—gallic, ferulic, *p*-coumaric, chlorogenic, and caffeic acids.

Extracts of soil from the litter zone and the grassland zone were tested against *Bromus rigidus* in the sponge assay. The extracts were made from soil taken in increment levels of 2 cm to a depth of 6 cm, and it was found that toxins were present in all three levels of soil from the litter zone and increased in amount with depth. No toxins were found in the grassland soil. Attempts to identify the toxins in the soil from the litter plot failed, but it was suggested that they might be tannins.

Del Moral and Muller (1970) found that herbs abound throughout groves of *E. camaldulensis* growing in sandy soils, and subsequent tests demonstrated that soils from such areas do not adsorb terpenes or phenolic inhibitors to the same degree as fine-textured soils. Moreover, they found that the toxins involved were degraded in soil more rapidly under aerobic than anaerobic conditions. Coarse-textured soils generally have considerably better aeration also, so perhaps the inhibitors that are adsorbed in a coarse soil are broken down faster.

Del Moral and Muller concluded that the zonation of herbs in and near *Eucalyptus camaldulensis* is primarily due to allelopathy, which is mitigated to some extent by other factors. They concluded further that both terpenes and phenolics are important phytotoxins produced by this species of *Eucalyptus*, and that the pattern of shifting of dominance with distance from the canopy indicates that terpenes are capable of inhibiting plants selectively. Phenolic acids act strongly where litter accumulates but, according to these investigators, they cannot materially influence the establishment of the bare zones or the inhibited grassland.

F. *Platanus occidentalis*

The landscape director at the University of Oklahoma told me several years ago that he was not able to get *Cynodon dactylon, Lolium multiflorum,* or *Poa pratensis* to grow under sycamore, *Platanus occidentalis,* even with repeated attempts and adequate irrigation and fertilization. Al-Naib (1968) investigated the problem and found extracts or decaying materials of leaves, fruits, and buds of sycamore to be inhibitory to growth of the above-mentioned grasses. This suggested that the bare areas under the sycamore trees might be due primarily to an allelopathic mechanism.

Subsequently, Al-Naib and Rice (1971) observed that virtually no herbaceous plants grow under sycamore trees in natural areas, except in the case of isolated trees in exposed areas where the fallen leaves are blown completely away from the area of the tree. A project was undertaken, therefore, to determine whether the bare areas under the sycamore in natural habitats were due primarily to competition for light, water, or minerals or to chemical inhibitors produced by the sycamore.

Stands of sycamore were selected in Pottawatomie County, Oklahoma for intensive studies. The area in which the stands were located had not been grazed for a considerable time period prior to the study. Very few species were found within the stands and individuals were scattered and had poor vitality (Fig. 34). Species in the stands included

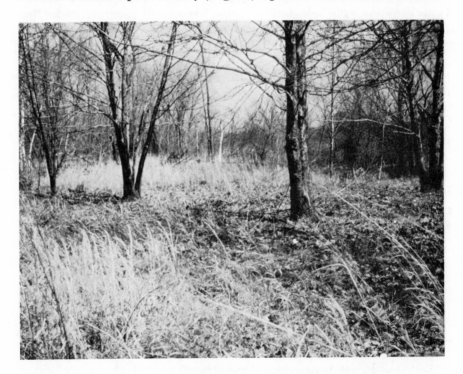

Fig. 34. View of sycamore stand showing bare area beneath canopy. (From Al-Naib and Rice, 1971.)

Ambrosia trifida var. *texana, Elephantopus carolinianus, Elymus virginicus, Spartina pectinata,* and *Symphoricarpos orbiculatus.* The following species were found away from the edge of the canopy and area of leaf fall and accumulation: *Andropogon glomeratus, Andropogon virginicus, Ambrosia psilostachya, Cynodon dactylon, Elymus virginicus, Panicum anceps, Panicum scribnerianum, Panicum virgatum, Setaria viridis, Symphoricarpos orbiculatus,* and *Tridens flavus.*

Sampling was accomplished by locating thirty 0.25 m² quadrats at the edge of the canopy, 30 quadrats 0.5 m outward from the first series, and 30 additional quadrats 0.5 m outward from the second series. All plants in the quadrats were clipped, separated by species, and oven-dried weights were determined. The weights of all species were found to be significantly lower in the quadrats at the edge of the canopy than in those farther away. The area immediately below the sycamore canopy was not sampled, as there was virtually no growth of herbaceous plants there.

Initial experiments were designed to determine if there were obvious differences in selected minerals, pH, or soil moisture under the sycamore canopy and away from the canopy in the dense herb zone. Analyses of total nitrogen, total phosphorus, and exchangeable and easily soluble copper, iron, and zinc indicated no differences in the two zones. The pH was virtually the same in the two zones also. Soil moisture was determined in the two zones in June, July, and August when it was most likely to be limiting to plant growth. It was measured in two levels, 0–15 cm and 15–30 cm, and was found to be greater under the canopy at both levels at all sampling periods (Table 34).

TABLE 34

Comparison of Soil Moisture under the Sycamore Canopy and Away from It in Summer of 1969 [a,b]

Depth of soil samples (cm)	Moisture (%)					
	June		July		August	
	Under	Outside	Under	Outside	Under	Outside
0–15	25.5	21.0 [c]	15.6	15.0	21.1	18.9 [c]
15–30	24.9	16.7 [c]	16.7	12.2 [c]	21.7	19.3

[a] Modified from Al-Naib and Rice (1971).

[b] Each value represents the average of ten soil samples.

[c] Difference from appropriate level under the canopy significant at 0.05 level or better.

TABLE 35

Effects of Shade on Growth of Herbaceous Species Associated with Sycamore [a]

	Mean oven-dried weight (gm/0.25 m^2)	
Species	In artificial shade	In full sunlight [b]
Ambrosia psilostachya	17.0	17.3
Andropogon glomeratus	34.8	35.9
Andropogon virginicus	23.1	24.6
Panicum virgatum	32.4	32.0
Setaria viridis	7.1	7.5

[a] Modified from Al-Naib and Rice (1971).
[b] No significant differences at 0.05 level.

Most of the species that did not grow under sycamore grew well under other nearby tree species where the light intensity as determined by measurements was just as low as under sycamore. Nevertheless, numerous shading devices designed to cast the same shade as the sycamore trees were placed in the herb area in the field in the spring of 1968. These were checked every week or two, but at the time chosen for sampling in October, they were found removed and destroyed by vandals. The exact locations could not be located because there were no noticeable differences in growth where they were located. The experiment was repeated again in 1969, and determination of oven-dried weights of species per unit area under the shading devices and in the open grassland indicated no significant differences (Table 35).

All evidence to this point indicated that competition for light, minerals, and water is probably not responsible for the failure of herbaceous plants to grow under sycamore trees. Moreover, we noted that growth of herbs did not occur or was inhibited anyplace where sycamore leaves were blown by the wind and accumulated in appreciable numbers away from the canopies of the stands. Experiments were thus undertaken to determine if allelopathy might be an important influence in the failure of herbs to grow well under the sycamore canopy and near it. Tests concerned effects of decaying sycamore leaves, leachates from living sycamore leafy branches, and soil collected under sycamore trees.

Field sampling of sycamore leaves on the ground after leaf fall indicated that there were 6.16 gm air-dried weight of sycamore leaves per 454 gm of soil to a depth of approximately 17 cm. In order to determine the effects of decaying sycamore leaves on selected test species, seeds of these species were planted in pots containing soil mixed with 1 gm air-dried ground leaf material per 454 gm of soil. Control pots contained 1 gm of air-dried peat moss per 454 gm of soil to keep the organic matter content the same. Fifty test seeds were planted in each pot with the exception of *Ambrosia psilostachya*, seedlings of which were transplanted from the field, because the seeds germinate very poorly even after cold treatment. All plants were kept under greenhouse conditions, and after germination was completed, the plants were thinned to the five largest plants per pot. The plants were allowed to grow for an additional 3 weeks, at which time they were harvested and oven-dried weights were determined. Decaying sycamore leaves inhibited seed germination and seedling growth of all test species (Table 36). These data indicate that leaves of sycamore contain toxins that are released into the soil during the decay process causing inhibition of herbaceous species present.

Leachate was obtained by spraying a fine mist of water over fresh, mature leafy sycamore branches, and this leachate was used to water

TABLE 36

Effects of Decaying Sycamore Leaves on Seed Germination and Seedling Growth [a]

Species	Experiment No.	Mean oven-dried weight of seedlings (mg)		Germination [c]
		Control	Test [b]	
Ambrosia	1	937.0	236.7	—
psilostachya	2	823.0	220.6	—
Andropogon	1	620.7	64.9	37
glomeratus	2	624.8	63.1	21
Andropogon	1	589.8	15.8	33
virginicus	2	566.4	15.9	25
Elymus	1	123.6	23.8	51
virginicus	2	128.3	27.2	62
Panicum	1	376.7	100.9	77
virgatum	2	355.5	30.0	88
Setaria	1	296.7	17.5	60
viridis	2	390.0	18.2	75
Tridens	1	944.6	67.0	56
flavus	2	905.5	54.5	52

[a] Modified from Al-Naib and Rice (1971).
[b] Dry weight significantly different from control at 0.05 level or better in all cases.
[c] Expressed as percent of control.

TABLE 37

Effects of Leaf Leachate of Sycamore on Germination and Seedling Growth [a]

Species	Experiment No.	Mean oven-dried weight of seedlings (mg)		Germination [b]
		Control	Test	
Ambrosia	1	937.0	385.5 [c]	—
psilostachya	2	823.0	321.5 [c]	—
Andropogon	1	181.8	178.2	70
glomeratus	2	157.7	92.0 [c]	63
Andropogon	1	283.4	201.8 [c]	77
virginicus	2	313.3	215.9 [c]	71
Elymus	1	102.5	100.5	97
virginicus	2	87.4	84.3	91
Panicum	1	155.3	150.3	95
virgatum	2	124.2	121.2	98
Setaria	1	296.7	187.5 [c]	64
viridis	2	329.9	232.5 [c]	52
Tridens	1	944.6	371.0 [c]	67
flavus	2	861.1	298.0 [c]	74

[a] Modified from Al-Naib and Rice (1971).
[b] Expressed as percent of control.
[c] Weight significantly different from control at 0.05 level or better.

pots of soil containing the same test species used in the previous experiment. Controls were irrigated with water that did not pass over sycamore leaves. Germination and growth were measured as before. The leachate reduced the percentage germination appreciably in all species except *Panicum virgatum* and *Elymus virginicus* (Table 37). The leachate also significantly reduced the oven-dried weights of all species except *Elymus virginicus* and *Panicum virgatum*. The failure of the leachate to inhibit germination and growth of *E. virginicus* seems significant in view of the fact that this species was one of few that grew at least sparsely under the canopy.

To determine effects of soil under the sycamore canopy on germination and growth of test species, soil minus litter was taken by means of a posthole digger, to prevent disturbing its vertical stratification, and placed directly in 4-inch plastic pots. Control soil was obtained in a similar way outside the canopy and away from the area of leaf fall. These soil collections were made in July when the sycamores were in full leaf and in November after the leaves and some fruits had fallen. The two soil collections were treated as separate experiments. Except for *Ambrosia psilostachya,* seedlings of which were again transplanted from the field, 50 seeds of each of the test species were planted in the pots and allowed to germinate. After the amount of germination was recorded, the five largest plants in each pot were allowed to grow for an additional 3 weeks. The oven-dried weights of the entire plants were then determined.

Soil from under the sycamore canopy significantly reduced both seed germination and oven-dried weights of all test species during both sampling periods (Table 38). The soil collected under the canopy in November caused a greater degree of inhibition of both germination and seedling growth than that collected in July. This was probably due to a greater accumulation of sycamore debris on the soil surface in November with the resultant leaching of substances from the debris into the soil.

Toxins produced by the leaves were identified as chlorogenic acid, scopoletin, and scopolin; those produced by the fruits as the same three plus isochlorogenic acid, band 510, neochlorogenic acid, and o-coumaric acid; and those present in leachate of leaves as chlorogenic acid and scopolin. All were found to be inhibitory to germination of

TABLE 38

Effect of Field Soils from the Sycamore Stand on Germination and Growth of Test species [a]

Species	Date soil taken	Mean oven-dried weight of seedlings (mg)		Germination [c]
		Control	Test [b]	
Ambrosia	July	365.2	275.0	—
psilostachya	November	312.1	196.1	—
Andropogon	July	453.8	38.3	57
glomeratus	November	543.8	32.0	31
Andropogon	July	176.0	25.8	34
virginicus	November	148.1	42.8	29
Elymus	July	78.4	39.0	62
virginicus	November	90.2	25.6	61
Panicum	July	140.2	16.6	77
virgatum	November	126.8	18.0	76
Setaria	July	281.5	113.2	39
viridis	November	253.0	40.0	28
Tridens	July	192.4	83.0	60
flavus	November	75.6	6.3	54

[a] Modified from Al-Naib and Rice (1971).
[b] Weight significantly different from control at 0.05 level or better in all cases.
[c] Expressed as percent of control.

seeds of a plant commonly used as a test species, *Amaranthus retroflexus*.

On the basis of the evidence obtained, Al-Naib and Rice (1971) concluded that the production of chemical inhibitors by sycamore is the basic cause of the failure of most herbaceous species to grow under sycamore trees or in areas where sycamore leaves accumulate. They concluded further that once the herbaceous species are slowed in germination and growth, even moderate competitive effects serve as a feedback mechanism which accentuates the retardation in growth.

G. *Celtis laevigata*

I observed over a period of several years on the University of Oklahoma campus at Norman that grasses and other plants did not grow under hackberry, *Celtis laevigata,* or under rough-leaved hack-berry, *Celtis occidentalis,* even though the lower branches were elimi-nated to a height of 5–6 m, which allowed full sunlight to penetrate entirely to the trunk during part of the day. This condition persisted even with addition of fertilizer and thorough watering. One of my graduate students and I found that this condition was present in natu-ral areas also, both in bottomland and in upland. Consequently, we investigated to determine what sort of interference on the part of the hackberry, *C. laevigata,* is responsible for the failure of herbs to grow under its canopy (Lodhi and Rice, 1971). *Celtis occidentalis* does not occur in natural areas near Norman, so only a few preliminary type experiments were run in connection with this species and material from campus trees was used.

A plot containing scattered hackberry and plum, *Prunus mexicana,* trees in a tall grass prairie area was established in the University of Oklahoma Grasslands Research Plots near Norman, Oklahoma. The grasslands plots are on a gently rolling upland with moderately deep sandy loam soil over a soft red sandstone bedrock. Vegetation of the area is tall-grass prairie that has been invaded by woody species since the elimination of burning and grazing starting in 1949. Dominant species in the plots are *Andropogon scoparius, A. gerardi, Panicum virgatum,* and *Sorghastrum nutans.* The growth of herbaceous spe-cies was observed to be considerably better under plum than hack-berry.

The herbaceous vegetation under several hackberry and several plum trees was sampled by means of clip quadrats. The plants were rated by species, oven dried, and weighed, and all four important .irie grasses were found to have significantly higher yields under plum trees than under hackberry trees. No differences were found, however, in yields around the two species away from their canopies.

Light intensities were measured several times during June and July at numerous positions under several plum and hackberry trees and the range of intensities under both species was found to be the same, 2600–3300 ft-c. Thus, differences in light competition could not be responsible for the differences in growth of herbs under the test and control (plum) trees.

Soil moisture, pH, texture, and several selected mineral analyses were made to see if the differences in vegetation under the plum and hackberry trees were due primarily to physical and chemical properties of the soil. Soil moisture was determined during 3 summer months by taking soil samples at each of two depths (0–15 cm and 15–30 cm). For physical and chemical soil analyses, soil samples minus litter were collected at the 0–30 cm level under hackberry and plum trees. Analyses were made of total nitrogen, total carbon, total phosphorus, and exchangeable and readily available iron, zinc, copper, and manganese.

There were no significant differences in pH, sand, silt, clay, organic carbon, or any of the mineral elements tested under plum and hackberry trees. Obviously, all essential elements were not quantified, but enough were measured to indicate that the reduction in herb growth under hackberry was probably not due to competition for minerals, and it obviously was not due to textural or pH differences.

Soil moisture was significantly higher under hackberry than under plum at both levels and all sampling times, so the reduction in herb growth under hackberry was obviously not due to competition for water.

Allelopathy was the only remaining mechanism of interference, and we investigated effects of decaying leaves, leachates of fresh leaves, and soil under hackberry versus that under plum on seed germination and growth of the four major prairie grasses.

To determine effects of decaying hackberry leaves on the test species, 30 seeds each of *Andropogon gerardi, A. scoparius,* and *Panicum virgatum* and large numbers of seeds of *Sorghastrum nutans* (to obviate poor germination) were planted in each test pot containing 1 gm of air-dried fresh hackberry leaf powder per 454 gm of soil. A similar number of seeds was planted in each control pot containing 1 gm of peat moss per 454 gm of soil in order to keep the organic matter content the same as in the test pots. Germination was determined after

2 weeks, and the plants were thinned to the four largest seedlings per pot. Seedlings were allowed to grow for 2 additional weeks and then harvested, oven dried, and weighed. The decaying leaves significantly inhibited germination and growth of all test species (Table 39).

Leaf leachate was obtained by use of artificial rain on freshly collected leafy hackberry branches, and the leachate was used to water test species in soil. Controls were irrigated with water that had not passed over hackberry leaves. The leachate was found to be inhibitory to all test species just as were the decaying leaves (Table 40). Apparently, toxins produced by hackberry leaves can leach out of living leaves into the soil, or they can be released by decay of the leaves. To determine the biological activity and stability of toxic compounds in the soil, soil collections were made in July and January, under hackberry (test) and plum (control). Collections were made with a sharpnose shovel, and the soil was transferred directly into the pots in order to disturb the profile as little as possible. Seeds of test species were placed in appropriate pots with 30 seeds per pot. Germination was determined at 2 weeks and dry weight at 4 weeks after planting.

The soil collected in July under hackberry did not significantly reduce seed germination or seedling growth (Table 41). However, the January sample significantly reduced seed germination and seedling growth of all test species. Apparently, the toxic compounds are more active in soil in late fall and winter after the accumulation of hack-

TABLE 39

Effects of Decaying Hackberry Leaves on Germination and Seedling Growth [a]

Species	Experiment No.	Mean oven-dried weight of seedlings (mg)		Germination [c]
		Control	Test [b]	
Andropogon gerardi	1	162 ± 8.3	116 ± 7.1	76
	2	165 ± 7.5	98 ± 7.9	68
Andropogon scoparius	1	167 ± 8.0	102 ± 8.2	72
	2	125 ± 8.8	87 ± 6.5	64
Panicum virgatum	1	203 ± 5.4	131 ± 8.7	64
	2	178 ± 7.7	129 ± 5.0	68
Sorghastrum nutans	1	195 ± 10.1	144 ± 7.2	—
	2	199 ± 6.9	128 ± 9.4	—

[a] From Lodhi and Rice (1971).
[b] Dry weight significantly different from control at .05 level in all cases.
[c] Expressed as percent of control.

...eaf Leachate of Hackberry on Germination and Seedling Growth [a]

Species	Experiment No.	Mean oven-dried weight of seedlings (mg)		Germination [c]
		Control	Test [b]	
Andropogon gerardi	1	201 ± 7.5	160 ± 6.6	21
	2	222 ± 7.6	141 ± 9.9	83
Andropogon scoparius	1	136 ± 9.3	85 ± 5.7	77
	2	110 ± 7.5	83 ± 4.4	69
Panicum virgatum	1	200 ± 10.1	164 ± 9.2	69
	2	201 ± 6.0	129 ± 8.5	73
Sorghastrum nutans	1	182 ± 9.4	145 ± 7.6	—
	2	199 ± 6.6	126 ± 9.5	—

[a] From Lodhi and Rice (1971).
[b] Dry weight significantly different from control at 0.05 level in all cases.
[c] Expressed as percent of control.

berry leaves and other plant parts on the soil surface. Without doubt, the levels of toxins in the soil under hackberry would still be high in March, when the grass species involved are just starting to renew growth, because low soil temperatures during the winter months would slow down oxidation or microbial degradation. Retardation of

TABLE 41

Effect of Field Soil from under Hackberry Trees on Germination and Seedling Growth [a]

Species	Date soil taken	Mean oven-dried weight of seedlings (mg)		Germination [c]
		Control	Test	
Andropogon gerardi	July 1969	177 ± 7.2	172 ± 7.1	92
	Jan. 1970	197 ± 7.4	122 ± 9.3 [b]	49
Andropogon scoparius	July 1969	111 ± 7.2	101 ± 6.4	84
	Jan. 1970	117 ± 7.7	91 ± 4.4 [b]	51
Panicum virgatum	July 1969	192 ± 8.2	182 ± 11.6	86
	Jan. 1970	193 ± 7.2	141 ± 5.4 [b]	47
Sorghastrum nutans	July 1969	144 ± 6.6	132 ± 5.6	—
	Jan. 1970	187 ± 6.7	121 ± 9.8 [b]	—

[a] From Lodhi and Rice (1971).
[b] Dry weight significantly different from control at 0.05 level.
[c] Expressed as percent of control.

growth of the herbs in the early part of the growing season probably causes increased inhibition due to competition. Of course, there would be an additional inhibitory effect due to the leachate from the leaves during rains, and thus toxins would continue to be renewed in the soil throughout the growing season. The dominant prairie grasses are perennials, which for the most part reproduce vegetatively, so inhibition of seed germination is probably chiefly important in preventing the invasion of the bare area under hackberry trees by annuals. Lodhi and Rice (1971) concluded on the basis of the evidence obtained that the paucity of herb growth under *Celtis laevigata* is primarily due to allelopathic effects of hackberry accentuated by competition.

Preliminary tests with aqueous extracts of fresh leaves indicated that *Celtis occidentalis* may produce higher quantities of toxins than *C. laevigata* (M. A. K. Lodhi, unpublished). If so, bare areas under *C. occidentalis* are probably due to an allelopathic mechanism, but this possibility needs to be thoroughly checked.

Lodhi and Rice (1971) identified the chief phytotoxins produced by *Celtis laevigata* leaves as scopolin, scopoletin, ferulic acid, caffeic acid, *p*-coumaric acid, and gentisic acid. All these were found to be very inhibitory to the germination of *Amaranthus palmeri* seeds.

H. *Miscellaneous Species*

Del Moral and Cates (1971) did a comprehensive and ingenious survey of the allelopathic potential of 40 species of ferns, conifers, and angiosperms of western Washington. The laboratory phase of the study involved the testing of leaves for volatile inhibitors and of leaves, litter, and bark (if present) for water-soluble inhibitors of root growth in seedlings of *Hordeum vulgare, Bromus tectorum,* and *Pseudotsuga menziesii.* The sponge and soil bioassay methods previously described were used (Muller *et al.,* 1964; Muller and del Moral, 1966). The results from all assays were combined to give an index of inhibition for each of the 40 species in the survey. A species was considered to induce significant inhibition if it had an index value of 20% or more.

The field phase of the survey involved the sampling of vegetation under the species involved in the survey and the separate sampling of vegetation adjacent to the survey species. Cover, frequency, and species composition were determined, and the coefficient of community was calculated for each species. A species was considered to demonstrate interference in the field if there was at least a 50% reduction in cover under it, the coefficient of community was less than 50%, and the species richness was less than 75% of that of the adjacent area in all samples.

Species were next categorized on the basis of results in the field and laboratory tests. Nine species were found to produce significant inhibition in the laboratory and interference in the field, and these were *Abies amabilis, Abies grandis, Abies procera, Picea engelmannii, Taxus brevifolia, Thuja plicata, Acer circinatum, Arbutus menziesii,* and *Rhododendron albiflorum.* Sixteen species produced significant inhibition but no field interference, five species produced no laboratory inhibition but showed interference in the field, and the rest (ten species) produced no inhibition and had no interference.

Del Moral and Cates (1971) concluded from the above that the interference (patterning) demonstrated by the nine species listed above was primarily due to allelopathy. They pointed out, however, that their results need to be examined further by testing inhibitory effects of the species on the native species influenced by the plants in question. In the case of the five species showing interference in the field and no inhibition in the laboratory, they suggested that the interference must be due to competition and not to allelopathy. Twenty-six species demonstrated little or no interference in the field.

The methodology used in this project appears to me to have excellent potential for surveys of allelopathic potential of species of woody plants in other areas.

Grodzinsky and Gaidamak (1971) observed that concentric zones of specific herbs are formed around scattered trees of *Pinus silvestris, P. strobus, Picea excelsa, Larix decidua, Thuja occidentalis, T. plicata,* and *Abies concolor* in parks in the Kiev and Chernigov regions of the U.S.S.R. They suspected that allelopathy was responsible for the patterns, and tests of aqueous extracts of the soil confirmed their suspicion. They subsequently quantified the phytotoxins in the upper layers of soil in the various herb zones. They found the concentration of phytotoxins was highest near the tree trunks and that a secondary peak occurred some distance beyond the crown of each tree. They consistently found the lowest concentration just outside the crown of each tree, and they termed this the neutral zone.

The neutral zone was occupied by characteristic herbaceous species such as *Urtica dioica, Chelidonium majus, Taraxacum officinale, Galium ruthenicum, G. intermedium, Veronica chamaedrys,* and *Leonurus quinquelobatus.*

Grodzinsky and Gaidamak (1971) found a similar neutral zone with a low phytotoxin content between beech–hornbeam (*Fagus–Carpinus*) forests and neighboring fescue–meadow grass associations in the Carpathian Mountains.

Parpiev (1971) investigated the relationships between shrubs and small trees in the middle Asian deserts and the herbaceous vegetation under the shrubs and trees. In one phase of his study, he tested extracts of seeds, fallen leaves, and leafy shoots of such woody species as *Haloxylon aphyllum, Salsola richteri, Populus pruinosa, Tamarix hispida,* and *Calligonum* spp. against seed germination of herbaceous species such as *Artemisia ferganensis* and *Chenopodium album,* which are common understory plants. He found that extracts of genetically and ecologically similar species of shrubs and small trees were favorable to germination of the seeds, but extracts of genetically and ecologically distinct species inhibited germination. Thus, patterning was strongly influenced by allelopathy.

Parpiev's results emphasize a very important point in the field of allelopathy, i.e., toxic interactions are generally much more likely to occur and to be more striking if species have only relatively recently been brought in contact with each other. This is probably the chief reason that introduced weeds and trees exhibit such striking allelopathic effects at times (e.g., *Eucalyptus* in California, pioneer weeds in old-field succession). Species that have evolved together for thousands of years in natural climax ecosystems are unlikely to retain strong allelopathic interactions.

8

Allelopathy and the Prevention of Seed Decay before Germination

I. DIRECT PRODUCTION OF MICROBIAL INHIBITORS BY SEED PLANTS

Probably one of the most critical points in the life cycle of many plants is seed germination. This is certainly the case with many annual plants, which include most cultivated plants, and is often true in the initial establishment and spread of many perennial plants. Lieth (1960) emphasized that reproduction from seed is very common even in a perennial grassland.

Almost every person who has planted seeds has experienced the loss of some due to decomposition by microorganisms. The incidence of decay is certainly influenced by environmental conditions in addition to internal conditions of the seeds. I suspect that most seeds that do not germinate rapidly after landing in soil would be decomposed before germination if they did not contain or produce microbial inhibitors, or, in other words, phytoncides. In fact, I suspect this may be one of the most consistent and important ecological roles of allelopathy in annual plants and many perennial plants growing in natural areas. According to Horton and Kraebel (1955), seeds of many annual herbs that are important in the fire cycle in California chaparral lie dormant for as long as 40–50 years. Many seeds lie dormant in the soil for several years even in humid and superhumid areas. It is very unlikely that seeds could remain in soil for even 2 years in many areas without being decomposed if they did not contain microbial inhibitors. Such a mechanism may not be as critical in crop plants because they have been selected over a long period of time for rapid seed

germination. Such seeds probably germinate rapidly enough generally that they do not allow time for decomposition. Another interesting
aspect of seed selection in cultivated plants is that dormancy mechanisms and germination inhibitors have generally been eliminated.
There is much clear evidence that many germination inhibitors in
seeds and fruits are compounds that are microbial inhibitors also, and
I will discuss this further later in this chapter.

Unfortunately, there is not a lot of direct evidence to support my
suggestion concerning the prevalence of microbial inhibitors in seeds,
but there is some, and there is much more indirect evidence that will
be discussed only briefly in this chapter. Even though the direct evidence for the role of allelopathy in the prevention of seed decay before germination is not great, I feel the importance of the phenomenon
warrants a separate chapter to emphasize it.

Ferenczy (1956) stated that Maksimov, in his plant physiology text
published in 1948 in the U.S.S.R., mentioned that certain seeds in the
swollen state are capable of germinating over years in the soil because
they discharge antimicrobial substances into their immediate environment. Evenari (1949) pointed out that seeds of *Brassica oleracea* contain a microbial inhibitor belonging to the mustard oils, and that the
resistance of crucifers to clubroot disease caused by *Plasmodiophora
brassicae* is attributed to their content of such oils. He stated further
that mustard oils and their vapors are highly toxic to different fungi in
concentrations as low as 10 ppm. He reported also that essential oils
have been used for a long time as disinfectants because of their pronounced antimicrobial action. According to Evenari, Focke reported
in 1881 that plants producing essential oils are protected against attacks by parasitic fungi. Another group of compounds found in many
seeds and toxic to numerous microorganisms is the alkaloid group
(Evenari, 1949). Many unsaturated lactones are potent antimicrobial
compounds, and these are common in seeds. Parasorbic acid found in
seeds of *Sorbus aucuparia*, and anemonin, protoanemonin, digoxige-
nin, gitoxigenin, and strophantidin are examples of unsaturated lactones that are strongly antimicrobial (Evenari, 1949). Evenari gave a
long list of species and plant parts demonstrated to produce or contain
seed germination inhibitors, and stated that these toxins are effective
against many kinds of processes, so it is probable that they affect one
or more very basic reactions common to all living organisms.

Many types of phenolic compounds occur in fruits and seeds also,
both as aglycones and as glycosides (Feenstra, 1960; Harborne, 1964;
Harborne and Simmonds, 1964; Henis *et al.*, 1964; Lane, 1965; Harris
and Burns, 1972). These include simple phenols such as catechol in

fruits of *Psorospermum* and *Citrus* (Harborne and Simmonds, 1964); glycosides of simple phenols, such as phlorin, a glycoside of phloro-glucinol, in *Citrus* fruits (Harborne and Simmonds, 1964); phenolic acids such as caffeic and chlorogenic acids in the seeds of sunflower (Lane, 1965); glycosides of phenolic acids such as glucosides of *p*-coumaric and caffeic acids that occur in seeds of *Linum* (Harborne, 1964); free flavonoids, such as tricin, in seeds of *Orobanche;* quercetin and myricetin in *Trifolium* seeds, casticin in seeds of *Vitex* (Harborne, 1964); anthocyanidins that are widely distributed in fruits (Harborne and Simmonds, 1964); glycosides of flavonoids, such as rutin, in seeds of *Brassica;* apigenin in celery seeds; two glycosides of kaempferol in *Solanum* seeds, numerous flavonoid glycosides in fruits of many spe-cies (Harborne, 1964); and tannins, both hydrolyzable and condensed, which are widespread in plants (Bate-Smith and Metcalfe, 1957) and which have been specifically identified in fruits and seeds (Henis *et al.*, 1964; Harris and Burns, 1970, 1972). Varga and Köves (1959) iden-tified several phenolic acids and gallotannins in dried fruits of 24 species of plants. Many more similar data are available, but these should emphasize the widespread occurrence of phenolics in seeds and fruits.

Much evidence has accumulated indicating that phenolic com-pounds of several types are important in the resistance of plants to infection by fungal, bacterial, and viral diseases (Schaal and Johnson, 1955; Kúc *et al.*, 1956; Cadman, 1959; Byrde *et al.*, 1960; Hughes and Swain, 1960; Farkas and Kiraly, 1962; Gardner and Payne, 1964). This evidence does not relate directly to the prevention of seed decay, but it certainly has an important indirect relation. The compounds have to be inhibitory to bacteria and fungi to prevent diseases caused by these organisms, so no doubt they inhibit growth of organisms involved in seed decay also.

Additional indirect evidence has been obtained in my laboratory that phenolics present in seeds and fruits might prevent seed decay. Representative compounds of all the types listed above have been found to be inhibitory to growth of several species of *Rhizobium, Nitrobacter,* and *Nitrosomonas* and to nitrification in soil (Rice, 1965a,b,c, 1969; Rice and Pancholy, 1973; E. L. Rice and S. K. Pan-choly, unpublished). I emphasize that this is very indirect evidence because the bacteria involved are not decay organisms. *Rhizobium* is not appreciably affected, however, by several antibiotics commonly used for medicinal purposes (E. L. Rice, unpublished), but still is strongly inhibited by many of the phenolic compounds. Three sensi-tivity disks of one of the tannins from *Euphorbia supina* virtually completely prevented the growth of *Rhizobium* over an entire 10 cm petri dish (Rice, 1969). Moreover, dishes containing three disks of this tannin never had any contaminants grow on them, even though they were opened many times in the laboratory over a period of several months (E. L. Rice, unpublished). Control dishes rapidly supported a dense growth of many bacterial and fungal contaminants.

Knudson (1913) found that *Aspergillus niger* and *Penicillium* sp. can use tannic acid, a hydrolyzable tannin, as a carbon source. He found only five other species of *Penicillium* and one of *Aspergillus* that could grow in the presence of a 5% solution of tannic acid, even with other carbon sources present. No other fungi were found that could grow in such a solution at all.

Benoit and his colleagues furnished further evidence for the effectiveness of tannins in preventing decay of organic material (Benoit and Starkey, 1968a,b; Benoit *et al.*, 1968). Benoit *et al.* (1968) found that purified wattle tannin reduced the decomposition of whole plant material from rye plants harvested at young, intermediate, and mature stages of growth by approximately 50% in a given time period. Benoit and Starkey (1968b) reported that purified wattle tannin slightly inhibited decomposition of polygalacturonic acid and pectin, but markedly inhibited decomposition of a plant hemicellulose preparation and cellulose. In a related project, Benoit and Starkey (1968a) found that wattle tannin reduced activity of polygalacturonase, cellulase, and urease. They concluded that inactivation by tannins of exoenzymes of microorganisms concerned with decomposition of large molecular weight compounds is an important part of the inhibitory effect of tannins on the decomposition of plant residues. This certainly would apply to decay of seeds, This could obviously be a very beneficial effect in the case of tannin-containing seeds, but it could be detrimental in decomposition and mineral cycling of high tannin-containing dead organic material. The latter phenomenon is probably a very important ecological role of allelopathy, but has hardly been touched in natural ecosystems.

The evidence presented in the past several paragraphs, although often indirect, does support the hypothesis that various types of phenolic compounds, when present in seeds, probably help prevent seed decay before germination. They probably play a similar role in many plants in natural areas, even when present only in the fruits.

Ferenczy (1956) performed a series of experiments directly concerned with microbial inhibition by intact seeds and fruits. Petri dishes containing a suitable solid medium with a pH of 7.0 were inoculated with a suspension of a test bacterium. After the surface of the medium was dry, a selected seed or fruit was half sunk into the culture medium. After 20 hours at 30°C, the dishes were examined for zones of inhibition of the test bacteria. Six different species of bacteria, which are common saprophytes in soil, but some of which are also parasitic on plants, were selected: *Bacillus cereus* var. *mycoides*, *B. megaterium* (strain 208), *B. subtilis*, *Aerobacter aerogenes*, *Erwinia carotovora*, and *Xanthomonas malvacearum*. Seeds and sometimes fruits of 512 species of plants belonging to 88 families were tested against all six species of bacteria. Seeds or fruits of 52 species belonging to 19 families were found to contain antibacterial compounds according to the test used. These compounds were localized in the seed coat and the external layer of the fruits, except in the species of *Fraxinus* where they occurred only in the embryo. Ferenczy (1956) stated that many seeds known to contain bacterial inhibitors, such as those of species of the Cruciferae, did not give positive results in his tests. Perhaps some chemical or mechanical activity has to occur in such cases before the toxins are released, or perhaps the toxins are produced only after microbial action on tissues of the seeds occurs (Farkas and Kiraly, 1962). Wright (1956) reported that white mustard seed (*Sinapis*) produced zones of inhibition on agar inoculated with *Bacillus subtilis* if the seed coats were not removed. She pointed out that these seeds, in addition, produce a diffusible antibacterial substance that is not present in the seed coats. Ferenczy (1956) found that some of the seeds and fruits were very inhibitory to fungi also, although no comprehensive tests were run against fungi.

Patrick and Koch (1958) reported that antifungal compounds are sometimes produced during the decomposition of certain plant residues in the soil. If these are produced in the vicinity of seeds, they could presumably aid in the prevention of seed decay.

Nickell (1960) tabulated all species of vascular plants reported to inhibit any or all of the following: gram-positive bacteria, gram-negative bacteria, fungi, mycobacteria, protozoa, phages, viruses, and yeasts. Yeasts, of course, are fungi but they are often listed separately in tests for antimicrobial substances. He found reports of active species in 157 families. Considering just those species in which the seeds were tested, he listed 50 species in 23 families which had antimicrobial activity (Table 42). Often other plant parts of several species in the same genera were found to have antimicrobial activity, but the seeds were not tested, and, of course, this was true of most genera. I suspect that in many species in which parts other than seeds have been shown to have antimicrobial activity, the seeds have similar activity.

Bowen (1961) reported that seed coats of sterilized seeds of the legumes, *Centrosema pubescens* and *Trifolium subterraneum,* were inhibitory to *Rhizobium* and other bacteria when placed on petri dishes inoculated with the bacteria. Fottrell *et al.* (1964) reported that myricetin, a flavonol, occurs in legume seeds and is toxic to *Rhizobium.* Work in my laboratory has demonstrated that myricetin is inhibitory to other bacteria also (E. L. Rice, unpublished).

Campbell (1964) reported a study on the viability of honey locust, *Gleditsia triacanthos,* seeds in relation to age, and some of his general observations are very appropriate here. He planted 20 seeds each year under similar conditions and checked on germination. When the seeds were 6 years old, four seeds failed to germinate and mold grew profusely on them. Hardly any mold grew on the 16 seeds that germinated, even though they were in close proximity to the seeds that molded. He found that very little mold grew on the germinating seeds for 18 years after collecting them. After that, abundant mold grew on all seeds. It appeared that an antifungal compound was present in viable seeds, which slowly lowered in amount with passing time. Dr. O. J. Eigsti (personal communication) told me that he has observed with watermelon (*Cucurbita*) seeds that viable ones will not mold, whereas the nonviable ones mold readily. It may be in some, or perhaps many species, that living embryos produce microbial inhibitors as Ferenczy (1956) suggested for *Fraxinus* spp. In other cases, it may be that the seeds decay before they are able to germinate if microbial inhibitors are not present in the seed coat, whereas those that have such inhibitors germinate successfully.

Henis *et al.* (1946) reported that aqueous extracts of carob, *Ceratonia siliqua,* pods inhibited *Cellvibrio fulvus, Clostridium cellulosolvens, Sporocytophaga myxococcoides,* and *Bacilus subtilis.* He found the carob pod to be rich in condensed tannins.

Smale *et al.* (1964) surveyed extracts of fruits (and other parts) of 125 species in 47 families for antibacterial activity against *Agrobacterium tumefaciens, Erwinia amylovora, E. carotovora, Pseudomonas syringae, Xanthomonas phaseoli, X. pruni,* and *X. vesicatoria* and for antifungal activity against *Aspergillus* sp., *Colletotrichum lindemuthianum, Endothia parasitica,* and *Monilia fruticola.* Many of the extracts were found to be inhibitory to one or more of the test microorganisms. Some inhibited only fungi, some only bacteria, and others both, among those extracts that had activity.

Lane (1965) investigated the dormancy mechanism in native *Helianthus annuus* seeds, and he suspected initially that some water-soluble inhibitor might be responsible for the dormancy. He devised

TABLE 42

Species with Seeds Demonstrated to Have Antimicrobial Activity against One or More of the Following: Bacteria Fungi, Mycobacteria, Protozoa, Phage, Virus, Yeast [a]

Family	Species [b]
Aceraceae	*Acer ginnala*
Betulaceae	*Betula populifolia*
Bignoniaceae	*Catalpa speciosa*
Caprifoliaceae	*Kolkwitzia amabilis*
Celastraceae	*Euonymus europaeus*
Compositae	*Ambrosia artemisiifolia*
	Eupatorium rugosum
	Lactuca floridana
	Prenanthes altissima
	Silphium terebinthinaceum
	Vernonia altissima
	Xanthium pennsylvanicum
Cruciferae	*Brassica japonica*
	Brassica oleracea
	Brassica rapa
	Cheiranthus allionia
	Cheiranthus cheiri
	Erysimum perofskianum
	Iberis sempervirens
	Lepidium hyssopifolium
	Malcomia maritima
	Matthiola bicornis
	Thlaspi arvense
Ericaceae	*Rhododendron maximum*
Guttiferae	*Garcinia morella*
Labiatae	*Agastache nepetoides*
	Ocimum basilicum
Lauraceae	*Persea americana*
Leguminosae	*Baptisia australis*
	Cargana microphylla
	Cassia absus
	Cassia fistula
	Cassia tora
	Cercis canadensis
	Crotalaria retzii
Lilaceae	*Allium cepa*
	Hosta japonica
Malvaceae	*Hibiscus mutabilis*
Meliaceae	*Melia azedarach*
Pedaliaceae	*Sesamum indicum*
Pinaceae	*Larix europaea*
	Picea abies

Table 42 (*continued*)

Family	Species [b]
Polygonaceae	*Rumex crispus*
Ranunculaceae	*Anemone canadensis*
Scrophulariaceae	*Calceolaria herbeohybrida*
	Clematis recta
	Verbascum blattaria
Solanaceae	*Solanum tuberosum*
Umbelliferae	*Angelica arguta*
Vitaceae	*Vitis labrusca*

[a] Selected from Table 1 of Nickell (1960).
[b] Nomenclature used as in Nickell (1960).

an apparatus to thoroughly leach the fruits and/or seeds. After leaching the seeds, he found that they still retained their dormancy, but molded and decayed rapidly when attempts were made to germinate them. On the other hand, if he exposed them to low temperatures for several weeks without any leaching, they did not mold and germinated well. Thus, these seeds contain water-soluble antimicrobial toxins. Leaching of the fruits, whether or not they contain seeds, caused them to mold and decay rapidly also when exposed to the conditions used for seed germination.

Harris and Burns (1972) investigated some factors affecting preharvest seed molding of grain sorghum, *Sorghum bicolor.* They observed the severity of seed molding of 49 hybrids at two locations in Georgia and rated the severity of molding on a scale of 1 to 5, with 1 showing little evidence of molding and 5 showing obvious grain deterioration. They found that consistent differences occurred between hybrids at the two locations, so correlations were run between tannin content of the seeds and the index of molding. The coefficient of correlation between tannin content and index of molding was −0.89 at one locality and −0.87 at the other, Moreover, 77.5% of the variability among hybrids for seed molding was accounted for by this relationship. Thus, it was concluded that high tannin content of the seed was the dominant inhibiting factor controlling preharvest molding.

Obviously, prevention of preharvest molding or decay of seeds is very important in agriculture in certain climates, and this is a different aspect of seed decay prevention than I have been emphasizing. Unquestionably, prevention of preharvest seed decay is important in natural ecosystems under some climatic conditions also. The importance of tannins in the case of grain sorghum indicates that similar microbial inhibitors are effective in prevention of both preharvest and postharvest seed decay.

II. PRODUCTION OF MICROBIAL INHIBITORS IN SEED COATS BY SOIL MICROORGANISMS

Wright (1956) inoculated seeds of white mustard, wheat (*Triticum*), and/or pea (*Pisum*) with either *Trichoderma viride, Penicillium frequentans, P. gladioli, Streptomyces griseus, S. venezuelae,* or *S. aureofaciens* and planted the inoculated seeds in two types of soil. *Trichoderma viride* produces the antibiotic gliotoxin in liquid culture; *Penicillium frequentans* produces frequentin; *P. gladioli* produces gladiolic acid; *Streptomyces griseus* produces streptomycin; *S. venezuelae* produces chloromycetin, and *S. aureofaciens* produces aureomycin. After a germination period of 6 or 7 days, the seed coats of mustard and pea seeds were removed and extracted, and the whole wheat seeds were extracted. The extracts were tested for antibiotic activity and the antibiotics were identified.

All three types of seeds inoculated with *Trichoderma viride* contained gliotoxin (Table 43). Pea seeds inoculated with *Penicillium frequentans* showed antifungal activity and yielded 1–1.5 μg frequentin per seed coat. Pea seeds inoculated with *Penicillium gladioli* were found to contain gladiolic acid, but the amount was not determined. The three actinomycetes, *Streptomyces griseus, S. venezuelae,* and *S. aureofaciens* failed to produce antibiotics when pea seeds were inoculated with them. When uninoculated pea seeds were planted in soil containing a natural strain of *Trichoderma viride*, the seed coats had

TABLE 43

Production of Gliotoxin in Wheat, Mustard, and Pea Seeds Inoculated with *Trichoderma viride* [a]

Seed	R_f value of active extract	Weight of gliotoxin/ seed coat (μg)
Wheat	0.84	0.02–0.03
Mustard	0.85	0.25
Pea	0.82	4.0
	R_f value of gliotoxin 0.85	

[a] From Wright (1956). Reproduced by permission of Cambridge University Press.

both antifungal and antibacterial activity and were found to contain gliotoxin.

The fact that antibiotics can be produced in uninoculated seeds if present in soil containing antibiotic-producing microorganisms adds still another dimension to the phenomenon of prevention of seed decay before germination. As I pointed out above, Wright (1956) found that mustard seed coats contain natural microbial inhibitors in addition to those produced by associated microorganisms.

III. CONCLUSIONS

The foregoing discussion indicates the important survival value of microbial inhibitors in seeds, and relatively strong evidence could be presented similarly for the presence and importance of such inhibitors in the outer parts of certain vegetative reproductive structures such as the scales of bulbs, the "peelings" of tubers, etc. Undoubtedly, there are strong evolutionary pressures operating in the selection of seeds and other reproductive structures containing effective antimicrobial toxins.

9

Impact of Allelopathy on Agriculture

I. PRODUCTION BY CROP PLANTS OF SUBSTANCES INHIBITORY TO OTHER CROP PLANTS

Since DeCandolle (1832) suggested that root exudates of certain weeds cause injury to some crop plants and that the soil sickness problem in agriculture might be due to exudates of crop plants, there have been several periods of considerable research activity in this field. One such period occurred in the early part of this century when Schreiner and his associates published numerous papers in which they presented evidence that soil sickness owing to single cropping is caused by the addition of toxins to the soil by the crop plants (Schreiner and Reed, 1907a,b, 1908; Schreiner and Shorey, 1909; Schreiner and Sullivan, 1909; Schreiner and Lathrop, 1911). Schreiner and Reed (1907b) pointed out that many kinds of microorganisms had been shown to produce waste products that are very inhibitory to themselves and often to other organisms. They reasoned that it is unlikely that a similar phenomenon does not happen in higher plants. They reported that a number of typically unproductive soils from different parts of the United States had been studied very carefully by the Bureau of Soils of the U.S. Department of Agriculture, and it had been demonstrated that many soils that were unproductive were not deficient in essential nutrients. For these reasons, numerous experiments were run to determine if such soils were unproductive because of the presence of toxins. Initial experiments in which wheat plants were grown in aqueous leachates of unproductive soils demonstrated that the plants grew more poorly in the leachate than in distilled water despite the presence of nutrients in the leachate. Moreover, if carbon black was added to the leachate and then filtered out, the leachate was no longer toxic, indicating that the toxins had been adsorbed by the carbon. Experiments were run next using a chemotropic response of roots to determine if substances exuded from living roots of various crop plants repel the roots. They concluded from their results that wheat roots exude materials that repel wheat, corn, cowpea, and oat roots and that oat roots exude materials which repel oat roots. Other results of Schreiner and his colleagues were discussed briefly in Chapter 2.

There were only scattered publications on the roles of allelopathy in agriculture for about the next 45 years (see Chapter 2). There has been extensive research activity in this area in the last decade and a half, much of it on production of toxins during decomposition of crop residues. This activity was probably stimulated by two earlier papers on effects of such residues by McCalla and Duley (1948, 1949). I will return to a discussion of crop residues in Section II.

Nielsen *et al.* (1960) investigated the effects of aqueous extracts of alfalfa hay (about 50% bloom); timothy hay (about 50% bloom); and mature corn stover, oat straw, and potato vines on seed germination and seedling growth of corn (*Zea mays*), soybeans (*Glycine max*), peas (*Pisum sativa*), oats (*Avena sativa*), alfalfa (*Medicago sativa*), and timothy (*Phleum pratense*). Dried and ground material was mixed with distilled water in a Waring blender for 10 minutes and filtered. This was used to water test seeds planted in quartz sand, and controls were watered with distilled water. The time required for germination, percentage germination after 7 days (10 days for *Phleum*), and root and shoot length were determined.

Alfalfa extract caused the greatest delay in germination of all species except one; germination of timothy was delayed the longest with timothy extract. Alfalfa extract significantly reduced the germination of alfalfa below that of the other extracts, and germination of timothy seeds was reduced by all crop extracts, but to a greater extent by alfalfa, timothy, and potato. No other germination effects were significant.

The extracts of alfalfa caused the greatest reduction in lengths of roots and shoots of all test species. Timothy extract was next in depressing root growth, and it affected shoot growth of all species except oats more seriously than did the extracts of oats, corn, or potatoes. Shoot growth of oats was affected least by the timothy extract. The sequence of extracts based on decreasing effectiveness in reducing shoot and root growth was alfalfa, timothy, corn, oats, and potato. The order of test species based on decreasing resistance to the toxic effects of the extracts was alfalfa, corn, soybeans, peas, oats, timothy. The roots were generally more strongly affected by the extracts than the shoots.

Nielsen *et al.* (1960) definitely demonstrated that certain crop plants contain water-soluble materials that inhibit seed germination and seedling growth of several crop plants. Unfortunately, it is very difficult to interpret such results from extracts in terms of plants growing in soil. Moreover, no tests were run in this investigation to determine if the results, or some of them, may have been due to osmotic concentrations of the extracts. Based on numerous other studies, I suspect they were not, but no one knows under the circumstances.

Börner (1960) reported that cold-water extracts of barley (*Hordeum*), rye (*Secale*), wheat (*Triticum*), and oats (*Avena*) inhibited root growth of wheat even in a concentration of plant material to water of 1:400. The inhibiting material was also detected in water extracts of soils containing different amounts of straw and root material. Börner identified ferulic, *p*-coumaric, vanillic, and *p*-hydroxybenzoic acids in aqueous extracts of the straw and alcoholic extracts of the roots. He found that a concentration of 10 ppm of each of these compounds in water culture inhibited growth of rye and wheat roots. Börner (1960) reported also that scopoletin is liberated from root hairs of living oat plants and that 3,4-dihydroxyflavone is excreted by living wheat and peanut (*Arachis hypogaea*) roots. He found scopoletin inhibited growth of oat and timothy roots at the low concentration of $3 \times 10^{-5} M$.

Grant and Sallans (1964) collected roots and tops of alfalfa, red clover, ladino clover, birdsfoot trefoil, timothy, brome grass, orchard grass, and reed canary grass in the late vegetative or early flowering stage. They dried the material, ground it, and made aqueous extracts, using 1 part of plant material to 20 parts distilled water. The mixture was placed in a Waring blender for 10 minutes and filtered, after which it was tested against seed germination and seedling growth of the same group of plants in germinating boxes.

Legume extracts lowered the percentage of germination in about half the tests, with the top extracts being generally more toxic than the root extracts. An exception to this was the extract of alfalfa roots, which severely reduced the germination of all four grass species and of red clover. Ladino clover top extract reduced the germination of all species tested except timothy and birdsfoot trefoil. Red clover extracts had the least effect on germination of any of the legume extracts.

In general, the grass extracts had less effect on germination than the legume extracts. The extracts of the tops had greater effects on germination again than did the root extracts. All of the grass top extracts lowered the germination of other grass species, but the reduction in germination of brome grass was not statistically significant in any case. Reed canary grass was the only species significantly affected by the grass root extracts. The only significant reductions in germination of legumes by grass extracts were the reductions in germination of ladino clover by the top extracts of timothy, reed canary, and orchard grass.

The extract of alfalfa roots reduced the shoot length of all species except timothy and alfalfa, and it severely retarded shoot growth of the other three legumes. The top extract of alfalfa had a generally similar, but less severe effect. The top extract of ladino clover reduced shoot growth in all species except timothy, but the root extract inhibited only the legumes. Birdsfoot trefoil had effects on shoot growth similar to ladino clover, and red clover did not affect shoot growth of the grasses, but reduced shoot growth of all legumes except alfalfa.

Extracts of the grasses generally had considerably weaker effects on shoot growth than the extracts of legumes. The root extracts had little effect at all, but the shoot extracts did reduce shoot growth in some cases.

Alfalfa extracts strongly inhibited root growth of all species and the root extract virtually prevented root growth of all species except alfalfa. The top extract had a similar effect on root growth of legumes, but inhibited the grasses less severely. Extracts of tops of ladino clover and birdsfoot trefoil strongly reduced root growth of all species. The root extract of birdsfoot trefoil had similar effects on all species, but root extracts of timothy and ladino clover reduced root length of only the legumes and reed canary grass. Red clover extracts inhibited root development of brome, reed canary grass, and all legumes except alfalfa, which was not affected by the top extract.

Grass extracts were generally less inhibitory to root growth than legume extracts, and top extracts were usually more effective than root extracts. The top extract of reed canary grass inhibited root development of all species, whereas the root extract had a significant effect only on brome grass, alfalfa, red clover, and birdsfoot trefoil. The top extract of timothy inhibited root growth of only brome grass, reed canary grass, alfalfa, and trefoil, and the root extract affected only alfalfa and trefoil. The root extract of brome grass inhibited root growth of brome and of all legumes except ladino clover, and its top extract inhibited all species except orchard grass and ladino clover. Orchard grass extracts were the least inhibitory of the grass extracts, the root extracts inhibiting root growth of trefoil only, and the top extracts inhibiting brome grass, orchard grass, reed canary grass, and trefoil.

Many of the extracts caused twisted roots, prevented root hair development, and, in the cases of top extracts of alfalfa and reed canary grass, killed the roots of test plants.

Grant and Sallans (1964) rated the species in the following order based on decreasing inhibition: alfalfa, birdsfoot trefoil, ladino clover, red clover, reed canary grass, brome grass, timothy, orchard grass. They listed alfalfa and timothy as the species least affected by the extracts and reed canary grass as the most susceptible to effects of the extracts. Overall, the top extracts were more inhibitory than the root extracts, except for alfalfa.

The investigation by Grant and Sallans had the same defects as that of Nielsen *et al.* (1960), but the results did support and extend those of Nielsen *et al.* (1960). Grant and Sallans pointed out the difficulty of extending their results to natural conditions, but they suggested that the suppression of root development of birdsfoot trefoil by all extracts might be indicative of the reasons for the difficulties experienced in obtaining good stands of birdsfoot trefoil. They suggested also that the pronounced inhibition of all species by alfalfa might help explain why alfalfa is considered a very aggressive species when grown with other forage crops. They reported that timothy and red clover are frequently planted together, and their data indicated that these species are quite compatible.

Kaurov (1970) investigated the growth of birdsfoot trefoil and yellow lupine in pure and mixed cultures and found that production per unit area was greater in mixed cultures than in a pure culture of either. He found also that birdsfoot trefoil was more active in absorption of radioactive phosphorus than lupine, and that migration of the ^{32}P from lupine to birdsfoot trefoil was more active than that from birdsfoot trefoil to birdsfoot trefoil. He concluded, therefore, that lupine in mixed cultures improves the condition of mineral nutrition of birdsfoot trefoil. There was no direct evidence here of any allelopathic effect, but evidence from other investigations suggests the possibility.

Pronin and Yakovlev (1970) reported that yields of fodder beans and maize increased in mixed cultures under both sterile and nonsterile conditions, and that this appeared to be connected with a favorable influence of root excretions of each plant on the other. They stated that under nonsterile conditions, the microorganisms of the root zone intensify the positive or negative influences of plants. The positive effects of the maize on the legume in this investigation indicated that more was involved in the interaction than just the improvement of nitrogen nutrition by the legume. The results in this case were certainly not due to allelopathy as I defined it earlier, but they do fit into

Molisch's (1937) implied use of the term, and the results definitely indicate mutual chemical interactions.

Lykhvar and Nazarova (1970) investigated the growth of several species of legumes and maize in pure and mixed cultures and reported that beneficial effects of legumes grown in mixed cultures with maize depend on specific varieties of the legume species. Many varieties gave detrimental results in mixed cultures indicating truly allelopathic effects. As a consequence of these experiments, new varieties of legumes were developed specifically for use in mixed cultures with maize or other crop or forage plants. This type of research appears to me to hold excellent promise in agriculture.

Gaidamak (1971) grew several crops of tomatoes and cucumbers in "gravel" culture using broken bricks as the substrate. He used fresh culture solution at the start of each new crop, but the same broken brick substrate. He analyzed the nutrient solutions used to grow the crops, and each solution contained amino acids, organic acids of an aliphatic series, phenolics, and several unidentified compounds. Most of the compounds had either a positive or negative effect when tested against the growth of certain test species. The solution used to grow the eighth crop of tomatoes contained additionally some unidentified toxins and phenolcarbonic acid which had strong inhibitory effects on test species.

Dadykin *et al.* (1970) studied the volatile secretions of several crop plants and found acetaldehyde, propionic aldehyde, acetone, methanol, ethanol, and other unidentified compounds in volatile secretions of beet, tomato, sweet potato, and radish leaves and carrot roots. Propionic aldehyde was found to have the greatest activity against test species in closed systems.

The investigations of allelopathic interactions of crop plants discussed so far have concerned effects of extracts, root exudates, and volatiles. Two other ways that toxins could be liberated from crop plants are by leachates of tops and decay or by leaching of residues. I discussed many ecologically meaningful experiments in Chapters 4, 6, and 7 in which leachates of tops of many species were shown to be toxic to many test species, but these did not concern crop plants. A few experiments on allelopathic effects of leachates have been conducted with crop plants.

Kozel and Tukey (1968) isolated a toxin from leachate of foliage of *Chrysanthemum morifolium* that completely inhibited the germination of lettuce seeds. It was apparently a phenolic compound and was a potent inhibitor of growth and development of chrysanthemum. Tukey (1969) stated that this species of chrysanthemum cannot be grown in the same soil for several years, apparently because of the accumulation of inhibitors.

Kozel and Tukey (1968) reported also that gibberellins leached from chrysanthemum plants may be stimulatory to stem elongation at one concentration and inhibitory to flowering at another concentration. Most growth-regulating compounds are, of course, inhibitory in some concentrations and stimulatory in others.

II. ALLELOPATHIC EFFECTS OF CROP RESIDUES ON CROP PLANTS

The majority of the investigations directly concerned with the roles of allelopathy in agriculture have involved effects of decomposing crop residues. This probably resulted from the expanding use of stubble mulch farming since the "dust bowl" days of the 1930's to control erosion by wind and water and the resulting decreases in crop yields in numerous instances (McCalla and Duley, 1948, 1949; Patrick and Koch, 1958; Guenzi and McCalla, 1962, 1966a,b; Norstadt and McCalla, 1963; Patrick et al., 1963; 1964; McCalla and Haskins, 1964; Guenzi et al., 1967; Patrick, 1971). It is obvious from the citations that most of this work has been conducted by McCalla and his colleagues in the U. S. Department of Agriculture and the University of Nebraska and by Patrick and his colleagues in the Canada Department of Agriculture.

McCalla and Duley (1948) reported that stubble mulch farming reduces the stand and growth of corn under some conditions, and they found that soaking corn seeds in an aqueous extract of sweet clover, *Melilotus alba,* for 24 hours reduced the subsequent percentage germination and growth of tops and roots on agar in petri dishes. Alfalfa extracts had less inhibitive effects, and wheat straw extracts either stimulated growth or caused no changes compared with the distilled water control. In a sequel to this project, McCalla and Duley (1949) placed soil from the Agronomy Farm at Lincoln, Nebraska on greenhouse benches and mulched some of it with wheat straw at the rate of 2–4 tons/acre and left some unmulched. They planted wheat seeds in both areas and kept the soil thoroughly wet by watering two or three times daily. This was done because the adverse effects of stubble mulching on corn were particularly striking during periods of wet, cool weather.

In three trials, the average percentage germination of corn in the mulched plots was 44, and in the unmulched was 92. The authors pointed out also that they had repeated this many other times in pot experiments with similar results.

Another phase of their investigation involved the soaking of corn grains in aqueous extracts of wheat straw or sweet clover for 24 or 48 hours and the placing of these on agar plates. In some instances, ammonium nitrate was added to the water in which the plant material was soaked to give a 0.5% solution. Some corn grains soaked in distilled water were placed on agar plates containing a 1% concentration of several organic nitrogen compounds. The water extract of sweet clover reduced the percentage germination and growth of corn roots, but the water extract of the wheat had little effect. The extract resulting from the wheat straw and ammonium nitrate reduced germination and growth markedly, and many of the roots grew upward. McCalla and Duley pointed out that there appeared to be an increased microbial growth with the added ammonium nitrate.

In the dishes containing organic nitrogen compounds, relatively high percentages of the corn roots grew upward, except on portions of the plates where there was limited bacterial growth because of the presence of fungi. Subsequent experiments indicated that the bacteria produced a gas under some conditions, causing the corn roots to grow upward, but the effects were not as striking as they were when the corn grains were in contact with the agar on which the microorganisms were growing. The percentage germination of corn was not affected by the microorganisms, but root growth was markedly affected in some cases.

The overall results seemed to indicate that the inhibitive effects of the mulch result from a combination of toxins present in the plant material plus toxins produced by microorganisms that are stimulated to grow more luxuriantly by material in the mulch.

Guenzi and McCalla (1962) collected crop residues in September from fields on the Agronomy Farm at Lincoln, Nebraska, air dried, and ground them to pass a 40-mesh screen. The materials consisting of wheat and oat straw, soybean and sweet clover hay, corn (maize) and sorghum stalks, and brome grass and sweet clover stems were extracted with hot and cold water using 1 part residue to 15 parts water. One-half of each water extract was autoclaved for 1 hour at 20-1b steam pressure. Additionally, wheat straw was extracted with ethanol, and the extract was separated into strong and weak acids, neutral, basic, and water-soluble compounds. The ethanol extracts were tested against seed germination and growth of wheat, whereas the hot- and cold-water extracts were tested for their effect on germination and growth of wheat, sorghum, and corn. The electrical conductivity of all water extracts was determined, and effects of KC1 solutions with the same conductivities were determined for all test species so that adjustments could be made for the salt content of the extracts. Moreover, the concentrations of reducing compounds were determined so that effects of glucose solutions with the same osmotic concentrations could be determined for all test species. It was found that the salt content would explain only 3–8% of the depressive effect of the water extracts, and even the highest osmotic concentration had only a very small depressive effect.

All residues were found to contain water-soluble substances that depressed plant growth of corn, wheat, and sorghum. The results of the tests against wheat are shown in Table 44. The general order of increasing toxicity was sweet clover stems, wheat straw, soybean hay,

TABLE 44

Influence of Water-Soluble Substances Extracted from Different Plant Residues on Germination and Growth of Wheat Seeds [a]

		Germination		Root growth		Shoot growth	
		AC [b]	No AC	AC	No AC	AC	No AC
Crop residues		Inhibition (%)					
Sweetclover stems	C [c]	−3 [e]	−8	58	7	24	21
	H [d]	−1	−8	51	12	10	10
Wheat straw	C	7	5	36	7	14	21
	H	−5	−5	18	36	7	28
Soybean hay	C	3	−3	80	30	66	45
	H	−1	−5	51	39	48	45
Oat straw	C	3	10	87	64	83	76
	H	−1	−3	84	45	79	62
Brome grass	C	1	3	71	55	48	59
	H	−1	27	71	62	52	78
Cornstalks	C	−7	89	75	87	62	93
	H	5	38	47	75	62	83
Sorghum stalks	C	9	100	87	100	86	100
	H	3	72	84	82	83	93
Sweetclover hay	C	64	3	95	82	90	83
	H	26	100	95	100	90	100
Mean	C	9.6	24.9	73.6	54.0	59.1	62.3
	H	3.1	27.0	62.6	56.4	53.9	62.4

[a] From Guenzi and Mc Calla (1962).
[b] AC, autoclaving for 1 hour at 20 lb. steam pressure.
[c] Cold-water soluble substances (extracted at 25°C).
[d] Hot-water soluble substances (extracted at 100°C).
[e] Negative sign indicates stimulation.

brome grass, oat straw, corn and sorghum stalks, and sweet clover hay. The nonautoclaved extracts of the residues inhibited seed germination and shoot growth more than the autoclaved extracts in most cases, but the autoclaved extracts were more depressive to root growth.

All five fractions derived from the ethanol extract of wheat straw contained substances toxic to growth of wheat seedlings. The water-soluble and strong acid fractions had the strongest depressive effects, and the basic fraction had the least effect. In a similar experiment in which corn was used as the test plant, the quantity of material from 2.3 gm of wheat straw completely inhibited growth of one corn seed. On this basis, Guenzi and McCalla estimated that this would be equivalent to about 101 lb of straw per acre, assuming a plant population of 20,000 plants per acre.

Norstadt and McCalla (1963) followed up the earlier investigation of McCalla and Duley (1949) in which it was suggested that effects of crop residues might be due to a combination of toxins from the residues and from microorganisms that were caused to grow more profusely by substances in the residues. Norstadt and McCalla used research plots, some of which were subsurface-tilled and some plowed during a 23-year period at Lincoln, Nebraska. A rotation of corn, oats, and wheat was followed in both types, and it was observed over this period that decreased yields and abnormal appearance of crops occurred in the subsurface-tilled (stubble-mulched) plots in the years with normal to above-normal precipitation. They isolated fungi from subsurface-tilled soil showing reduced growth and cultured them in potato dextrose broth. Corn seeds were soaked in the broth for 6 hours and placed in petri dishes between double layers of filter paper moistened with a little of the broth. The percentage germination and lengths of roots and shoots were determined after 3 days. In a group of 91 isolates, 14 reduced germination to 50% or less, whereas distilled water control usually had better than 90–95% germination.

One fungus, which produced a toxin that was particularly potent against growth of corn plants, was identified as *Penicillium urticae.* Norstadt and McCalla (1963) identified the toxin as patulin and compared its inhibitory effect on Cheyenne wheat with 2,4-dichlorophenoxyacetic acid (2,4-D), coumarin, and indole-3-acetic acid (IAA). Germination, expressed as percentage of the control, which occurred in a 50 ppm solution, was as follows: 2,4-D, 40; coumarin, 80; IAA, 85; and patulin, 85. The concentration required to reduce root length to 50% of the control was 2,4-D, 1 ppm; coumarin, 9 ppm; IAA, 25 ppm; and patulin, 20 ppm. Shoot growth was reduced to 50% of the control by 63 ppm of IAA, 20 ppm of coumarin, 40 ppm of patulin, and 7.5 ppm of

2,4-D. Thus, it was found that patulin is a pretty potent inhibitor of growth in higher plants in addition to its known inhibitory effect on fungi. Patulin was subsequently found to be inhibitory to Cheyenne wheat seedlings in sand and two kinds of soil.

McCalla and Haskins (1964) reported that in a later test of 318 fungi isolated from soil in stubble-mulched plots at Lincoln, Nebraska, 52 produced toxins that reduced shoot growth of corn by 50% or more, and 167 produced toxins that reduced root growth of corn by a comparable percentage. These fungi were not identified, nor were the toxins. Several fungi produce patulin (Norstadt and McCalla, 1963), and many fungi produce other substances toxic to growth of higher plants (McCalla and Haskins, 1964). According to McCalla and Haskins (1964), Krasilnikov found 5–15% of 1500 cultures of actinomycetes tested to be inhibitory to growth of higher plants, about one-third of the 300 or more cultures of non-spore-forming bacteria and 20–30% of the spore-forming bacterial cultures. The possibility is very good, of course, that crop residues would encourage the growth of many of these organisms.

Guenzi and McCalla (1966a) identified and quantified five phenolic acids in mature plant residues of oats, wheat, sorghum, and corn. These five compounds were *p*-coumaric, syringic, vanillic, ferulic, and *p*-hydroxybenzoic acids. *p*-Coumaric acid was present in the greatest amounts. Both acid and base hydrolyses were used to free the acids from the bound form, and higher concentrations were found in alkaline hydrolysates, indicating an ester type linkage. All five acids were shown to be inhibitory to growth of wheat seedlings.

Guenzi and McCalla (1966a) estimated on the basis of usual yields of the four crop plants at Lincoln that the following amounts of *p*-coumaric acid would be added in pounds per acre in the residue: 89 by sorghum, 72 by corn, 8 by wheat, and 23 by oats. They pointed out that even though these acids are mostly bound in the residues, there should be periods during decomposition when rather large amounts could be released in the immediate vicinity of the residue and be sufficiently high to affect plant growth.

The next project undertaken by Guenzi and McCalla (1966b) was the extraction, identification, and quantification of phytotoxins in soil from stubble-mulched and plowed plots at Lincoln, Nebraska. They used a number of solvent systems and techniques for extracting and separating the toxins. One method employed sodium pyrophosphate (0.1 M) for 2 hours at room temperature, centrifugation, and extraction successively with diethyl ether at pH 12, pH 7, and pH 1. The extracted material in each case was dried and different concentrations in water were tested against germination and growth of wheat. All fractions from the stubble-mulched soil were found to be inhibitory, but the acid fraction was most inhibitory.

Another technique involved extraction with acetone for 2 hours at room temperature, partial evaporation, centrifugation, evaporation to dryness, followed by separation of toxic fractions on a column of Woelm neutral alumina using eight eluting solvents. The material obtained by the acetone extraction and the fractions separated on the column were tested against germination and growth of wheat. All fractions were found to be inhibitory to growth of shoots and roots of wheat seedlings in some concentration, but effects on germination were slight.

Four solvents were used to extract phenolic acids from the soil in the stubble-mulched and plowed plots: sodium pyrophosphate (0.1 M), 2 N HCl, 2 N NaOH, and a 0.1% aqueous solution of CaO. The soil (top 3 inches) was extracted for 4 hours at room temperature, centrifuged, filtered, the filtrate was acidified to pH 2, recentrifuged, and the resulting filtrate was extracted with diethyl ether. The ether was concentrated and phenolics were separated by paper chromatography and quantified. Five phenolic acids were identified, and they were the same ones identified previously in the residue (Table 45). The amounts shown in the table were determined from the NaOH extraction because only three of the phenolic acids—p-coumaric, p-hydroxybenzoic, and vanillic acids —were detected in the other three

TABLE 45

Concentration of Phenolic Acids from a 2N NaOH Extract of a Sharpsburg Plowed and Subtilled Soil, with Each Value Being a Mean of Three Replicates [a]

	Concentration			
	Subtilled		Plowed	
Acid	ppm [b]	% of OM [c]	ppm [b]	% of OM
Ferulic	7.6 ± 4.0	0.021	3.7 ± 1.5	0.010
p-Coumaric	14.4 ± 2.3	0.040	9.4 ± 2.9	0.026
Syringic	T [d]		T	
Vanillic	1.5 ± 0.7	0.004	1.5 ± 0.5	0.004
p-Hydroxybenzoic	1.2 ± 0.3	0.003	1.3 ± 0.1	0.003

[a] From Guenzi and McCalla (1966b).
[b] ppm calculated on the oven-dried weight of soil.
[c] OM, organic matter.
[d] T represents <1 ppm.

extracts, and they were present in concentrations of less than 1 ppm. One interesting result was the fact that ferulic acid was twice as high in concentration in the stubble-mulched as in the plowed plot. *p*-Coumaric acid was approximately 50% higher also in the subtilled plot (Table 45).

Guenzi and McCalla (1966b) pointed out that the concentrations of phenolic acids were relatively low compared with those required to inhibit growth of plants. They emphasized, however, that concentrations would unquestionably be higher in localized areas around fragments of residues. Moreover, they pointed out that there are apparently many phytotoxic substances present in low concentrations in soil, and these would probably have synergistic effects on plant growth, particularly under suboptimum growing conditions.

Guenzi *et al.* (1967) investigated changes in phytotoxic activity of water extracts of residues of corn, wheat, oat, and sorghum residues during decomposition in the field during a 41-week period. Wheat was used as the test plant in most assays, but wheat and corn were both used in the initial test of mature residues at harvest time. Nine varieties of wheat straw were tested at harvest time against wheat. The varieties used were Nebred, Warrior, Cheyenne, Ponca, Yogo, Wichita, Pawnee, Bison, and Omaha. The extract of Ponca wheat straw was found to have a significantly greater depressive effect on germination of wheat than any of the extracts of other wheat varieties, but there were no differences among other varieties. The extract of Nebred wheat straw was significantly less toxic to root growth of wheat than extracts of other varieties, and there were no significant differences among other varieties. Extracts of the different wheat varieties varied greatly, however, in their depressive effects on shoot growth of wheat, ranging from 11% for Nebred to 36% for Omaha, and many of the differences were statistically significant.

Changes in toxicity of the extracts of residues during decomposition in the field varied considerably depending on the type of residue (Table 46). The toxicity of extracts of wheat straw remained about the same through the first 4 weeks of decomposition, but virtually all toxicity had disappeared by 8 weeks. The greatest toxicity in the extract of oat straw residue occurred at harvest time and essentially all inhibitory activity was gone after 8 weeks of decomposition as in wheat. The extracts of sorghum residues increased in toxicity up to 16 weeks of decomposition during the 1963 season, but showed a generally slow decline in activity during decomposition in the 1964 season. Toxicity of extracts of corn residues remained high during 22 weeks of decomposition, but decreased rapidly thereafter.

TABLE 46

Wheat Seedling Growth in Response to Water-Soluble Phytotoxic Materials from Crop Residues in the Field at Different Periods of Decomposition during 1963 [a,b]

Period of decomposition (weeks)	% of growth inhibition [c]			
	Wheat straw		Oat straw	
	Roots	Shoots	Roots	Shoots
0	14 ‡	11 †‡§	49§	43 ‡
1	7 †‡	16‡§	33 ‡	51 ‡
2	9 ‡	12 †‡§	34 ‡	50 ‡
4	8 ‡	18 §	6 *†	18 †
8	−5 *	9 *†‡	−4 *	5 *
12	−7 *	5 *	−1 *	6 *
16	−2 *†	8 *†‡	−4 *	2 *
35	8 †‡	5 *	2 *	11 *†
41	12 ‡	6 *†	14 †	5 *

	Sorghum residue		Corn Residue	
	Roots	Shoots	Roots	Shoots
0	37 †	59 ‡	25 ‡	49 ‡
1	43 †	57 ‡	20 †	31 †
2	43 †	58 ‡	24 ‡	40 †
4	53 ‡	53 ‡	43 ‡	53 ‡
8	62 ‡	54 ‡	24 ‡	37 †
12	64 ‡	67 §	10 *†	40 †
16	85 §	77 ‖	11 *†	35 †
22	40 †	40 †	19 †‡	35 †
28	11 *	23 *	6 *	21 *

[a] Modified from Guenzi *et al.* (1967).

[b] Each value is a mean of three replicates.

[c] Selections within individual crop residues and in the same column which have a symbol (*,†,‡,§,‖) in common do not differ in the character measured at the 5% probability level. Negative sign indicates an increase over the untreated.

Martin and Rademacher (1960b) incorporated fresh rape roots in soil and planted wheat seeds in this and similar soil without the rape roots. They found that the wheat seedlings were inhibited at first, but after 4 days, growth was stimulated.

Patrick and Koch (1958) did a comprehensive investigation of the effects of decomposing residues of timothy, corn, rye, and tobacco on respiration of tobacco seedlings using manometric techniques. Their study included effects of different conditions of decomposition on the toxicity of the residues also. They obtained soil and plant material for their experiments from the Science Service field plots at Harrow, Ontario, Canada. The four crops listed above were grown separately in the plots for at least 2 consecutive years.

Plant materials were collected at three different stages of growth: young, intermediate, and nearly mature. The young stage was collected 5–6 weeks after planting; the intermediate was collected 6–8 weeks after planting; and the mature was collected 10–14 weeks after planting. In the last stage, the corn and tobacco plants were still green in color, whereas the rye and timothy were only partly green. Entire plants were collected, the roots were cleansed of soil, and the plants were cut into pieces about 1 inch long. They were either used immediately or air dried and stored for future use.

Decomposition experiments involved addition of 250 gm fresh weight (or 60 gm air-dried weight) of plant material to 1000 gm of fresh soil obtained from the field plot in which the particular plant had grown. All controls consisted of similar soil obtained from plots in which no plants were allowed to grow for 2 years and to which no plant material was added. In each case, the soil or soil plus thoroughly mixed plant material was added to 1 gallon sterile glazed crocks. In some pots, sufficient water was added to saturate the soil, but in others the excess water was allowed to drain away until field capacity was attained. The pots were covered with aluminum foil and allowed to stand for 0–30 days at a temperature range of 60°–70°F. In other cases, similar soil or plant and soil mixtures were autoclaved for 40 minutes at 18 lbs/in² pressure in cotton-plugged Erlenmeyer flasks, after which they were allowed to set under the same conditions as previously described.

At various times soil in some of the flasks and pots was extracted with water for 15–20 minutes, centrifuged, the liquid was filtered through Seitz filters to remove soil particles, microorganisms, and plant debris; and the filtrates were tested for phytotoxic effects usually within 5 days after preparation. The assay involved the placing of 6-day-old sterile tobacco seedlings (var. Harrow Velvet) in the filtrates or sterile 0.01 M phosphate buffer for 16 hours at 20°C, after which the seedlings from the filtrates were washed in sterile distilled water and placed in sterile 0.01 M phosphate buffer also. The respiration rates of the various sets of tobacco seedlings were then determined by the Warburg method.

Additionally, effects of the various filtrates on germination and growth of tobacco, barley, and timothy seed and seedlings were determined in petri dishes.

Patrick and Koch (1958) found that substances were formed during the decomposition of residues of all four species which were inhibitory to respiration in tobacco seedlings (Table 47). Moreover, they found that greater inhibition occurred if decomposition took place under saturated soil conditions. This indicated either that different kinds of toxins were produced or that concentrations were greater under saturated conditions, according to Patrick and Koch. Another possibility could be that the toxins produced were destroyed faster under aerobic conditions.

Additional experiments were run in which the soil moisture conditions were varied. In one case, decomposition was carried out for 15–20 days in soils at field capacity, followed by saturation. In another type of experiment, the soil was kept saturated for 15–20 days, followed by a period at field capacity. It was found that extracts made after decomposition for 15–20 days at field capacity followed by flooding for only 3–5 days were very toxic. On the other hand, it was found that if decomposition was carried out under saturation conditions

TABLE 47

Oxygen Uptake of Tobacco Seedlings as Affected by the Products of Decomposition of Plant Residues in Soils Held at Saturation and at Field Capacity [a]

| Plant material added to soil | After 20-day decomposition period at | | | |
| | Saturation | | Field capacity | |
	pH range [b]	O_2 uptake [c]	pH range	O_2 uptake
Soil only	6.4–6.6	128	6.4–6.6	131
Timothy	4.8–5.2	18	5.9–6.4	90
Rye	5.3–5.8	45	6.0–6.6	104
Corn	4.9–5.4	28	6.0–6.5	99
Tobacco	5.5–5.9	68	6.9–7.5	112

Control 125 ($\pm$ 8) [d]

[a] From Patrick and Koch (1958). Reproduced by permission of the National Research Council of Canada from the *Can. J. Bot.* **36,** 621–647.

[b] pH range after the 20-day decomposition period; pH of each extract was adjusted to 5.3 prior to testing.

[c] O_2 uptake, in μl of O_2 after 6 hours at 20°C, of 50 Harrow Velvet tobacco seedlings. In each instance the tobacco seedlings were exposed for 16 hours to the various extracts and then returned to phosphate buffer (pH 5.3) before their O_2 uptake was determined, Each figure is based on the average of four different decomposition series for each of which three determinations of four replicates each were made.

[d] O_2 uptake, in μl of O_2 (after 6 hours at 20°C) of comparable seedlings preexposed (16 hours) to 0.01 *M* phosphate buffer solution, based on the average of 12 determinations.

for the same period and then changed to field capacity, the toxicity decreased slowly and was reduced by half 10 days after the return to the drier conditions.

Results of experiments in which plant materials of different ages were decomposed under saturation conditions for various periods of time were striking (Table 48). The period of time required for toxic substances to be formed was markedly affected by the stage of maturity of the plant residues added to the soil. When residues from young plants were added, toxic substances were produced relatively early in decomposition, but these substances were inactivated relatively early also. When materials from mature plants were added, a longer period of decomposition was required for toxic substances to be formed, but the toxicity remained high for a longer period. In all cases, the toxic substances disappeared much more rapidly from tobacco than from timothy, rye, and corn.

Patrick and Koch (1958) did experiments to determine the relation-

TABLE 48

Effect of Plant Maturity and Period of Decomposition on Relative Toxicity of the Resulting Products [a]

Age of plant material added to soil	Type of plant	Decomposition period (days) at 60–70°F						
		0	5	10	15	20	25	30
Young (5 to 6 weeks after planting)	Soil only	− [b]	−	−	−	−	−	−
	Timothy	−	+ [b]	++	+++	++	−	−
	Rye	−	−	+	++	+	−	−
	Corn	−	−	+	++	+	−	−
	Tobacco	−	−	+	+	−	−	−
Intermediate (6 to 8 weeks after planting)	Soil only	−	−	−	−	−	−	−
	Timothy	−	+	+++	+++	++	+++	++
	Rye	−	+	++	+++	+++	++	++
	Corn	−	−	++	+++	++	+++	++
	Tobacco	−	−	+	+++	++	−	−
Mature (10 to 14 weeks after planting)	Soil only	−	−	−	−	−	−	−
	Timothy	−	−	−	++	++	+++	+++
	Rye	−	−	−	+	++	+++	++
	Corn	−	−	−	+	++	+++	+++
	Tobacco	−	−	−	+	++	++	−

[a] From Patrick and Koch (1958). Reproduced by permission of the National Research Council of Canada from the *Can. J. Bot.* **36**, 621–647.

[b] Toxicity rating: −, nontoxic: extracts which inhibit respiration of 6-day-old tobacco seedlings by less than 19%; +, ++, and +++ are mild, intermediate, and highly toxic, producing inhibition of respiration of 20–40%, 41–60%, and 61–95%, respectively.

ship between the degree of toxicity of the various extracts and their pH. In these experiments, they determined the pH of the soil extracts before addition of the plant residue, immediately afterward and at subsequent 5-day intervals, along with assays of toxicity. In any case, they found no appreciable change in pH immediately after addition of the residues and no toxicity. The pH of some extracts shifted from the 6.2–6.9 range to the 4.8–5.9 range in 5 days of decomposition. Corresponding with this change was an increase in toxicity of the extracts. Overall, they found a high degree of consistency between the relative toxicity of extracts and their pH. These experiments did not enable Patrick and Koch to determine whether the toxicity effect was due solely to pH or whether a low pH resulting from the residues caused more toxins to be produced. To determine which was true, they ran a series of experiments using different extracts and buffers in which the pH of aliquots of each was adjusted from 4.6 to 7.6. They used an extract of fallow soil containing no decomposing plant residues, a highly toxic extract of soil containing plant residue previously assayed, an extract from decomposition that was previously found to be nontoxic, and a 0.01 M phosphate buffer. After the pH's of each were adjusted in the range indicated, each aliquot was assayed for inhibition of respiration of tobacco seedlings in the usual way. The results made it clear that the toxicity of the solutions was not due to acidity. Thus, they concluded that the toxic substances involved are produced chiefly under acid conditions, but once formed are inhibitory over a fairly broad range of pH's.

Tests of extracts of soil with plant residues which was autoclaved before setting for 15 days indicated that very little production of toxins had occurred. If the autoclaved flasks were kept for as long as 25 days, extracts of the soil were inhibitory, with most of them reducing oxygen uptake of tobacco seedlings by as much as 35%. Patrick and Koch inferred from these results that decomposition of the plant residues is necessary for toxins to be produced, and that some of the soil organisms must become reestablished in autoclaved flasks that set longer than 15 days.

Extracts were made directly from the plant residues after grinding them to a fine powder, and these extracts were tested in the tobacco bioassay. No inhibiting effects were found. This was an interesting result because several workers have demonstrated that extracts of timothy, rye, and corn are toxic to seed germination and seedling growth of several species of crop plants (Nielsen *et al.*, 1960; Guenzi and McCalla, 1962, 1966a; Grant and Sallans, 1964; Guenzi *et al.*, 1967). Perhaps the toxins that affect seed germination and seedling growth are different from those that affect respiration of tobacco seedlings. Patrick and Koch (1958) did not think so, however, because they tested extracts of soil containing plant residues against germination and growth of tobacco, barley, and timothy and found that only the extracts that inhibited uptake of oxygen in tobacco seedlings inhibited growth of seedlings. The answer to this dilemma is still not apparent.

Patrick and Koch (1958) reported that when tobacco seedlings were placed in some of the toxic extracts, the apical meristem region soon turned brown, whereas in other toxic extracts the zone of elongation turned brown while the apical meristem remained white. All the toxic extracts inhibited root hair formation also, and root hairs were less abundant than on controls.

In discussing the increased production of toxins in poorly drained and acid soil, Patrick and Koch pointed out that initially all their soils were only weakly acid, and some were only temporarily saturated. Thus, they felt that localized zones probably occur in most soils where ideal conditions exist at least briefly, especially in the neighborhood of pieces of plant residue. They felt it was especially significant also that the roots of seedlings appeared to be most sensitive to the toxins produced by decomposing residues. They would have a good chance of contacting localized zones of toxin production in the soil. They suggested also that there is a strong likelihood that any condition causing a reduction in respiratory activity of seedlings is also likely to cause some retardation of all the physiological functions, with corresponding inhibiting effects on many processes associated with growth and development.

Patrick *et al.* (1964) cited evidence for the fairly rapid breakdown of many phytotoxins in soil and pointed out that many persons feel they have no important effects as a result. They emphasized that the amount of inactivation is often balanced by new production and that the effective quantity is the difference between the amount produced and the amount destroyed.

Patrick *et al.* (1963) extended the investigations of Patrick and Koch (1958) to field studies in the Salinas Valley, California. Plant-residue-containing soils were obtained from fields treated in the conventional way by growers. In some fields, cover crops of barley, rye, or wheat with or without vetch and averaging 10–15 tons per acre of green plant material had been disked or plowed under. This was done just before the plants came into full head. In other fields, broadbeans, sudan grass, or remnants of a commercial crop of broccoli had been plowed or disked under. Sampling was done periodically, and consisted of collecting composite samples of plant residue with the surrounding soil.

The samples were divided into three fractions: soil and residue in the relative proportions found in the field, soil after all recognizable plant residues were removed, and plant residue free from soil. Each fraction was extracted with water in a fashion similar to the method of Patrick and Koch (1958). When the extraction was completed, the pH and electrical conductivity were determined. The latter was done because the salt content increases in most fields under irrigation, and controls were run containing a mixture of salts in water to give the same electrical conductivity. This enabled the effects of the salts to be balanced out in the test samples. Tests of phytotoxicity were run by determining the effects of test and control extracts on seed germination and seedling growth of lettuce. In some cases, broccoli, white beans, and tobacco were used to see how results compared.

The extracts of soil and residue in the proportions found in the field and of soil after the residue was removed showed low toxicity in the tests, whereas the residue had an appreciable depressive effect on root growth of lettuce. The results for the residue extracts and controls are shown in Table 49. Soil immediately adjacent to residue and extracts of similar soil were bioassayed and found to be inhibitory to root growth of lettuce.

Overall, extracts of decomposing field residues of barley, rye, broccoli, broadbean, wheat, vetch, and sudan grass were found to be toxic to lettuce seedlings.

Patrick et al. (1963) found that the salinity of surface layers of soil was increased during decomposition of plant residues, and that the injurious effects of the decomposition products were increased with increasing salinity.

Careful observations were made of lettuce and spinach plants growing in the fields to determine whether the stunting, uneven growth, and root injury often observed in the Salinas Valley could be attributed to decomposition products. Trenches were dug to observe roots, and it was found that roots in contact with or close to fragments of decomposing plant debris often had discolored or sunken lesions where the roots contacted the debris. In addition, there were many instances of browning of the apical meristems and other injuries.

Patrick et al. (1963) clearly demonstrated that toxic decomposition products of plant residues are produced under field conditions. Apparently, the toxins do not move far from the loci of production, however, and it appears that the extent of root injury and the total effect on the

TABLE 49

**Effect of Water Extracts of Field Soil and Decomposing Plant Residues
on Germination and Growth of Lettuce [a]**

Plant residue	Time of decomposition in field (days)	Average length (mm) of radicles	
		Plant [b] residue	Control [c]
Barley	0–3 [d]	15.3	21.8
	10–13	10.1	21.7
	15–18	13.6	19.8
	20–23	9.3	20.1
	23–26	14.6	19.6
Rye	10–13	14.1	19.5
	14–17	12.0	20.2
	23–26	13.1	21.0
	29–32	19.5	19.3
Wheat	17–20	14.1	19.6
	22–25	10.1	20.8
Vetch	5–8	17.0	20.0
	23–26	17.6	21.0
Broccoli	0–3	12.2	20.2
	20–23	8.1	19.8
Sudan grass	10–13	17.9	20.1

[a] Modified From Patrick *et al.* (1963).

[b] Average of 20 lettuce seedlings after 100 hours in water extract; tests run at room temperature (68°–75°F); tests with each extract replicated 4 times. Electrical conductivity of extracts adjusted to 1.5–1.8 mmho/cm at 25°C; pH 7.0–7.5.

[c] Water containing equal amounts of NaCl, Na_2SO_4, $MgSO_4$, and $CaCl_2$ salts adjusted to give the above-mentioned conductivity readings and pH.

[d] Two–five fields were sampled at each period; and for brevity, the decomposition periods were grouped in 3-day ranges.

plant would depend on how frequently the growing root system encounters plant residue fragments when the accompanying decomposition products are toxic. These workers concluded that one of the most important roles of the toxins produced is in the etiology of root disease, and this will be discussed briefly in another section of this chapter.

Patrick (1971) reported that toxins identified by gas chromatography from decomposing rye residue were acetic, butyric, benzoic, phenylacetic, hydrocinnamic, 4-phenylbutyric, and ferulic acids. There were five additional peaks that were not identified, but did not appear to be fatty acids.

III. ALLELOPATHIC EFFECTS OF WEEDS ON CROP PLANTS AND VICE VERSA

A. Effects of Vegetative Plants

DeCandolle (1832) suggested that root exudates of thistles (*Cirsium*) injure oat plants in the field, root exudates of *Euphorbia* and *Scabiosa* injure flax, and *Lolium* root exudates injure wheat. Surprisingly, there has been little research effort exerted since that time concerning possible allelopathic effects of weeds on crop plants. There has been considerable research on such effects of weeds in natural plant communities and some of these results will be mentioned briefly later.

It has been known for many years that the yield of flax is greatly reduced when even a small percentage of flax weed, *Camelina alyssum*, is growing among the flax plants. Grümmer and Beyer (1960) found no toxic root excretions, but the leaves were found to be the source of potent plant inhibitors. Using artificial rain, flax plants in close proximity to *Camelina* plants produced 40% less dry matter than the controls in which the same amount of water was added directly to the soil. The experimental setup was such that no competition was involved.

Kohlmuenzer (1965b) reported that water extracts of tops of *Galium mollugo* in dilutions from 1:1 to 1:100 of plant material to water inhibited germination of wheat by 18–100% and inhibited 19–42% of radish, *Raphanus sativus* var. *radicula*. Dilutions of 1:10 to 1:500 retarded the growth of seedlings of cultivated sunflower, *Helianthus annuus*, by 10–100%. Development of onion, *Allium cepa*, bulbs and roots was markedly inhibited also by similar extracts. Dilutions of 1:5 and 1:10 caused necrosis of meristematic tissues of onion.

Dzubenko and Petrenko (1971) investigated the interactions between two weed species, *Chenopodium album* and *Amaranthus retroflexus*, and two crop species, *Lupinus albus* and *Zea mays*, in laboratory and greenhouse experiments with water and sand culture. They reported that root excretions of the crop plants inhibited growth of the weeds and increased their catalase and peroxidase activity. Exudates of the roots of the weed species, however, stimulated growth of the cultivated plants.

Bieber and Hoveland (1968) tested water extracts of several weed species against seed germination of crownvetch, *Coronilla varia*, and other selected crop species and found that extracts of *Lepidium vir-ginicum, Oenothera biennis,* and *Digitaria sanguinalis* were very toxic. Water extract of *Lepidium* inhibited seed germination also of *Festuca arundinacea, Trifolium incarnatum, Lespedeza cuneata,* and *L. striata* at a concentration of 1:150 (w/v). *Lepidium* residues in-corporated into soil for 10 weeks were toxic to germination of crownvetch seed also.

Neustruyeva and Dobretsova (1972) reported that wheat, oats, peas, and buckwheat suppress growth, accumulation of above-ground bio-mass, and leaf surface of lambs quarter, *Chenopodium album.* Oats have a marked effect that peaks at flowering time. In studying the mechanism of action, it was found that oats do not decrease the uptake of nitrogen, phosphorus, and potassium by *Chenopodium* as buck-wheat does, in spite of the fact that oats have a much greater inter-ference. It was concluded from the overall results that oats exert an allelopathic effect in addition to their competitive role. This con-clusion was supported by Markova (1972) who found that oats sup-pressed the growth of *Erysimum cheiranthoides* in both laboratory and field tests owing at least in part to an allelopathic mechanism.

Bell and Koeppe (1972) pointed out that growth and yield reduc-tions of corn by infestations of giant foxtail, *Setaria faberii,* have been well documented, and the reductions have always been ascribed to competition without any efforts to determine if allelopathic effects might be involved also. They decided, therefore, to investigate the effects of root exudates of giant foxtail on corn under conditions in which competition was not involved. The same kind of experimental staircase setup was used by Bell and Koeppe as described in Chapter 4 in connection with the investigation of Wilson and Rice (1968) on the allelopathic effects of root exudates of *Helianthus annuus.*

Experiments were run by Bell and Koeppe (1972) to investigate the following: (1) effects of exudates of giant foxtail seedlings started at the same time on the staircase as the corn seedlings, (2) effects of exudates of mature living giant foxtail plants, (3) effects of leachates of roots of dead giant foxtail plants, and (4) effects of material leached from whole plant residue of giant foxtail which was cut up and in-corporated in pots alternating with pots of test corn plants on the staircase setup. Their results indicated that exudates of seedlings of giant foxtail did not affect growth of corn plants, but exudates of ma-ture giant foxtail roots, leachates of dead roots, and leachates of giant foxtail whole plant residue significantly inhibited growth in height, accumulation of dry weight, and accumulation of fresh weight of corn plants (Fig. 35). They found that the time required for effects to ap-

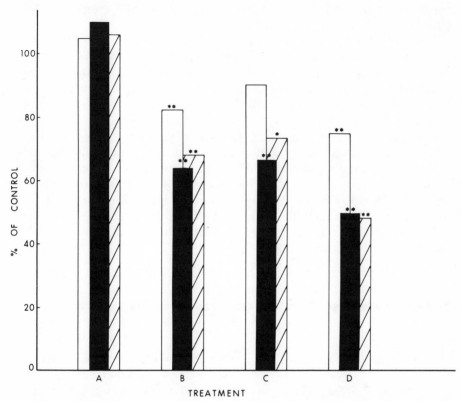

Fig. 35. Allelopathic influence of *Setaria faberii* on *Zea mays*. Height (white bars), fresh weight (black bars), and dry weight (hatched bars) are presented as a percentage of the control after 1 month's association. Treatments included corn seedlings (A) started together with giant foxtail seedlings; (B) growing with mature live giant foxtail; (C) growing with whole dead giant foxtail plants; and (D) growing in contact with the material leached from giant foxtail residue which was cut and incorporated into the sand culture pots. ∗, Significant difference from control at 0.05 level; ∗∗, significant difference from control at 0.01 level. [From Bell and Koeppe (1972). *Agronomy J.* **64**, 321–325.]

pear differed with exudate of living roots and leachate of residue. The exudate limited growth of the corn plants from the outset of the experiment, whereas the effects of the residue were not apparent for approximately 1 month after the start of the experiment. Bell and Koeppe pointed out that when competition was removed from the giant foxtail–corn interference, the inhibition of corn growth dropped from 90 to 35% when compared with weed-free controls. They concluded that the 35% reduction in corn growth under these conditions could be attributed only to allelopathic compounds carried by the circulating solutions.

Bell and Koeppe (1972) suggested that inhibitory effects of crop plants on weed seedlings may be potentially as real as the selective inhibitory responses in the reverse direction and that such phytotoxic compounds might in fact act as natural herbicides. Certainly, the results of Dzubenko and Petrenko (1971) previously discussed support this suggestion.

I discussed a great deal of evidence in Chapters 4 and 7 which demonstrated clearly that many species of weeds produce toxins that leach out of living tops or residues, exude from living roots, volatilize from living plants, are released by decomposition of residues, and are very inhibitory to other weedy species and often to themselves. I feel it is highly likely that these same toxins would affect many crop plants, and similar sorts of comprehensive investigations should be undertaken to test this important possibility.

B. Weed Seeds versus Crop Seed Germination and Vice Versa

Gressel and Holm (1964) investigated the effects of aqueous extracts of weed seeds on germination of seeds of eight crop species belonging to five families. Seeds of 13 weed species representing nine plant families were employed: *Abutilon theophrasti. Amaranthus retroflexus, Ambrosia artemisiifolia, Barbarea vulgaris, Brassica juncea, Chenopodium album, Datura stramonium, Digitaria sanguinalis, Echinochloa crusgalli, Eragrostis cilianensis, Polygonum pennsylvanicum, Portulaca oleracea,* and *Setaria lutescens*. The crop species employed were alfalfa, cabbage (*Brassica oleracea*), carrot (*Daucus carota*), pepper (*Capsicum frutescens*), radish, timothy, tomato (*Lycopersicum esculentum*), and turnip (*Brassica rapa*).

The extracts were made by grinding seeds with distilled water at the rate of 1 gm of seed to 16.7 ml of water, centrifuging, and filtering. The extracts were then tested in petri dishes against germination of crop seeds. One hundred and eight combinations were assayed, and more than half of these inhibited germination. Gressel and Holm stated that they tested many varieties of tomatoes, peppers, and carrots and found that some varieties were unaffected, whereas other varieties were highly susceptible. They found that seed lots of the same crop variety harvested in different years differed also in their sensitivity to the extracts.

When intact weed seeds were placed on filter paper disks with crop seeds, but not in direct contact, inhibitions in germination and seedling growth of crop species resulted again in many cases.

In another type of experiment, Gressel and Holm (1964) added extracts of weed seeds to sterilized and unsterilized soil in which seeds of crop species were planted. They found that emergence was delayed and seedling growth was inhibited in both the sterile and nonsterile soil. They found that the incorporation in soil of intact *Abutilon* seeds with tomato seeds significantly inhibited elongation of the tomato seedlings. This was repeated in field experiments with similar results.

Subsequent fractionation of *Abutilon* seeds indicated that the inhibitors in seeds of that species came primarily from the embryo and endosperm. Analysis of the extract of *Abutilon* seeds indicated that the amino acids present fully accounted for the inhibition elicited by the extract. Inhibitors in the other weed seeds were not identified.

Unfortunately, very little effort has gone into investigating the effects of crop seeds or crop plants on germination of weed seeds and growth of weed seedlings. Funke (1941) pointed out that beet seeds produce substances which inhibit growth of *Agrostemma githago*, but not that of *Sinapis alba*. He investigated numerous other instances of selective toxicity also and concluded that such activity explains the exclusive presence of certain weed species in cultivated fields. The possible tremendous economic importance of this phenomenon causes Funke's suggestion to warrant much more careful research.

Lazauskas and Balinevichiute (1972) tested excretions from seeds of hairy vetch, *Vicia villosa*, against seed germination and seedling growth of *Polygonum persicaria, Plantago lanceolata, Raphanus raphanistrum, Agrostemma githago, Rumex crispus, Galeopsis tetrahit, Vicia cracca, Convolvulus arvensis, Centaurea cyanus, Sinapis arvensis, Stellaria media, Spergula arvensis,* and *Matricaria inodora.* They found that germination and, particularly, seedling growth were markedly inhibited in many tests.

Prutenskaya (1972) reported that germinating seeds of millet, wheat, oats, vetch, maize, and buckwheat stimulated germination of *Sinapis arvensis* seeds, whereas germinating barley seeds inhibited germination of *Sinapis* seeds. The substances produced by the various crop seeds were separated by paper chromatography, and it was found that the compounds which stimulated or inhibited germination of *Sinapis arvensis* seeds were produced during germination.

IV. ALLELOPATHY VERSUS NITROGEN FIXATION

A. Inhibition of *Rhizobium* and Nodulation of Legumes

A great many investigations concerning the chemical inhibition of *Rhizobium* by microorganisms and higher plants and the chemical inhibition of nodulation of several crop species of legumes by higher plants were discussed in Section III of Chapter 4. These will not be covered again here, but I feel it is important to emphasize that many common species of weeds in cultivated fields have been shown to chemically inhibit growth of *Rhizobium* in cultures, and to markedly inhibit nodulation of legumes and hemoglobin synthesis in the nodules when the legumes are growing in soil. Beggs (1964) described a widespread practical problem in grasslands in New Zealand because of the inhibition of nodulation of overseeded *Trifolium* spp.

B. Inhibition of Free-Living Nitrogen Fixers

This topic was also discussed in Section III of Chapter 4. The evidence concerning the importance of free-living nitrogen fixers in agriculture is less definite than for symbiotic nitrogen fixation. Certainly, the blue-green algal nitrogen fixers are important in some specialized crops such as rice. Whatever their importance, many weed species have been demonstrated to chemically inhibit *Azotobacter* and various nitrogen-fixing blue-green algae (Rice, 1964, 1965a,b,c, 1969, 1972; Rice and Parenti, 1967; Blum and Rice, 1969; Parks and Rice, 1969). Iuzhina (1958) also found several bacterial species in soil of the Kola Peninsula in the U.S.S.R. which were antibiotic to *Azotobacter*.

V. ALLELOPATHY AND SEED GERMINATION OF CROP PLANTS

A. Inhibitors of Seed Germination

This topic has been discussed in several sections in this chapter in relation to crop plants, and in Chapters 4, 6, 7, and 8 in relation to many weedy species. Evenari (1949) gave a long list of species that have been shown to produce inhibitors of seed germination, and among these were numerous species of crop and forage plants. Le-Tourneau *et al.* (1956) gave a list of weeds and crop plants inhibitory to the germination of wheat seeds. Varga and Köves (1959) reported the presence of germination inhibitors in fruits of many species of plants. Massart (1957) found germination inhibitors in the glomerules of beet.

Germination inhibitors are often present in seeds of plants in natural habitats and these have important survival value (Went, 1948; Went and Westergaard, 1949; Koller, 1955a,b). Crop seeds, on the other hand, have been selected for rapid germination and for elimination of dormancy mechanisms. There are still some crop seeds, however, that contain substances that inhibit their own germination relatively strongly. No doubt some weak inhibitors occur in many of them. Mosheov (1937) and Miyamoto *et al.* (1961) demonstrated that some wheat seeds contain germination inhibitors. Lahiri and Kharabanda (1962–1963) reported the presence of potent, water-soluble, heat-stable seed germination inhibitors in the glumes of three forage species, *Lasiurus sindicus, Cenchrus ciliaris,* and *C. setigerus.* The inhibitors caused important practical problems in the establishment of these forage species after seeding in India. Logan *et al.* (1968) reported a germination inhibitor in the seedcoat of sericea, *Lespedeza cuneata.* They suggested that the inhibitor might be responsible for the slow germination and poor seedling establishment often encountered with this species.

B. Inhibitors of Preharvest Seed Germination

Under certain climatic conditions, seeds often germinate before harvest, or subsequent to cutting and shocking and before threshing for storage. This can result in a considerable economic loss. Apparently very little research has been done to minimize this condition. Harris and Burns (1970) investigated the relationship between the tannin content of the seeds of several grain sorghum, *Sorghum bicolor,* hybrids and preharvest germination. They found a strong negative correlation, indicating that the tannins were good inhibitors of preharvest seed germination. Tannins, like many other phenolic compounds, are strong inhibitors of growth as well as germination and are potent microbial inhibitors also. No doubt there are many other important examples of preharvest seed germination inhibitors, and I feel much more research is needed in this area in many parts of the world.

C. Inhibitors of Preharvest and Postharvest Seed Decay

Prevention of preharvest seed decay is very important in agriculture in certain climatic conditions (Harris and Burns, 1972) and is probably important in natural ecosystems under some conditions also. Prevention of postharvest seed decay is extremely critical in many species in natural ecosystems, as I pointed out in my discussion of this subject in Chapter 8. It is apparently less critical in crop species because the seeds have usually undergone rigorous selection by man over a long period of time for rapid germination and no dormancy. No doubt prevention of decay after planting is still of considerable importance in some crop plants. Unquestionably, the high tannin content of some hybrid sorghum varieties, which prevents preharvest seed germination and decay, would also prevent postharvest decay.

VI. THE ROLES OF ALLELOPATHY IN PLANT INFECTION

A. The Promotion of Infection

Patrick *et al.* (1964) pointed out that many plant pathologists feel that toxins play causal roles in some, if not most, plant diseases. The toxins involved are generally thought to be produced by the pathogenic microorganisms involved in the diseases. Cochrane (1948) suggested, however, that some root rots are initiated by the direct toxic action of plant residues. Considerable evidence was obtained by Patrick and his colleagues to support the suggestion (Patrick and Koch, 1958; Patrick *et al.*, 1963, 1964; Patrick, 1971). In field studies in Salinas Valley, California, Patrick *et al.* (1963) observed that discolored or sunken lesions were often present on roots of lettuce or spinach plants where the roots grew in contact with or in close proximity to fragments of plant residues. When isolations were made from the lesions, no known primary pathogen was consistently obtained, and the microorganisms most frequently found were common soil saprophytes. They concluded that the toxins produced by the decomposing residues conditioned roots to invasion by various low-grade pathogens.

Toussoun and Patrick (1963) found that the root rot of bean caused by *Fusarium solani* f. *phaseoli* was greatly increased if the bean roots were exposed to toxic extracts from decomposing plant residues before inoculation with the pathogen. Patrick and Koch (1963) reported that the extent and severity of black root rot of tobacco caused by *Thielaviopsis basicola* were much greater when the tobacco roots were exposed to toxic extracts of decomposing plant residues prior to inoculation. Moreover, they found that the pathogen was equally destructive to susceptible and resistant varieties of tobacco after treatment of roots with the toxic extracts.

Thus, another dimension is added to the harmful effects of phytotoxins on plants.

B. Resistance to Infection

The role of allelopathy as it relates to disease resistance of plants was discussed briefly in Chapter 2, Section III and Chapter 8, Section I. Many plants have been found to produce compounds, either prior to or after infection by certain pathogens, that make the plants resistant to diseases caused by the pathogens (Schaal and Johnson, 1955; Kúc *et al.*, 1956; Kúc, 1957; Clark *et al.*, 1959; Buxton, 1960; Byrde *et al.*, 1960; Condon and Kúc, 1960; Hughes and Swain, 1960; Farkas and. Kiraly, 1962; Minamikawa *et al.*, 1963; Gardner and Payne, 1964). Many of the same compounds, which have been implicated in other aspects of allelopathy, have been reported to be important in many instances in the resistance of plants to diseases.

As early as 1911, Cook and Taubenhaus found that tannins are very inhibitory to many parasitic fungi and suggested that they may be important in the resistance of some plants to fungal infection. According to Cruickshank and Perrin (1964), Maranon reported that strains of *Oenothera* sp. resistant to *Erysiphe polygoni* had higher tannin contents than susceptible strains. Cadman (1959) found that raspberry leaves contain a substance that prevents the infection of plants by viruses when it is mixed with the inoculum. He decided on the basis of several tests that the substance was a tannin. Somers and Harrison (1967) reported that certain wood tannins are very inhibitory to spore germination and hyphal growth of *Verticillium albo-atrum*, especially the condensed tannins. They suggested that the tannins may be important, therefore, in host resistance to *Verticillium* wilt disease.

Johnson and Schaal (1952) reported a good correlation between scab (caused by *Streptomyces scabies*) resistance of several potato varieties and the phenolic content of the peels of their tubers as indicated by the ferric chloride test. They suggested that the chief compound involved is chlorogenic acid. Other workers have been unable to repeat their results, however (Farkas and Kiraly, 1962). Kúc *et al.* (1956) found that slices of potato tubers (var. Netted-Gem) inoculated with *Helminthosporium carbonum* produced appreciable amounts of chlorogenic and caffeic acids subsequent to the infection. Both compounds were found to be inhibitory to growth of *H. carbonum*, with caffeic acid being most inhibitory. The combined activity, however, could not account for the total activity of the crude potato extract. Cysteine, which was present in the extract, gave a pronounced synergistic effect when added to either caffeic or chlorogenic acid. Later, Clark *et al.* (1959) found an amino acid addition product of chlorogenic acid in the peel of two varieties of potatoes, Russet and Netted-Gem. This compound is highly toxic to race 1 of *Helminthosporium carbonum*.

One of the best-known examples for the protective role of phenolics formed prior to infection is that of onion in relation to infection by *Colletotrichum circinans* (Farkas and Kiraly, 1962). The resistance of onion varieties is correlated with the red or yellow pigmentation of the bulb scales. The pigments are flavones and anthocyanins, which are not inhibitory to the pathogen, but protocatechuic acid and catechol occur along with them. These phenols are water soluble, and they diffuse from the dead cell layers of the scales and inhibit spore germination and hyphal penetration of the pathogen. Apparently, cases of preformed resistance factors are rare (Farkas and Kiraly, 1962; Cruickshank and Perrin, 1964).

There are many examples of the production of protective compounds subsequent to infection, similar to that reported by Kúc *et al.* (1956) and described above. Only a few will be discussed, however. Hughes and Swain (1960) reported a 10- to 20-fold increase in concentration of scopolin and a 2 - to 3-fold increase in chlorogenic acid in potato tuber slices infected with *Phytophthora infestans*. The tremendous increase in scopolin caused a blue fluorescent zone around the infected area. Cruickshank and Perrin (1964) stated that increases in concentrations of phenolic substances have been reported around lesions resulting from the infection of rice leaves by *Piricularia oryzae* and *Helminthosporium* sp., the infection of leaves of *Paulownia tomentosa* by *Gloeosporium kawakamii*, the infection of the leaves and peel of apple by *Venturia inaequalis* and *Podosphaera leucotricha*, and the infection of sweet potato roots by *Ceratocystis fimbriata*. Minamikawa *et al.* (1963) found that two coumarins, umbelliferone and scopoletin, increase markedly due to infection of sweet potato roots by *C. fimbriata*. Farkas and Kiraly (1962) found that resistant wheat–rust combinations also accumulate phenolics more rapidly than susceptible combinations. After a thorough review of pertinent literature, Farkas and Kiraly (1962) concluded that a pronounced, postinfectional rise in concentration of phenolics is one of the best-documented characteristics of resistance to fungus diseases. They pointed out that this has also been demonstrated for some bacterial and virus diseases. Cruickshank and Perrin (1964) reported that significant increases in concentrations of scopoletin, kaempferol, quercetin, caffeic acid, chlorogenic acid, and isochlorogenic acid have been associated with virus activity in various hosts. They stated also that coumarin has been shown to inhibit reproduction of tobacco mosaic virus.

According to Farkas and Kiraly (1962), hypersensitivity is one of the most important types of defense reactions of plant tissues to diseases caused by rusts, mildews, *Phytophthora*, and some viruses. This reaction consists of the rapid death of a few cells in highly resistant varieties, thus confining the pathogen to a restricted area. The breakdown of cellular structure apparently results from an excessive oxidation of polyphenols.

Cobb *et al.* (1968) suggested that several monoterpenes produced by *Pinus ponderosa* may play a part in its resistance to infection by *Fomes annonus* and *Ceratocystis* spp., especially in conjunction with accumulation of phenolics.

According to Cruickshank and Perrin (1964), Muller and Borger proposed the "phytoalexin theory" of disease resistance in 1939, i.e., that a compound designated as a phytoalexin, which inhibits the development of the pathogen, is formed or activated only when the parasite comes in contact with the host cells. This theory differs from the previously discussed concept in that the phytoalexins are thought to be unusual metabolites not found at all in uninfected tissues. By 1964, five phenolics and one nonphenol were identified as apparent phytoalexins (Cruickshank and Perrin, 1964): (1) ipomeamarone, isolated from sweet potato roots infected with *Ceratocystis fimbriata* and identified as a furanoterpenoid; (2) orchinol, isolated from orchid tubers infected with *Rhizoctonia repens* and identified as 2,4-dimethoxy-7-hydroxy-9,10-dihydrophenanthrene; (3) 3-methyl-6-methoxy-8-hydroxy-3,4-dihydroxyisocoumarin, isolated from carrot root tissue inoculated with *Ceratocystis fimbriata*; (4) pisatin, isolated from pea pods inoculated with *Monilinia fructicola* and identified as 3-hydroxy-7-methoxy-4′,5′-methylenedioxychromanocoumarin; (5) phaseollin, isolated from French bean pods infected with *Monilinia fructicola* and identified as 7-hydroxy-3′,4′-dimethylchromenochromanocoumarin; and (6) trifolirhizin, isolated from roots of red clover (not inoculated, but not under aseptic conditions) and identified as a glucoside of an isoflavonoid. Cruickshank and Perrin (1964) illustrated the structures of all these proposed phytoalexins. The phytoalexin theory has failed to gain wide acceptance, as indicated by the fact that Farkas and Kiraly (1962) did not even mention the theory or the identified phenolic phytoalexins in their rather comprehensive review of the role of phenolic compounds in disease resistance.

The importance of disease resistance in basic ecology and agriculture is certainly unquestioned. The evidence is clear that many of the same toxins that have been implicated in other phases of allelopathy are important in protecting plants against diseases. In fact, it appears that some of the same compounds may be involved in various allelopathic effects against microorganisms from the period before seed germination, through seed germination, plant growth, reproduction, and seed maturation.

C. General Microbial Inhibitors in Plants

This subject has been discussed briefly elsewhere in this book and was covered fairly thoroughly in Section I of Chapter 8. I will only say at this point that large numbers of plant species have been analyzed for the presence of inhibitors of many kinds of microorganisms, both pathogenic and nonpathogenic (Osborn, 1943; Cavallito and Bailey, 1944; Cavallito et al., 1944, 1945; Lucas and Lewis, 1944; Seegal and Holden, 1945; Gottshall et al., 1949; Lucas et al., 1951; Frisbey et al., 1953, 1954; Lucas et al., 1955; Ferenczy, 1956; Wright, 1956; Nickell, 1960; Dominguez et al., 1964; Henis et al., 1964; Rice, 1964, 1965a,b,c, 1969, 1972; Mallik, 1966; Mathes, 1967; Rice and Parenti, 1967; Blum and Rice, 1969). Many hundreds of species were found to have antimicrobial activities, but a number of the results were concerned with human pathogens and have little relevance to agriculture directly. Many of the results were relevant to agriculture, and to plant growth and development in general, and were discussed elsewhere. The above list was not meant to be exhaustive.

VII. RELATED PHENOMENA THAT ARE NOT STRICTLY ALLELOPATHIC

The chemical makeup of forage or crop plants often has striking effects on the digestibility and nutritional value of the plants to ruminants because of the effects of certain toxins on microorganisms in the rumen of the animals (Smart et al., 1961; Nagy et al., 1964; Hungate, 1966; Sidhu and Pfander, 1968; Harris et al., 1970; Bauchop, 1971;

Cummins, 1971). Smart *et al.* (1961) found that compounds in extracts of sericea leaves were polyphenolic in nature and inhibited the activity of rumen cellulase. The cellulase is produced, of course, by microorganisms in the rumen.

Nagy *et al.* (1964) reported that the essential oils of *Artemisia tridentata* are inhibitory to several bacterial species. Moreover, when they added essential oils of *A. tridentata* to alfalfa hay substrate in deer, sheep, or cattle rumen fluids in artificial rumen systems, the rate of short-chain fatty acid production was markedly depressed.

Sidhu and Pfander (1968) reported that some samples of orchard grass, *Dactylis glomerata,* resulted in poor growth, death loss, and stiffness when fed to lambs. They extracted orchard grass hay with three different solvent systems and tested substances obtained against cellulose digestion in an artificial rumen system using alfalfa hay as the substrate. Toxins were present in each of the extracts which reduced cellulose digestion by 8.5%, and the investigators concluded that more than one metabolic inhibitor was present in orchard grass. They also found a cellulose digestion-permitting factor in orchard-grass hay, and when they removed it, the digestibility of the residue of orchard-grass hay was reduced about 50%.

Harris *et al.* (1970) and Cummins (1971) found that the tannin content of sorghum grain and forage affected their digestibility. This effect is no doubt due to the pronounced antimicrobial action of tannins plus the direct effect of tannins in precipitating proteins.

Koths and Litsky (1962) investigated the antibiotic activity of certain bacterial cultures for the control of poultry pathogens in soils of poultry yards. It seems to me that there is real promise in this sort of research, not only from the standpoint of production of antibiotics by other microorganisms, but also from that of production of antimicrobial substances by higher plants.

Another important agricultural phenomenon related indirectly to allelopathy is the resistance of certain plants to attack by predators. Todd *et al.* (1971) found that the resistance of barley to the greenbug, *Schizaphis graminum,* is related to the amounts of phenolic and flavonoid compounds and related substances in the barley plants. Many of the same compounds found to be important in this resistance have been shown to be potent phytotoxins also. Morgan and Collins (1964) reported that certain organic treatments, including changes due to crop rotation, helped control soil populations of *Pratylenchus penetrans,* a nematode.

A short related discussion concerning plant–animal chemical interactions is included in Chapter 15.

10

Impact of Allelopathy on Horticulture and Forestry

I. ROLES IN HORTICULTURE

A. Introduction

I have arbitrarily divided this discussion of allelopathy in plants propagated by man for his use into its roles in agriculture, horticulture, and forestry. My goal has been to include crop and forage plants under agriculture, ornamentals and fruit producers under horticulture, and lumber producers under forestry. There are obviously many other categories that could be included such as floriculture, viticulture, etc. Nevertheless, I hope my intent is clear.

In the early part of this century, Pickering (1917, 1919) observed that apple trees were injured by interference from grass. He thought at first that the effects were due to competition for minerals or exclusion of oxygen from the tree roots by the grass. After experimentation, he ruled out these factors as causes. He next investigated the possibility that the grass was producing a toxin. He planted grass in a tray completely separated from the container in which the apple seedlings were growing, and allowed drainage from the soil in which the grass was growing to flow into the container of apple seedlings. Despite the fact that no competition was allowed, the apple seedlings were inhibited, indicating that allelopathy was responsible for the interference.

Walnut trees have been known for many years to produce a toxin injurious to apple trees (Massey, 1925; Schneiderhan, 1927). In fact, Schneiderhan (1927) reported that the toxin sometimes kills neighboring apple trees.

Krylov (1970) reported that cultivation of potatoes in the space between rows of young apple trees results in accumulation of toxins that inhibit tree growth. These toxins cause the total nitrogen content in the roots and tops to decrease, and they also cause a change in the composition of proteins in the bark. The amount of soluble albumins rises, and the quantity of residual proteins drops. The toxins interfere with photosynthesis in the apple trees also.

There has been surprisingly little research on allelopathic phenomena in ornamental plants. This is particularly strange in view of the fact that many gardeners and greenhouse workers are very much aware of many of these problems. I have had greenhouse supervisors tell me that they have to discard soil in which they have grown stock, *Malcomia maritima*. Some have told me that all sorts of crucifers poison soil so that plants do not grow satisfactorily afterward, including the crucifers. The prevalence of such ideas makes it seem desirable for considerable research to be done in this area.

I mentioned the work of Kozel and Tukey (1968) in the previous chapter in which they found that *Chrysanthemum morifolium* produces a potent phytotoxin that leaches from the leaves and is very inhibitory to the growth and development of chrysanthemum. Tukey (1969) stated that chrysanthemum cannot be grown in the same soil for several years, apparently because of the accumulation of inhibitors in the soil.

Oleksevich (1970) reported that barberry, horse chestnut, rose, lilac, viburnum, fir, and mockorange have considerable allelopathic activity. He found that they inhibit neighboring plants and cause soil toxicity. He stated that barberry produces a large amount of berberine, an alkaloid, which is a strong inhibitor of growth and development.

Podtelok (1972) tested water extracts of the roots of *Acer campestre, A. platanoides, A. pseudoplatanus, A. tataricum, A. laetum, A. turkestanicum, A. ginnala, A. negundo, A. saccharinum, Quercus robur,* and *Fraxinus excelsior* against seedling growth of these species. He found that the extracts had considerable inhibitory activity, and he arranged them in a series from most active to least active. He suggested that the allelopathic activities should be considered in selecting mixtures of these species for ornamental or forest plantings.

Grafting and budding are rarely considered in discussions of allelopathy, but Molisch (1937), in his classic book on the subject, discussed some of the chemical interactions that occur under such circumstances. He pointed out that one can obtain a dwarf tree by grafting a luxuriant growth form such as the tall growing pear onto the stock of a quince. In such a case, the quince limits the luxuriant growth of the pear tree. He reported also that such a tree fruits in 4 years or earlier and is less hardy and has a shorter life span than a pear grafted on a pear stock. Molisch pointed out that other dwarf trees, such as apple, peach, plum, and almond, behave similarly.

Tukey (1969) also discussed several important allelopathic responses in horticulture resulting from grafting or budding. Among these were dwarfing; resistance to diseases; changes in time of maturation of fruits; and changes in size, color, and quality of fruits.

Molisch (1937) discussed a great many experiments he performed, which demonstrated that fruits of apple, pear, and related plants produce a volatile compound, ethylene, that diffuses away from the fruits and affects other plants in striking ways. He pointed out that ethylene influences the growth in length and thickness of seedlings, hastens the ripening of fruit in amazing ways, promotes proliferation of lenticels, hastens callus formation and leaf fall, prevents the negative geotropic curvature of hypocotyls, and cancels epinastic curvatures.

B. The Peach Replant Problem

The problem of replanting fruit trees following the removal of old orchards has been recognized as a hazardous one for many years in the United States and Europe (Klaus, 1939; Proebsting and Gilmore, 1941; Koch, 1955). The problem is usually species specific, and other plants grow well in the same soil. This replant problem has been reported for apples, grapes, cherries, plums, peaches, apricots, and citrus (Proebsting and Gilmore, 1941; Patrick *et al.*, 1964). Comprehensive investigations covering possible competitive and allelopathic interference have been carried out apparently only for peaches, apples, and citrus.

According to Koch (1955), aboveground symptoms of affected peach replants are usually retarded growth, eventual stunting, and different degrees of intercostal chlorosis. The roots display different degrees of discoloration and necrosis with brown lesions invariably occurring on otherwise white lateral roots. Occasionally, the effect is so severe that the peach replants die. Koch pointed out also that the effects on the roots show up rapidly, often within 24 hours after emerging from the parent root tissue.

According to Proebsting and Gilmore (1941), a survey of the peach-growing districts in California indicated varying success of replanted orchards, from almost complete failure to complete success. The differences in response could not be correlated with climate, soil texture, or obvious cultural practices. Consequently, they undertook a thorough investigation covering the following possible causes for the failure of replants: (1) depletion of common nutrients either by the preceding orchard or by soil organisms using root residues as a source of energy, (2) depletion of minor elements, (3) diseases carried over from the previous orchard, and (4) direct toxicity of the roots or their decomposition products.

They laid out several fertilizer plots in districts where the peach replant problem was most serious. These involved addition of varying amounts of ammonium sulfate, potassium sulfate, superphosphate, manganese, zinc, copper, vitamin B_1, indolebutyric acid, indolepropionic acid, and peat moss. None of these eliminated the basic problem, although minor responses did occur in some cases.

Proebsting and Gilmore (1941) pointed out that certain diseases, such as crown gall caused by *Pseudomonas tumefaciens,* could be important factors in some failures; however, they found many cases of subnormal development where the peach trees were completely free of pathogens. Thus, they concluded that nutrition and disease must play only minor roles in the peach replant problem.

Subsequent experiments were designed by Proebsting and Gilmore to determine if an allelopathic mechanism might be involved in the peach decline. Initially, peach seedlings were grown in 5-gallon cans in the greenhouse either in screened soil from a peach orchard exhibiting the trouble or in screened soil from adjacent land not previously in peaches. No significant differences in growth of the seedlings were obtained. However, when 500 gm of peach roots were added to virgin soil in the same containers, definite growth inhibition resulted. The total average shoot length per control tree was 481 cm versus 326 cm for the test, and the average weight per control tree was 102.5 gm versus 53.7 gm for each test tree.

In another experiment, almond, apricot, and myrobalan seedlings were planted in a field where peaches had been removed, with peach seedlings planted as checks. The myrobalan seedlings made very strong growth, growth of almond and apricot was satisfactory, but that of peach seedlings was very poor.

An apricot orchard, made up of alternating rows on apricot and peach roots, was planted following the removal of a 40-year-old peach orchard. The apricot trees on apricot roots showed strikingly better growth than the apricot trees on peach roots, when normally peach roots give trees of just as good vigor. The effect was still apparent when the trees were 9 years old.

In another experiment, bark and wood of peach roots were separated, dried, and ground. The ground material was added in varying amounts to peach seedlings in 3-gallon sand cultures. Usually, 10 gm of bark added around the root area and next to the stem killed the seedlings in 4–5 days.

In one experiment, seven types of tests were examined in sand culture plus the control: (1) ground root bark, (2) ground root bark plus an equivalent amount of ground peat moss, (3) ground root wood, (4) material extracted from root bark with alcohol, (5) root bark residue after alcohol extraction, (6) water extract of root bark, (7) root bark residue after water extraction, and (8) just sand as control. Seedlings were planted in all, and a complete nutrient solution was supplied. All test material caused injury to tops and roots of the peach seedlings except the root bark residue after alcohol extraction.

Amygdalin is known to be present in root bark of peach, so an experiment was run in which 1 gm of amygdalin was added to 250 ml of nutrient solution and applied once or twice a week to trees in sand. No injury occurred. When the same amount of amygdalin was applied along with a trace of emulsin, however, injury was severe. Two such treatments 3 days apart killed the trees in 30 to 40 days after the first treatment. Emulsin digests the amygdalin to benzaldehyde and hydrogen cyanide, so Proebsting and Gilmore tested the effects of benzaldehyde and potassium cyanide in amounts ranging up to 1 gm of benzaldehyde per week in two treatments and 0.1 gm of potassium cyanide once a week. The benzaldehyde had little effect, but the 0.1 gm dosage of potassium cyanide caused severe injury to the peach seedlings.

Proebsting (1950) reported a carefully documented case history of the peach replant problem based on field observations at Davis, California. Two rows of apple trees and two rows of Lovell peach trees planted in 1922 were removed in 1942, and all four rows (22 trees per row) were planted with Faye Elberta peach seedlings. These were observed and measured each year for 6 years, and it was apparent by the end of the first year that the trees succeeding apples were making better growth than those succeeding peaches. At the end of the sixth growing season, the average circumference of the trees following apples was 58.2 cm, whereas it was only 42.4 cm for peach trees following peaches. At that time, the average yield in pounds per tree was 216.4 after apples and 118.8 after peaches.

Havis and Gilkeson (1947) did an investigation similar to the sand culture experiment of Proebsting and Gilmore (1941). The materials added to the sand medium were (1) oven-dried (80°F) ground root bark of peach, (2) root bark frozen in carbon dioxide and then ground, (3) whole small fresh roots frozen in carbon dioxide and then ground, and (4) whole fresh roots of various sizes cut into pieces not over 0.75 inches long. The plants used were 1-year Lovell seedlings budded to Elberta in the first experiment, and, in the second, two types were used: (1) Elberta budded on Lovell stocks and (2) Elberta seedlings. The duration of each experiment was 7 months. They reported that there was no evidence at any time in either experiment of toxic effects from any of the materials added.

Koch (1955) gave a thorough review of evidence for the peach replant problem and of efforts to determine the cause. He reported that the cause had been attributed to insects, nutritional disturbances, spray residues, phytotoxins, and nematodes. He suggested that a coordinated research effort covering several possibilities should be carried out. Such an effort was initiated by the Canada Department of Agriculture and carried on over a period of several years (Patrick, 1955; Ward and Durkee, 1956; Mountain and Boyce, 1958; Mountain and Patrick, 1959; and others).

Patrick (1955) investigated the role of toxins in the peach replant problem. He was chiefly interested in how toxins arise, whether or not microorganisms are necessary for their production, and whether they are due entirely to amygdalin. In his first series of experiments, he used soil obtained from site (under peach trees) and intersite areas in an orchard in which the replant problem was evident. The soil was passed through a screen to remove all pieces of roots, stones, and other foreign material. The peach root residue used was obtained from roots of 2-year-old Lovell peach seedlings grown in typical peach soil with no previous peach history. The smaller roots were gound to a coarse powder, and the bark was removed from the larger roots and ground to a coarse powder. The woody parts of the larger roots were not used.

The residues were added to site and intersite soil at the rate of 1–5% (w/w). Some of the samples were autoclaved in 15 lb/in² pressure for 20 minutes. The flasks containing the soil were incubated for several days at 25°C. The soil was extracted with water, the water was filtered through cheesecloth and then through a Seitz filter. The extracts were then tested against respiration of Lovell peach seedling root tips using the Warburg technique.

The rates of breakdown of amygdalin in the various substrates were determined by use of sodium carbonate picric acid papers to detect HCN. This compound is produced along with benzaldehyde when amygdalin is digested. Results of these tests indicated that microorganisms are necessary for decomposition of the amygdalin because no HCN was produced when the soil was autoclaved (Table 50). It appeared that the soil from the site areas contained a higher proportion of microorganisms capable of hydrolyzing amygdalin than soil from the intersite area because breakdown of the amygdalin began more rapidly in the site soil. Similar results were obtained when pure amygdalin was added to the soils at the rate of 0.25%. The addition of pure amygdalin, of course, eliminated the possibility of introducing into the soil samples specific microorganisms occurring with the peach root residues.

The water extracts of soil samples incubated with peach root residues or amygdalin were very inhibitory to respiration in peach roots (Table 51). The inhibition increased with increasing amounts of residue and with time of incubation of the soil and residue up to 3 or 4 days from the start. Again, it was evident that the production of toxic substances from amygdalin or root residue depended on the presence of microorganisms capable of utilizing the amygdalin. Sour cherry root residue either stimulated respiration or had virtually no effect depending on the time of incubation. Later experiments in which 10% root

TABLE 50

Relative Ability of Soil Microorganisms in Various Soils to Decompose the Amygdalin in Peach Root Residues [a]

2% Peach root residues added to fresh soil samples from	Test for CN after incubation at 25°C for			
	24 hours	48 hours	96 hours	240 hours
Old peach site area (soil under stump and around roots)	++++ [b]	++++	++++	++
Intersite area (10 feet from site)	++	+++	+++	++
Old site area (autoclaved)	− − −	− − −	− − −	−
Sour cherry orchard	++	+++	+++	++
Compost soil	− − −	− − −	− − −	+
Muck soil	− − −	− − −	− − −	+

[a] From Patrick (1955). Reproduced by permission of the National Research Council of Canada from the *Canadian Journal of Botany* **33**:461–486.

[b] Amount of CN produced determined by the intensity of red color of the Na picrate paper ½ hour in the reaction flask: ++++, intense red color—strong CN production; +++ and ++, decreasing intensity of red color—diminishing amounts of CN produced; +, pale orange color—weak CN production; − − −, yellow color of Na picrate paper—no CN produced.

TABLE 51

The Influence of Incubation Time, Soil Type, and Other Factors on the Relative Toxicity of the Resulting Soil Leachates as Determined by the Intensity of Their Inhibiting Effects on the Respiration of Excised Peach Root Tips [a]

Incubation time (hours) at 25°C before extracts made	Peach root residue (2%) [b]	Peach root residue (5%)	Substances added to old peach orchard soil (site area)				
			0.25% Amygdalin		Peach soil autoclaved		Sour cherry root residue (2%)
			Site area soil	Intersite area soil	Peach root residue (2%)	Amygdalin (0.25%) [c]	
	Percent total inhibition (or stimulation) of respiration in 5 hours at 20°C [c]						
60	48	—	51	—	—	—	—
70	60	—	55	—	8	10 stim.	8 stim.
100	40	78	72	—	6	15 stim.	—
150	—	68	82	7 stim.[d]	3 stim.	7 stim.	15 stim.
200	—	59	73	19 stim.	—	—	2
300	—	—	74	14	—	12	—

[a] Modified from Patrick (1955). Reproduced by permission of the National Research Council of Canada from the *Can. J. Bot.* **33**, 461–486.

[b] Amount of peach root residues, amgdalin or other root residues, calculated as percent by weight of the total soil contents of the flask added to each flask.

[c] Percent total inhibition of respiration in 5 hours of 15 excised peach root tips placed in the various soil–water leachates (containing varying amounts of the decomposition products of the substances indicated) was calculated in the usual manner using as check (or normal respiration rate) the respiration of identical root tip samples placed in soil–water leachates containing none of these products.

[d] If total O_2 uptake was greater than that of the check it was calculated as percent total stimulation of respiration.

residues of tobacco or pepper were added to site soil indicated that these residues stimulated respiration of peach roots.

Experiments were run to determine the effects on respiration of benzaldehyde and cyanide, which, along with glucose, are the breakdown products of amygdalin. Amygdalin, emulsin, and a combination of these were tested also. It was found that amygdalin or emulsin individually had no effect on respiration, but markedly inhibited respiration of peach roots when combined. Calcium cyanide added to site soil was found to result in extracts that were very inhibitory to respiration also. Benzaldehyde in water was very inhibitory to respiration in peach roots, with a dilution of 1:5000 (w/v) causing some inhibition.

Patrick (1955) cut down some 14-year-old peach trees and established plots that included the former location of a tree plus the surrounding 10 feet. Some were fumigated with ethylene dibromide, others with methyl bromide, and some were not fumigated. Lovell peach seedlings about 5 months old were planted 1 foot apart in all plots. Populations of nematodes and microorganisms were determined throughout the following growing season. The peach seedlings in the site areas showed poor growth in both fumigated and unfumigated plots, whereas seedlings 4 feet beyond the site in the intersite area grew well. There was slight improvement in growth in the fumigated site areas, but the contrasts with intersite areas were still great. It was concluded, therefore, that nematodes or other organisms which would have been greatly reduced by the soil fumigants were not responsible for all the stunting in the site areas. As much as 40% inhibition of respiration in peach roots resulted from water leachates of soil in the fumigated site areas.

Roots of 4-week-old intact peach seedlings were placed in water extracts of soil from site areas, and after 3–7 days, the seedlings showed wilting symptoms and drying of leaves starting from the bottom of the plant. The meristematic regions of the roots turned brown also. All these symptoms also appeared in seedlings placed in a 1:2000 dilution of benzaldehyde in water, whereas no injurious effects appeared even after 2 weeks in extracts of soil from intersite areas.

A large number of microorganisms capable of utilizing amygdalin were isolated from peach root agar inoculated with soil from the site areas in old peach orchards. Both fungi and bacteria were involved, but few actinomycetes were able to grow on the media containing only peach root residue or amygdalin as a carbon source. Many more organisms capable of utilizing amygdalin were isolated from site soil than from intersite soil.

Patrick (1955) concluded that whenever amygdalin and micro-organisms capable of utilizing it are present in soil, soluble toxic substances highly detrimental to living peach roots are likely to be produced in that soil. The amounts of these toxins and, thus, the degree of toxicity produced, would depend on the amount of old peach roots remaining in the soil after the old trees have been removed as well as on their amygdalin content. The toxic effects would be greatest for the first year or two after the trees are removed and should gradually diminish. Patrick pointed out that this diminishing toxicity would explain, at least in part, the frequent observation that the replant problem diminishes 2 or 3 years after removal of the old trees.

Because Patrick's (1955) research demonstrated that amygdalin is the source of phytotoxins produced from peach root residues, Ward and Durkee (1956) determined amounts of this glycoside in various parts of 2- and 3-year-old Lovell peach seedings and in roots of several varieties of peach trees of different ages. They found that concentrations varied some with different trees of the same variety and age and that amygdalin occurs in leaves, stems, and roots (Table 52). The stems have the lowest concentration followed in increasing amounts by leaves and roots. The roots had their highest concentration in the spring, whereas the tops had their highest concentration in the fall. The concentration of amygdalin was highest in the root bark.

Sampling was not adequate to draw definite conclusions, but the concentrations of amygdalin in the root bark of the single trees tested

TABLE 52

Amygdalin Content of Two-Year-Old Lovell Peach Seedlings [a]

Date of sampling	Tree	Amygdalin (mg/gm dry weight)			
		Leaves	Stem, branches, twigs	Large roots	Small roots
June 25, 1954	A	7.4	4.9	41.5	53.8
June 25, 1954	B	7.1	4.7	39.8	36.6
October 22, 1954	C	13.0	9.3	15.5	22.8
October 22, 1954	D	18.3	9.3	32.8	37.8
October 22, 1954	E	16.9	4.8	21.4	26.1

[a] From Ward and Durkee (1956). Reproduced by permission of the National Research Council of Canada from the *Can. J. Bot.* **34**, 419–422.

of the varieties Yunnan and Shalil were considerably lower than in any of the other varieties. These two varieties are somewhat resistant to the replant problem.

Mountain and Boyce (1958) investigated the relation of nematodes, and particularly *Pratylenchus penetrans,* to the growth of young peach replants in old peach orchards. They found that the first roots produced by the young trees are attacked within a relatively short time by *P. penetrans,* which is an endoparasite. It propagates rapidly in the newly formed succulent tissues, and, during the early spring period, degeneration of the root system sometimes becomes evident. The populations drop rapidly, however with the advent of higher soil temperatures. As populations of *P. penetrans* decrease, ectoparasitic nematodes with stylets capable of penetrating into the conducting elements of the roots appear. During the second year, the endoparasites continue to decrease and the ectoparasites increase.

Mountain and Boyce (1958) concluded that the precise role of *P. penetrans* in the peach replant problem is not clear, despite the fact that relatively large populations appear to be connected with the failure of replanted trees. They suggested that this nematode, and others, may be related to the problem in one or both of the following ways: (1) the nematodes may create infection courts for certain bacteria and fungi of peach soils, thus affording opportunity for production of toxins through the breakdown of amygdalin, and (2) the nematodes may be pathogens whose parasitic activities profoundly affect plant growth directly.

Mountain and Patrick (1959) extended the work of Mountain and Boyce (1958) and reported that *Pratylenchus penetrans* hydrolyzes amygdalin directly by its own enzymes and indirectly through mechanical damage of the host's root cells. This allows host emulsin and substrate to get together and produce phytotoxins.

Patrick *et al.* (1964) summarized the results of all research on the peach decline problem by stating that, although many questions still remain, the evidence suggests that, regardless of the causal organisms involved, the production of toxic substances through the hydrolysis of amygdalin appears to be the main mechanism involved in peach root degeneration. They pointed out that any lesion-producing agency that can rupture or penetrate root cells can cause the release of phytotoxins and produce root damage. These agencies include nematodes, fungi, insects, and physical factors. In addition to the production of toxins from living roots, microorganisms release them from peach root residues also. Thus, it appears that allelopathy is the primary cause of the peach decline problem.

C. The Apple Replant Problem

Börner (1959) reported that nurserymen in Germany encounter the replant problem with apple trees after cultivation of apples for even 1 or 2 years, and they find it essential to plant apple seedlings in soils that have never before been used to grow apples. The symptoms of affected apple trees are retarded growth and shortened internodes, resulting in a rosettelike appearance. In addition, the roots are often discolored, and growth of the tap root is reduced. Börner pointed out that many causes had been suggested, including nutrition, nematodes, and toxins. He stated that Fastabend had found that chopped apple roots or water leached through affected soils produced the toxicity symptoms when added to virgin soil in which apple seedlings were growing.

Börner (1959) decided to study further the effects of apple root residues on growth of apple seedlings and to identify the toxins. Siberian crabapple, *Malus baccata,* seedlings were grown in solution culture with root bark from a 16-year-old apple tree, *Malus sylvestris* (var. Stayman Winesap), added in amounts of 0.2, 1, and 10 gm per 500 ml of solution. After 33 days, the plants were harvested and various kinds of measurements were made (Table 53). The tops and roots were markedly inhibited, especially the roots, even at a concentration of only 0.2 gm per 500 ml of solution. Preliminary tests indicated that one or more phenolic compounds were present in the flasks with bark.

TABLE 53

Influence of Root Bark of a 16-Year-Old Apple Tree on the Growth of
Apple Seedlings in Water Culture [a,b]

Growth response	Growth with S.E. in flask (500 ml) containing different amounts of bark			
	0 gm bark	0.2 gm bark	1.0 gm bark	10.0 gm bark
Number of leaves	13.0 ± 0.9	9.8 ± 0.8	7.8 ± 0.9	No growth
Length of stem (cm)	16.1 ± 3.4	10.7 ± 2.8	4.1 ± 0.3	No growth
Length of root (cm)	19.4 ± 0.6	9.9 ± 0.7	5.7 ± 0.3	No growth
Dry weight of leaves (mg)	715.0 ± 65.9	337.5 ± 69.5	141.3 ± 29.9	No growth
Dry weight of stem (mg)	220.0 ± 57.2	110.0 ± 35.8	35.0 ± 6.4	No growth
Dry weight of roots (mg)	155.0 ± 9.6	96.3 ± 7.1	70.0 ± 9.3	No growth

[a] From Börner (1959).
[b] Duration of experiment was 33 days.

The phenolics were extracted with ether, chromatographed on paper, and identified as phlorizin, phloretin, p-hydroxyhydrocinnamic acid, phloroglucinol, and p-hydroxybenzoic acid.

Börner decided next to determine if the same phenolics could be detected in soil to which he added apple roots. In this experiment, he added 25 gm of air-dried apple roots of small diameter to 500 gm of soil, followed by sufficient distilled water to moisten the soil. At intervals of 1–3 days, sufficient water was added to the soil to leach through it for 2 hours. At each time, the leachate was extracted with ether, and the phenolics were separated by paper chromatography and identified.

When the soil was leached immediately after adding the apple roots, only phlorizin was found in the leachate. Soil leached 1–2 days later yielded phlorizin, phloretin, p-hydroxyhydrocinnamic acid, and phloroglucinol. After 8–13 days, only the last two compounds were present in the soil. The only compound detected in the earlier water culture experiment and not in soil was p-hydroxybenzoic acid.

Roots of two apple species were extracted with ethanol in a Soxhlet apparatus, and the extracts were chromatographed. Phlorizin was the only phenolic previously identified that was found, indicating that it was the only one of the five that is a natural constituent of apple roots. Börner concluded, therefore, that the others are microbial decomposition products of phlorizin. He did find the flavonoid glycoside quercitrin in the root extract of a 16-year-old tree in addition to phlorizin.

In another experiment, Börner (1959) added 1 or 2 gm of pure phlorizin to 100 gm of soil. Some phlorizin was sterilized in an autoclave and some was not, and all was subsequently allowed to stand at 22°C. Every 24 hours at first, and later every 2–3 days, 10 gm of soil were extracted with ethanol in a Soxhlet apparatus for 1 hour, and the phenolic compounds were identified in each lot. The same five phenolic compounds were found after a period of time, as in the original experiment in which apple root bark was added to nutrient solution, if the soil was not sterilized. Sterilized soil continued to contain only phlorizin. From the sequence of events, Börner concluded that phloretin, p-hydroxyhydrocinnamic acid, phloroglucinol, and p-hydroxybenzoic acid are decomposition products of phlorizin and that the decomposition is accomplished by microorganisms. He inferred also that the sequence of decomposition is as follows.

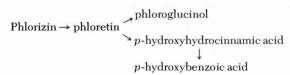

He demonstrated as well that species of *Aspergillus* and *Penicillium* isolated from apple root residues are able to decompose phlorizin in the same way.

Phlorizin and the four phenolics resulting from its decomposition were tested in solution culture against growth of apple seedlings. All five compounds inhibited growth of at least some parts of the apple seedlings. Root growth and dry weight of leaves were most strongly affected, and phlorizin and phloretin appeared to be most inhibitory. However, after a while, other decomposition products were present in these flasks.

Börner's overall conclusion was that the importance of the identified phytotoxins in the apple replant problem depends on (1) the physiological effectiveness of the toxins, (2) their concentrations in the soil of orchards, and (3) the ability of microorganisms to destroy them.

Holowczak *et al.* (1960) reported that numerous isolates of *Venturia inaequalis* were able to decompose phlorizin to glucose and phloretin, and phloretin to phloroglucinol and *p*-hydroxyhydrocinnamic acid.

Börner (1963a,b) later found that *Penicillium expansum* isolated from soil in an apple orchard produced patulin and an unidentified phenol when growing in soil containing leaf and root residues of apple. Patulin is a potent phytotoxin, as indicated previously (Norstadt and McCalla, 1963).

Berestetsky (1970, 1972) investigated the apple replant problem in the U.S.S.R. and concluded that the inhibition of apple seedlings in old apple orchards is due at least in part to decomposition products of root residues. When he inoculated these root residues with *Penicillum claviforme* and *P. martensii,* phytotoxic substances were produced.

Williams (1960) listed numerous phenolic acids and flavonoid glycosides produced by leaves, bark, and fruit of apple trees, and most are known phytotoxins under experimental conditions. Nobody has investigated these in relation to the apple replant problem, although they may be important.

The apple replant problem is certainly not completely solved, but present evidence indicates that allelopathic mechanisms, perhaps at more than one level, are very important in the problem and may be the primary cause.

D. The Citrus Decline and Replant Problem

After citrus trees have been grown on some soils for several years, the yields begin to diminish, the trees become less thrifty, abnormal

occurs, and new growth is slow in spite of standard fertilizer
.. pest-control practices and generally good management (Martin,
1948). When young citrus trees are replanted in such groves, growth is
very slow compared with that of similar young trees in noncitrus soil.

Preliminary soil-fumigation experiments conducted by Martin
(1948) caused him to suspect that some kind of soil biological factor
was at least partly responsible for the replant problem. He pointed out
that the chief microbiological agents in the soil which might affect
citrus growth are nematodes, chiefly *Tylenchulus semipenetrans*, path-
orgenic microorganisms, and saprophytic organisms. Martin decided,
therefore, to determine if the fungus flora is different in citrus soils
than in noncitrus soils. He obtained soil samples at various depths
from many old citrus groves and similar numbers and kinds of samples
from noncitrus areas at intervals of 4–6 months over a 2-year period.
These were plated out, and numbers and types of saprophytic fungi
were determined by the dilution technique.

Sixty-three species of fungi were found in old citrus soil and 52 in
noncitrus soil. More than half of these were only encountered occasionally. Usually, the commonly encountered species were found in
both types of soil. *Torula* sp. 1 was found only in noncitrus soil, however, and *Pyrenochaeta* sp. and an unidentified fungus (D_1) were
found only in old citrus soil. Although *Fusarium* spp. were found in
both types of soil, they occurred in much greater numbers in old citrus
soil.

On the basis of additional work, Martin (1950a) listed the most abundant species of fungi in old citrus soil in order of decreasing number
as *Fusarium solani, Pyrenochaeta* sp., fungus D_1, blue-green peni-
cillia, *Aspergillus versicolor,* and *Penicillium nigricans.* He tested
many fungi singly and in combinations against germination of sweet
orange seeds and development of the seedlings using ground citrus
roots mixed in quartz sand as the medium for seed germination and for
growth of the inoculated fungi. Most of the fungi tested had very little
effect on seed germination or seedling growth of orange.

Cylindrocarpon radicicola caused the decay of 80% of the orange
seeds and infected the roots of all seedlings that developed. *Fusarium
oxysporum* exerted a similar effect except that more seeds germinated. In the *Fusarium solani* cultures, 67% of the seeds germinated,
and the root tips of all seedlings except one became infected. In the
presence of *Phyrenochaeta* sp., 73% of the seeds germinated. Fungus
D_1 alone had little effect, but this species in combination with *Pyrenochaeta* sp. and *Fusarium solani* inhibited germination and caused
decay of all but one of the 60 seeds tested. This also happened when

Fusarium solani and *Pyrenochaeta* sp. were combined. Martin concluded, therefore, that the type of fungus population developing as a result of prolonged growth of citrus on the same soil may be partly responsible for decay of citrus feeder roots and for the reduced growth of citrus in second or third plantings in the same soil.

Martin *et al.* (1953) fumigated old citrus and noncitrus soils in the greenhouse and the field using five different fumigants. In greenhouse studies, orange seedlings were planted 6 weeks after fumigation. The plants were harvested after 9 months, weighed, and leaves and feeder roots were ground and analyzed for 18 mineral elements. Leaves collected from orange and lemon trees in the field plots were analyzed for eight elements. Growth of sweet orange seedlings was markedly improved in old citrus soil that was fumigated in greenhouse studies, and marked improvement of growth of both lemon and orange trees in old groves occurred in field plots that were fumigated. In some cases growth was nearly doubled.

Citrus seedlings grown in old citrus and noncitrus soils were not significantly different in chemical composition. Fumigation did not change the level of any nutrient from a deficiency to a sufficiency level, with the possible exception of manganese in a few tests. Moreover, fumigation of noncitrus soils produced similar chemical changes in the citrus plants, but did not increase growth, and growth of citrus seedlings in nonfumigated noncitrus soils was better than that in fumigated old citrus soils. Martin *et al.* (1953) inferred from this evidence that the increased growth in old citrus soils after fumigation must have been caused by destruction of detrimental soil organisms and not by changes in the nutrient status of the soils.

Martin *et al.* (1956) fumigated two kinds of old citrus and noncitrus soils in pots in the greenhouse and then inoculated the soil in the pots with one fungal species or a combination of species. Sweet orange seedlings were than planted in the pots and allowed to grow for 6–9 months. The soil was sampled periodically also for kinds of fungi present. They found that destruction of the existing population in old citrus soil resulted in about as good orange seedling growth as in noncitrus soil. Reinoculation of the fumigated soils with selected fungi did not have much influence on seedling growth either in most cases. The one exception was inoculation with *Thielaviopsis basicola*, which greatly reduced growth of orange seedlings in two types of soils. The reduction in growth with this fungus was less when it was combined with some other fungi, such as *Penicillium nigricans* or *Stachybotrys atra*.

Martin and Ervin (1958) grew 12 different legume companion crops ith sweet orange seedlings in old citrus soil, and all but one study decreased growth of the orange seedlings. A 1-year rotation to a different crop increased growth considerably when sweet orange seedlings were subsequently planted in the soil. Grasses appeared to be most effective, but they did not cause growth of orange seedlings to even approach that of seedlings in noncitrus soil. Of 22 kinds of organic materials added to old citrus soil, only one increased growth of sweet orange seedlings, and that was pine needles. Martin and Ervin did not comment on the possible reason for the stimulation by pine, but it may have been due to inhibition of microorganisms by the condensed tannins in pine needles (Rice and Pancholy, 1973). This would certainly agree with previous conclusions of Martin and his colleagues that certain microorganisms in old citrus soils are responsible for the citrus replant problem.

The design of all experiments conducted by Martin and his co-workers was such that they could conclude only that certain microorganisms (particularly fungi) are apparently responsible for the poor growth of citrus in old citrus soils. Unfortunately, nothing definite could be concluded as to how the detrimental microorganisms reduce the growth of citrus seedlings. There were some implications that the effects might be due to infection of the roots by certain fungi, but no clear evidence for inferring it. I have seen no suggestion regarding the possibility that the fungi might be producing phytotoxins, either directly or by decomposition of some specific compound in citrus roots. The basic question, therefore, as to the primary cause of the citrus decline and replant problem seems to me to be wide open. However, on the basis of research on production of toxins from other plant residues, it seems likely to me that phytotoxins are produced by microbial action from citrus residues and that allelopathy is involved to some extent, therefore, in the citrus replant problem and may be the primary cause. Obviously, much research remains to be done before this can be substantiated.

II. ROLES OF ALLELOPATHY IN FORESTRY

The widespread occurrence of woody species that are allelopathic to other species and sometimes to themselves (see Chapters 5, 6, 7, 8, and Section I of this chapter) makes it seem highly likely that allelopathy is very important in forestry. Unfortunately, very little research has been done in this area relating specifically to forestry, and I feel this should be remedied.

Brown (1967) observed that even on a similar site, jack pine (*Pinus banksiana*) stands ranging from a few stems to 1000 or more per acre may be found within a few yards of each other. He observed that ground cover plants showed similar extremes in density. Measurements of soil texture, available minerals, depth of water table, waterholding capacity, soil acidity, root competition, slope exposure, microclimate, and seed dispersal did not reveal differences that explained the differences in the jack pine stands. Moreover, there were no differences in logging or fire history, so Brown investigated the possibility of naturally occurring, biologically active materials on jack pine seed germination and growth.

Water extracts of 56 species of plants commonly associated with jack pine were used as the moistening medium for germination of seeds in the laboratory. Nine of the extracts were found to inhibit significantly the germination of jack pine seeds (Table 54). Two species of *Prunus* completely inhibited germination, and two species of *Solidago* and *Salix pellita* almost completely inhibited it. There was no relationship to the pH of the extract because the range of pH's of the noninhibiting extracts was greater than the range of inhibiting ones.

Three species that inhibited jack pine seed germination under laboratory conditions, six that showed no influence, and two that stimu-

TABLE 54

Germination of Jack Pine Seeds in the Presence of Inhibitory Plant Extracts [a]

Species	Plant part extracted	pH of extract	Percent germination after 14 days [b]
Boletus edulis	Fruiting bodies	—	37
Cladonia cristatella	Plants	5.1	24
Sphagnum capillaceum	Plants	4.6	22
Salix pellita	Leaves	6.2	9
Prunus pumila	Leaves	—	0
Prunus serotina	Leaves	6.2	0
Gaultheria procumbens	Leaves	6.3	21
Solidago juncea	Flowers	—	11
Solidago juncea	Leaves	5.0	9
Solidago uliginosa	Leaves	—	2
Control (average)	—	—	82 [c]

[a] From Brown (1967).
[b] Significant at 1% level according to Student's t test.
[c] Range 62–93%.

lated germination were selected for field studies by Brown (1967). A virtually pure stand of each was selected, several plots were laid out, plants were clipped to a height of 1–2 inches, the surface was tilled slightly with a rake, and four seeds of jack pine were planted per 0.04 m^2 with a total of 400 seeds in each cover type. All species that consistently inhibited germination of jack pine seeds in laboratory tests did so in the field. The two species that were stimulatory in the laboratory allowed high germination rates in the field also, but the neutral species in laboratory tests gave variable results in the field, with some inhibiting germination and some having little effect. Brown's experiment did not permit any conclusion concerning the role of allelopathy in the subsequent growth of seedlings. There were definite interference effects by several of the cover species, however.

D. L. Hymes and J. M. Parks (personal communication) tested water extracts of freshly fallen leaves of 30 woody forest species from Tech Mountain near Montgomery, West Virginia against the free-living nitrogen fixer, *Azotobacter chroococcum*, and against the symbiotic nitrogen fixer, *Rhizobium leguminosarum*. They found that the extracts had very little effect on *Azotobacter*, whereas extracts of 11 species inhibited *Rhizobium*, some markedly.

In the introduction to this chapter, I discussed the research of Podtelok (1972), and it is certainly pertinent to this section also. Mirchink (1972) found a large number of fungi that produce citrinin, patulin, penicillic acid, and rubrotoxin in podzolic, soddy podzolic, and gray forest soils in the U.S.S.R. He identified the toxins by UV spectra and paper chromatography. He stated that all four compounds are toxic to higher plants, and the first three are antimicrobial also. Affected plants have higher respiratory rates and various synthetic processes are inhibited also during the early stages of plant growth. Mirchink concluded that microorganisms play important roles in forests through the production of such phytotoxins.

The investigation by del Moral and Cates (1971) in Washington forests discussed in Section III of Chapter 7 certainly is applicable here also.

11

Plant Parts That Contain Inhibitors and Ways in Which Inhibitors Enter the Environment

I. PARTS KNOWN TO CONTAIN INHIBITORS

This chapter deals only with inhibitors *in* higher plants but includes inhibitors *of* microorganisms. Although most of the information has been covered in the previous chapters, I feel a concise summary is worthwhile for reference purposes, and only the six major organs of plants are considered. The only citations listed are those in which the specific organs under discussion were tested separately, and no effort is made to include all citations possible. There are many papers concerning work with combinations of plant parts, such as shoots of grasses or plant residues in which various plant parts were combined for testing, but these are not included under any category. Evenari (1949) gave a rather complete list of citations indicating plant parts known to produce inhibitors of seed germination. I have chosen, therefore, to cite only selected papers prior to 1949 not cited by Evenari.

A. Stems

Stems have not been tested separately by many workers, but some stems have been shown to contain inhibitors, and in some instances they are the chief source of toxicity (Gottshall *et al.*, 1949; Lucas *et al.*, 1951; 1955; Frisbey *et al.*, 1953, 1954; Nickell, 1960; Guenzi and McCalla, 1962; Rice, 1964; Abdul-Wahab and Rice, 1967; Wilson and

Rice, 1968; Parks and Rice, 1969; Ballester and Vieitez, 1971; Vieitez and Ballester, 1972; Bell and Muller, 1973).

B. Leaves

Leaves seem to be the most consistent source of inhibitors, and most investigators have tested them, at least in combination with some other parts. They have been shown specifically by many workers to contain toxins (Osborn, 1943; Cavallito and Bailey, 1944; Lucas and Lewis, 1944; Gray and Bonner, 1948a; Evenari, 1949; Gottshall *et al.*, 1949; Lucas *et al.*, 1951, 1955; Bennett and Bonner, 1953; Frisbey *et al.*, 1953, 1954; Mergen, 1959; Nickell, 1960; Jameson, 1961; Dominguez *et al.*, 1964; Muller and Muller, 1964; Muller *et al.*, 1964; Reid, 1964; Rice, 1964, 1965a,b, 1969; C. H. Muller, 1965; W. H. Muller, 1965; Abdul-Wahab and Rice, 1967; Brown, 1967; Wilson and Rice, 1968; del Moral and Muller, 1969, 1970; McPherson and Muller, 1969; Parks and Rice, 1969; Schlatterer and Tisdale, 1969; Al-Naib and Rice, 1971; Ballester and Vieitez, 1971; Olsen *et al.*, 1971; Rasmussen and Rice, 1971; Chou and Muller, 1972; Vieitez and Ballester, 1972; Bell and Muller, 1973; Rice and Pancholy, 1973).

C. Roots

Roots have generally been found to contain fewer and generally less potent or at least smaller amounts of inhibitors than leaves, but this is sometimes reversed. Many workers have assayed roots separately, and many roots have been found to contain inhibitors (Bonner and Galston, 1944; Evenari, 1949; Goodwin and Kavanagh, 1949; Gottshall *et al.*, 1949; Lucas *et al.*, 1951, 1955; Frisbey *et al.*, 1953, 1954; Eberhardt, 1954; Goodwin and Pollock, 1954; Börner, 1959, 1960; Nickell, 1960; Grant and Sallans, 1964; Rice, 1964, 1972; Wilson and Rice, 1968; Parks and Rice, 1969; Podtelok, 1972; Robinson, 1972; Rice and Pancholy, 1973).

D. Flowers or Inflorescence

Only a small number of investigators has assayed flowers or inflorescences specifically for the presence of inhibitors, but nevertheless we know now that many flowers contain high concentrations of toxins (Gottshall *et al.*, 1949; Lucas *et al.*, 1951; 1955; Frisbey *et al.*, 1953, 1954; Nickell, 1960; Lahiri and Kharabanda, 1962-1963; Rice, 1964; Brown, 1967; Wilson and Rice, 1968; Ballester and Vieitez, 1971; Vieitez and Ballester, 1972).

E. Fruits

From the standpoint of allelopathy, fruits have been generally neglected, much as have stems and flowers. Some investigators have surveyed fruits of large numbers of families and species, however, for the presence of inhibitors of seed germination and microorganisms, so we know that toxins are present in many fruits (Elmer, 1932; Evenari, 1949; Gottshall *et al.*, 1949; Lucas *et al.*, 1951, 1955; Frisbey *et al.*, 1953, 1954; Ferenczy, 1956; Massart, 1957; Varga and Köves, 1959; Nickell, 1960; Manasse and Corpe, 1965; Grodzinsky, 1967; Al-Naib and Rice, 1971).

F. Seeds

Seeds have been widely assayed for the presence of inhibitors of seed germination and microorganisms, so we know that many of them from a great number of families and species do contain inhibitors (Osborn, 1943; Evenari, 1949; Gottshall *et al.*, 1949; Lucas *et al.*, 1951, 1955; Frisbey *et al.*, 1953, 1954; Ferenczy, 1956; Nickell, 1960; Bowen, 1961; Miyamoto *et al.*, 1961; Fottrell *et al.*, 1964; Gressel and Holm, 1964; Henis *et al.*, 1964; Lane, 1965; Logan *et al.*, 1968; Harris and Burns, 1970, 1972; Lazauskas and Balinevichiute, 1972; Prutenskaya, 1972).

II. WAYS IN WHICH INHIBITORS GET OUT OF PLANTS

A. Volatilization

Considerable research has been done on the emanation of volatile inhibitors from plants since Elmer (1932) demonstrated that volatile substances from apples inhibit growth of potato sprouts. McKnight and Lindegren (1936) and Walton *et al.* (1936) reported that vapors from garlic are bactericidal to organisms such as *Mycobacterium cepae.*

Salvia leucophylla, S. mellifera, and *S. apiana* have been shown to produce potent volatile inhibitors of other higher plants and of some microorganisms (C.H. Muller, 1965; W. H. Muller, 1965; Muller and Muller, 1964; Muller *et al.,* 1964). Numerous species of sagebrush, including *Artemisia californica, A. cana, A. arbuscula, A. frigida, A. nova,* and *A. tridentata,* produce volatile essential oils that markedly inhibit certain bacteria in addition to seed germination and seedling growth of many species (Muller *et al.,* 1964; Nagy *et al.,* 1964; Asplund, 1969). Volatile inhibitors of seed germination and seedling growth are produced also by *Heteromeles arbutifolia, Lepechinia calycina, Prunus ilicifolia, P. lyoni,* and *Umbellularia californica* (Muller, 1966).

The genus *Eucalyptus* has long been known to produce several volatile terpenes, and several of these have been shown to be very toxic to seed germination and seedling growth of numerous species of plants (del Moral and Muller, 1970). Baker (1966) demonstrated that volatile growth inhibitors are produced by *E. globulus* and that they are more inhibitory to growth of *Cucumis* roots than to *Eucalyptus* roots and hypocotyls. Del Moral and Muller (1970) found that fresh leaves of *E. camaldulensis* produce large amounts of several volatile terpenes that are toxic to plant growth, but litter, bark, and roots do not emit significant amounts.

Neill and Rice (1971) found that volatile inhibitors are produced by fresh leaves of *Ambrosia psilostachya* and suggested that these may play an important role in old field succession. They did not identify the inhibitors, but most, if not all, species of *Ambrosia* are known to produce several sesquiterpene lactones (Geissman *et al.,* 1969), and these may be the inhibitors. Other species of *Ambrosia* should be tested for the production of volatile inhibitors, and those produced by *A. psilostachya* should be identified.

Dadykin *et al.* (1970) reported that leaves of beet, tomato, and sweet potato and roots of carrot produce several volatile plant inhibitors in a closed system, but it was not demonstrated that these have any effect under field conditions.

Bell and Muller (1973) found that *Brassica nigra* produces potent volatile toxins, but their experiments indicated that these toxins are not responsible for the failure of annual grasses to grow in the patches of *Brassica* in California grasslands.

In general, it appears that volatile inhibitors may be most significant ecologically under arid and semiard conditions.

B. Leaching

At least some biologists have been aware of the leaching phenomenon since early in the eighteenth century, and many kinds of inorganic ions, elements, and compounds as well as organic compounds have been identified in the leachate of plant foliage (Tukey, 1966, 1969, 1971). In fact, Lee and Monsi (1963) reported that they found a statement by Banzan Kumazawa in some ancient Japanese documents about 300 years old that rainwater or dew from leaves of *Pinus densiflora* is harmful to crops underneath. There is no question, therefore, that plants are leaky systems even when alive and more so after death. Factors affecting the leaching of materials from leaves were discussed by Tukey (1969, 1971). In this discussion of the release of inhibitors by leaching, I am going to cite primarily those investigations in which the actual leachate of living plants or of plant material was tested for toxicity. The fact that phytotoxins have been demonstrated in extracts of various plant parts does not mean that they will leach or exude from the plant. Of course, water-soluble toxins that are still present after death of a plant part generally can leach out.

In addition to the volatile inhibitors produced by *Artemisia*, at least *A. absinthium* (Bode, 1940; Funke, 1943) and *A. tridentata* (Schlatterer and Tisdale, 1969) produce water-soluble toxins that leach from living or dead leaves. This is true also of *Eucalyptus globulus, E. camaldulensis* (del Moral and Muller, 1969, 1970), and *Ambrosia psilostachya* (Neill and Rice, 1971).

Leachates of living and/or dead leaves of the following species have been shown to contain growth inhibitors: *Encelia farinosa* (Gray and Bonner, 1948a,b); *Juglans* spp. (Bode, 1958); *Camelina alyssum* (Grümmer and Beyer, 1960); *Arctostaphylos uva-ursi, Melilotus alba, Juglans nigra* (Winter, 1961); *Crysanthemum morifolium* (Kozel and Tukey, 1968); *Helianthus annuus* (Wilson and Rice, 1968; Rice, 1971a); *Rhus copallina* (Blum and Rice, 1969); *Atriplex polycarpa* (Cornelius, 1969); *Comptonia* sp. (Fraser, 1969); *Adenostoma fasciculatum* (McPherson and Muller, 1969); *Rhus glabra* (Parks and Rice, 1969); *Platanus occidentalis* (Al-Naib and Rice, 1971); *Celtis laevigata* (Lodhi and Rice, 1971); *Sporobulus pyramidatus* (Rasmussen and Rice, 1971); *Euphorbia supina, Aristida oligantha, Bromus japonicus* (Rice, 1971a); *Arctostaphylos glandulosa* (Chou and Muller, 1972); and *Brassica nigra* (Bell and Muller, 1973).

Leachates of the following miscellaneous plant parts have also been shown to contain inhibitors: seeds of 12 weed species (Gressel and

Holm, 1964—see Section III,B, Chapter 9 for list of species—all used in intact seed test except *Eragrostis cilianensis*), apple root residue (Börner, 1959), dried fresh rape roots (Martin and Rademacher, 1960b), top residue of *Avena fatua* (Tinnin and Muller, 1971), wheat straw (McCalla and Duley, 1949), bark of *Malus* sp. and *Aesculus hippocastanum* (Winter, 1961), and stems of *Brassica nigra* (Bell and Muller, 1973). Perhaps all tests of aqueous extracts of residues belong here, but I have chosen not to include them (see Chapter 9).

C. Exudation from Roots

Since the comprehensive investigation of Lyon and Wilson (1921) demonstrated that roots of several crop plants exuded large amounts of organic compounds even under sterile conditions, numerous persons have found that many kinds of organic compounds are exuded by living roots of many species (Lundegardh and Stenlid, 1944; Fries and Forsman, 1951; Eberhardt, 1954; Katznelson *et al.*, 1955; Petrii and Chrastil, 1955; Rovira, 1956, 1965, 1969, 1971; Martin, 1957; Samtse-vich, 1968). It has been shown very clearly also that numerous kinds of organic compounds can exude from roots of donor plants and can be taken up by adjacent plants (Grodzinsky, 1969; Rovira, 1969; Ivanov and Yakobson, 1970; Foy *et al.*, 1971). Factors affecting the rates and amounts of root exudation were discussed by Rovira (1969, 1971).

In cases in which no radioactive tracers have been introduced into the plant or no unusual compound has been applied or injected, it is very difficult, even under axenic conditions, to determine which com-pounds that appear outside the roots are actually exuded from them and which ones result from the sloughing off of outer cells. Under nonsterile conditions, the problem is worse because new compounds can result from the metabolic activity of microorganisms. Con-sequently, one is forced to use the term root exudate in a broad sense in most applications to allelopathy. Generally, it is used in such cases to refer to inhibitors resulting from the presence of living roots where no leachates, volatiles, or residues from the tops of the plants are present. This is the way I will use the term in the rest of this section. Woods (1960) reviewed the literature on phytotoxic root exudates, but he used the term more broadly than even I have defined it.

There have been only relatively few investigations in which inhib-itory root exudates have been clearly demonstrated, even on the basis of my broad definition. Several crop plants including wheat, oats, corn, and cowpeas were demonstrated by Schreiner and Reed (1907b) and Schreiner and Sullivan (1909) to produce inhibitory root exudates, and since that time only a few other crop plants have been added to the list: guayule (Bonner and Galston, 1944), a non-nodulating soybean (Elkan, 1961), and cucumbers and tomatoes (Gaidamak, 1971). Thus, this appears to be a fruitful area for future research.

Fortunately, there have been several noncrop species that have been shown to produce toxic root exudates: *Sorghum halepense* (Abdul-Wahab and Rice, 1967); *Araucaria cunninghamii, Pinus elliottii, Flindersia australis* (Bevege, 1968); *Ambrosia psilostachya* (Rice, 1968; Neill and Rice, 1971); *Euphorbia supina* (Brown, 1968; Rice, 1968); *Helianthus annuus* (Rice, 1968; Wilson and Rice, 1968); *Aristida oligantha* and *Bromus japonicus* (Rice, 1968); *Digitaria sanguinalis* (Rice, 1968; Parenti and Rice, 1969); *Sporobolus pyramidatus* (Rasmussen and Rice, 1971); *Setaria faberii* (Bell and Koeppe, 1972); and *Calluna vulgaris* (Robinson, 1972).

D. Decay of Plant Material

The problem of determining whether inhibitors already present are being released from plant material by decay is very difficult, if not impossible, to solve. There is always the possibility that certain microorganisms are changing nontoxic compounds to toxic ones as in the case of amygdalin in peach residues (Patrick, 1955), or that they are synthesizing inhibitors as in the production of patulin by *Penicillium urticae* growing on wheat straw residue (Norstadt and McCalla, 1963), the production of patulin and a phenolic inhibitor by *Penicillium expansum* growing on apple residue (Börner, 1963a,b), or the production of other inhibitors by microorganisms decomposing residues of various crop plants (Patrick and Koch, 1958; Patrick *et al.*, 1963). Moreover, water-soluble inhibitors should easily leach out of plant residues after death when the various membranes generally lose their differential permeability. There are, of course, many potent inhibitors, such as most flavonoids (aglycones), which are only very slightly soluble in water, and these are probably released only by decomposition. I will cite below only those investigations in which growth inhibition was demonstrated after incorporation of plant residues in the substrate and in which the inhibitors were not shown to result from the activity of microorganisms. This does not mean, of course, that future research will not demonstrate that they are produced by microorganisms. I have cited work on apple residues below because phlorizin is present in the residue and is released by decay as well as by leaching, and it is inhibitory to apple seedlings. It is known, of course, that several other inhibitors are produced by decomposition of the phlorizin by microorganisms (see Chapter 10, Section I,C).

In spite of the restrictions I have placed on the inclusion of citations, there are several species of plants in which growth inhibitors have been shown to be released from their residues during decay. These include wheat and oats (Börner, 1960; Guenzi *et al.*, 1967); barley and rye (Börner, 1960); corn and sorghum (Guenzi *et al.*, 1967); apple (Börner, 1959); *Artemisia absinthium* (Funke, 1943); *Agropyron repens* (Welbank, 1960); *Sorghum halepense* (Johnson grass, Abdul-Wahab and Rice, 1967; Parks and Rice, 1969); *Helianthus annuus* (Rice, 1968; Wilson and Rice, 1968; Parks and Rice, 1969); *Euphorbia supina* (Brown, 1968; Rice, 1968); *Ambrosia psilostachya* (Rice, 1968; Parks and Rice, 1969; Neill and Rice, 1971); *Rhus glabra, Erigeron canadensis, Chenopodium album, Aristida oligantha,* and *Andropogon scoparius* (Parks and Rice, 1969); *Sporobolus pyramidatus* (Rasmussen and Rice, 1971); *Platanus occidentalis* (Al-Naib and Rice, 1971); *Celtis laevigata* (Lodhi and Rice, 1971); *Typha latifolia, T. angustifolia, Heleocharis palustris, Schoenoplectus lacustris,* and *Acorus calamus* (Szczepańska, 1971); *Glyceria aquatica* (Szczepańska, 1971; Szczepański, 1971); *Setaria faberii* (Bell and Koeppe, 1972); *Andropogon virginicus* (Rice, 1972); and *Brassica nigra* (Bell and Muller, 1973).

Even if questionable examples are eliminated, there is definite evidence that at least some inhibitors get out of plants by each of the four methods discussed. In most of the examples cited, much work still needs to be done to clarify the exact sources and identities of the effective inhibitors.

12

Chemical Nature of Inhibitors

I. INTRODUCTION

My goal in this chapter is to discuss the different types of organic compounds that have been identified as inhibitors produced by microorganisms or higher plants. I have no intention of naming every individual compound that has been implicated in an inhibitory role. It would be a tremendous task to discuss all antibiotics and marasmins (Chapter 1, Section II) that have been identified, so I will discuss only certain representative ones. I do plan to be a bit more comprehensive in discussing the phytoncides and kolines that have been identified from higher plants.

I do not plan to discuss the detailed biosynthesis of the various types of inhibitors either, although this is a fascinating area. Most chemical inhibitors are compounds that have been termed secondary substanes by Fraenkel (1959) and Whittaker and Feeny (1971) because they are of sporadic occurrence and thus do not appear to play a role in the basic metabolism of organisms. There are many thousands of such compounds, but only a limited number of them have been identified as toxins involved in allelopathy. Whittaker and Feeny (1971) stated that, with few exceptions, the secondary compounds could be classified into five major categories: phenylpropanes, acetogenins, terpenoids, steroids, and alkaloids. They pointed out further that the phenylpropanes and alkaloids originate from a small number of amino acids, and the rest originate generally from acetate. The flavonoids, of course, are hybrids in this scheme, as the authors pointed out, because one ring arises from phenylalanine and the other from an acetate origin (see Section II in this chapter).

The term acetogenins is attractive because it conveniently includes all the diverse secondary compounds that arise from acetate. Unfortunately, it does not help much in indicating chemical similarities. I have chosen, therefore, to devise a system that has 14 categories plus a catchall category (miscellaneous). Most antibiotics, marasmins, phytoncides, and kolines which have been identified fit in one of the 14 chemical categories, but a few do not. The categories are given in capital letters in Fig. 36, and the known or suspected metabolic pathways are indicated based on Neish (1964), Brown (1964), and Robinson (1963). It is evident from the diagram that the inhibitors arise either through the acetate or the shikimic acid pathway. Several types of inhibitors that originate from amino acids actually come through the acetate pathway. These include some of the amino acid and polypeptide inhibitors, some of the alkaloids, probably some of the sulfides, and the purines and nucleosides (Robinson, 1963; Neish, 1964, Whittaker and Feeny, 1971). The other types of inhibitors that originate from amino acids apparently arise from phenylalanine or tyrosine, and these compounds are formed from shikimic acid.

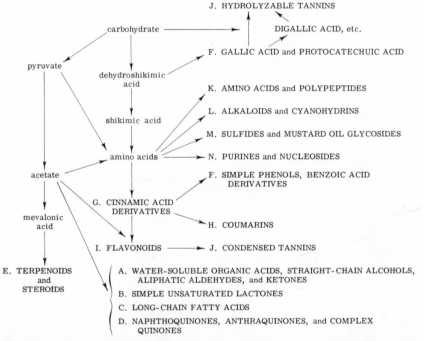

Fig. 36. Probable major biosynthetic pathways leading to production of the various categories of allelopathic agents. Letters refer to subheadings under which categories are discussed in next section of this chapter.

II. TYPES OF CHEMICAL COMPOUNDS IDENTIFIED AS INHIBITORS

A. Simple Water-Soluble Organic Acids, Straight-Chain Alcohols, Aliphatic Aldehydes, and Ketones

Evenari (1949) pointed out that the concentrations of several organic acids, such as malic, citric, acetic, and tartaric acids, in fruits are often high enough to inhibit seed germination. He also stated that unripe grains of corn and unripe seeds of peas will not germinate because of the presence of acetaldehyde.

Three organic acids, malonic, citric, and fumaric, are exuded from seeds of *Pinus resinosa* and inhibit germination of the zoospores and growth of *Pythium afertile* (Agnihotri and Vaartaja, 1968). Acetaldehyde, propionic aldehyde, acetone, methanol, and ethanol are emitted as volatile growth inhibitors by beet, tomato, sweet potato, and radish leaves and by carrot roots in closed systems (Dadykin *et al.*, 1970). Prutenskaya *et al.* (1970) determined that several organic acids are among the toxins produced from decomposing soybean residues. According to Gaidamak (1971), several organic acids of an aliphatic series are exuded as toxins by roots of cucumber and tomato plants.

Patrick (1971) reported that acetic and butyric acids are among the toxins produced during decomposition of rye residues.

B. Simple Unsaturated Lactones

There are, of course, many types of lactones of varying complexity, but I am including in this category only the simple ones that arise from acetate. The more complex ones, such as the coumarins and cardiac glycosides (steroids), will be discussed in later categories.

Parasorbic acid (Fig. 37) was identified from the fruits of *Sorbus aucuparia* and is very inhibitory to seed germination and seedling growth and also is antibacterial (Evenari, 1949). The aglycone of ranunculin (Fig. 37), protoanemonin, is also inhibitory to seed germination and to many bacteria. This compound is produced by several species of the Ranunculaceae (Evenari, 1949).

Several well-known antibiotics, such as patulin (Fig. 37) and penicillic acid, (Fig. 37) are simple lactones (Evenari, 1949; Neish, 1964). All are, of course, inhibitory to at least some microorganisms, and patulin

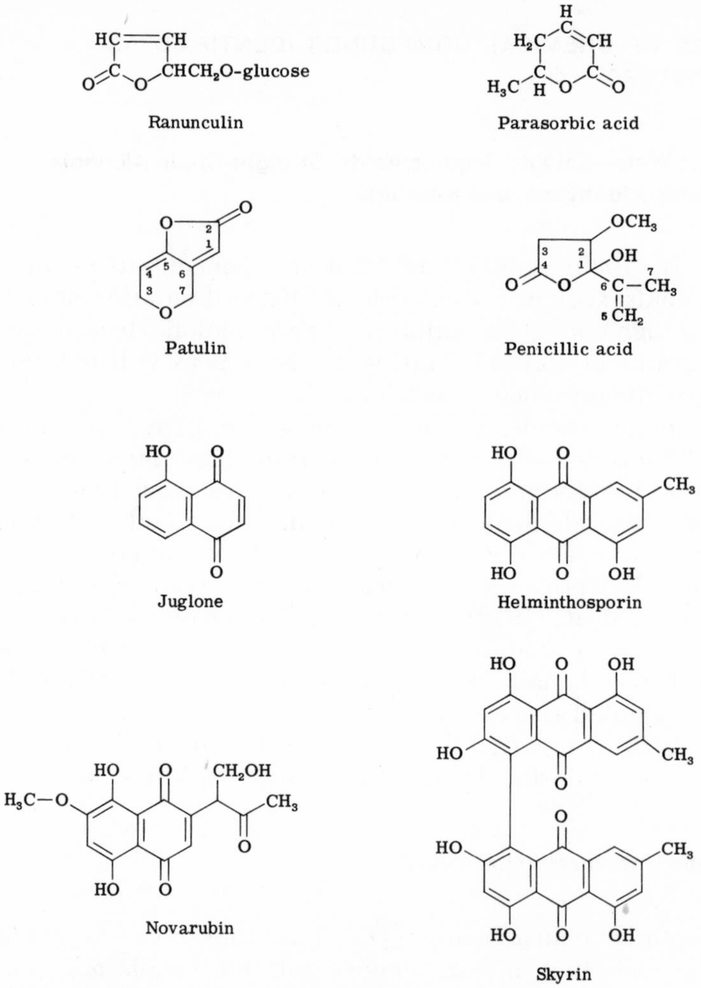

Ranunculin

Parasorbic acid

Patulin

Penicillic acid

Juglone

Helminthosporin

Novarubin

Skyrin

Fig. 37. Representative simple unsaturated lactones, naphthoquinones, and anthraquinones that have been implicated in allelopathy.

is very inhibitory to higher plants (Norstadt and McCalla, 1963). Patulin is produced by a number of fungi, according to Norstadt and McCalla (1963), and they found that *Penicillium urticae* produces large amounts when growing on wheat straw residue. Börner (1963a,b) reported that *Penicillium expansum* produces significant amounts of patulin during decomposition of apple root and leaf residues, and he feels this may be important in the apple replant problem as previously indicated (Chapter 10).

Penicillic acid is produced by *Pennicillium cyclopium* (Neish, 1964) and probably by other species.

C. Long-Chain Fatty Acids

According to Proctor (1957) there is considerable evidence that many long-chain fatty acids are inhibitory to bacteria and fungi. I have found very few examples, however, of the possible role of such compounds in allelopathy. Proctor (1957) concluded that the inhibitor produced by *Chlamydomonas reinhardi,* which is very toxic to another alga, *Haematococcus pluvialis,* (see Chapter 3) is probably a long-chain fatty acid or a mixture of such acids. He tested eight of these acids, nonanoic, decanoic, lauric, myristic, palmitic, stearic, oleic, and linoleic, and found all to be inhibitory to *Haematococcus* and other algae.

According to Proctor (1957), Spoehr concluded that the algal inhibitor chlorellin produced by *Chlorella* is a mixture of photooxidized unsaturated fatty acids. Unfortunately, none of the ecologically important antibiotics from the algae has been unequivocally identified to my knowledge, and this needs to be done.

D. Naphthoquinones, Anthraquinones, and Complex Quinones

This group of quinones is thought to be formed by-head-to-tail condensation of acetate units with decarboxylation, reduction, and oxidation reactions occurring in addition to cyclization (Robinson, 1963; Neish, 1964). The evidence for this method of formation of the anthraquinones is good (Neish, 1964), but the evidence for the formation of naphthoquinones by this method is not firm (Robinson, 1963).

Juglone, a potent toxin from walnut trees, was identified by Davis (1928) as 5-hydroxynaphthoquinone (Fig. 37). This is the only inhibitor produced by higher plants which is definitely known to be a naphthoquinone. Wilson and Rice (1968) found a naphthalene derivative of some kind in the leachate of leaves of *Helianthus annuus.* They suggested that it might be some sort of derivative of α-naphthol, but were not sure, so its identity needs to be determined. Novarubin (Fig. 37) is a marasmin produced by the pathogenic fungus, *Fusarium solani,* and it has been isolated from various cultures of the fungus and from diseased pea plants (Owens, 1969). It causes diseased plants to wilt.

Numerous anthraquinones are produced by higher plants and by fungi (Harborne and Simmonds, 1964). I know of none, however, in the higher plants which has been identified as an inhibitor of importance in allelopathy. Several antibiotics and marasmins have been identified as anthraquinones, however (Neish, 1964; Owens, 1969). The antiobiotic, helminthosporin (Fig. 37), produced by the fungus, *Helminthosporium graminium*, is one example (Neish, 1964). Skyrin (Fig. 37) is a dianthraquinone marasmin produced by the chestnut blight fungus, *Endothia parasitica*, and it changes water permeability of cells at the low concentration of $10^{-6}M$ (Owens, 1969).

The tetracycline antibiotics, such as aureomycin, are dimeric quinones and are even more complex than skyrin (Whittaker and Feeny, 1971). Aureomycin is produced by *Streptomyces aureofaciens* (Wright, 1956).

E. Terpenoids and Steroids

The terpenoids and steroids have basic skeletons derived from mevalonic acid or a closely related precursor (Robinson, 1963). They are built up of 5-carbon isoprene or isopentane units linked together in various ways and with different types of ring closures, functional groups, and degrees of saturation. According to Robinson (1963), the term terpenoids is preferred over terpenes because the former includes all compounds built of isoprene units regardless of the functional groups, whereas the latter refers only to hydrocarbons. The basic types of terpenoids are the monoterpenoids (C_{10}), sesquiterpenoids (C_{15}), diterpenoids (C_{20}), triterpenoids (C_{30}), and tetraterpenoids (C_{40}).

Higher plants produce a great variety of terpenoids (Robinson, 1963), but only a small number of them has been shown to be involved in allelopathy. Microorganisms do not appear to produce large numbers and varieties of terpenoids, but certain fungi do produce terpenoids and mixed terpenoids which are important as marasmins (Owens, 1969).

The monoterpenoids are the major components of the essential oils of plants (Robinson, 1963), and they are also the predominant terpenoid inhibitors that have been identified from higher plants. Sigmund (1924) reported that several monoterpenoids from essential oils are inhibitory to seed germination and to certain bacteria. Evenari (1949) suggested that the monoterpenoids and aromatic aldehydes may be chiefly responsible for the inhibitory activity of essential oils.

Camphene, camphor, cineole, dipentene, α-pinene, and β-pinene were identified by Muller and Muller (1964) as the volatile inhibitors produced by *Salvia leucophylla*, *S. apiana*, and *S. mellifera* (Fig. 38). Camphor and cineole were found to be most inhibitory to root growth of test seedlings, and these two terpenes were later identified in the air around *Salvia* plants in the field (C. H. Muller, 1965). Asplund (1968) investigated the relationship between the structure of ten monoterpenes and the inhibition of germination of radish seeds. The compounds tested were (+)camphor, (−)camphor, (+)pulegone (Fig. 38), (−)borneol, 1,8-cineole, limonene (Fig. 38), α-phellandrene (Fig. 38), *p*-cymene, α-pinene, and β-pinene. Those compounds with a functional ketone group, the two camphors and pulegone, were much more inhibitory than all the others. The least inhibitory was β-pinene followed by 1,8-cineole, and the rest were similar in activity.

Cineole, α-phellandrene, α-pinene, and β-pinene are volatile inhibitors produced by *Eucalyptus camaldulensis*, and cineole and α-pinene are apparently most important in the allelopathic activity of this species because these were found to be adsorbed on the soil in the field in significant amounts (del Moral and Muller, 1970).

Artemisia absinthium produces three sesquiterpene inhibitors, β-carophyllene (Fig. 38), bisabolene (Fig. 38), and chamazulene (Grümmer, 1961). *Ambrosia psilostachya* and *Ambrosia acanthicarpa* produce several sesquiterpenes, at least some of which may be inhibitory (Miller *et al.*, 1968; Geissman *et al.*, 1969). This has not been definitely demonstrated, but Neill and Rice (1971) did show that *Ambrosia psilostachya* produces volatile inhibitors, and it is possible that these inhibitors are the sesquiterpenes.

White and Starratt (1967) isolated a phytotoxic compound, which they named zinniol (Fig. 38), from cultures of *Alternaria zinniae*. It is not strictly a terpenoid, but it does have an isoprene side chain. This fungus causes leaf and stem blight of zinnia, sunflower, and marigold, and Owens (1969) suggested that zinniol is possibly the marasmin responsible for the stem withering, chlorosis, and leaf-tip curling characteristic of the disease. White and Starratt found that the compound also inhibits seed germination and has weak activity against fungi and bacteria.

The sesquiterpenoid, helminthosporal (Fig. 38), is a marasmin produced by the fungus, *Cochliobolus sativus*, which causes common root rot of cereals (Owens, 1969). Ophiobolin (Fig. 38) is a mixed terpenoidlike compound that is apparently a marasmin produced by *Cochliobolus miyabeanus* which causes a leaf spot of rice (Owens, 1969). Alternaric acid (Fig. 38) is a lactone with a long terpenoid side chain, and it is thought to be a secondary determinant of the early

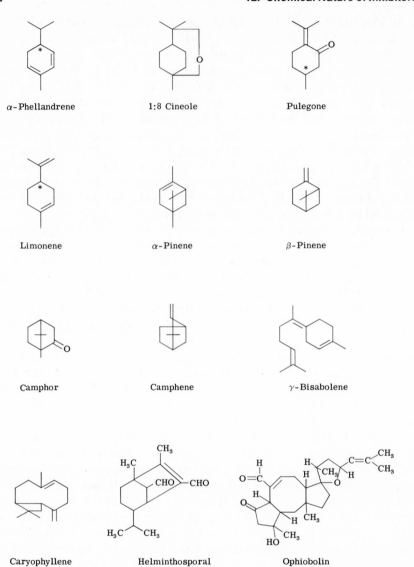

Fig. 38. Some terpenoids, steroids, and compounds with isoprenoid side chains which have been implicated in allelopathy. (Helminthosporal, ophiobolin, alternaric acid, zinniol, and ascochitine after Owens, 1969.)

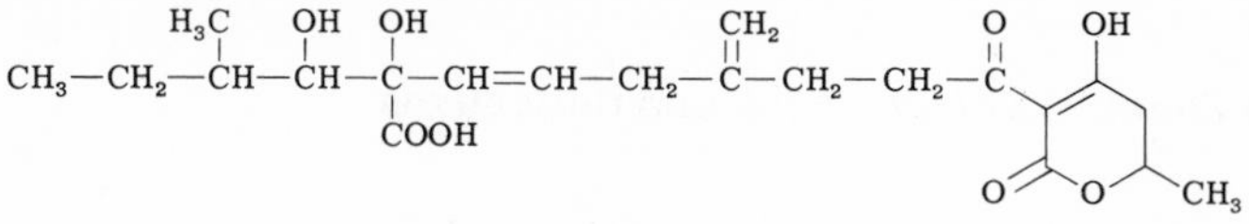

H₃C   OH OH   CH₂   O   OH

CH₃—CH₂—CH—CH—C—CH=CH—CH₂—C—CH₂—CH₂—C

COOH   O   O   CH₃

Alternaric acid

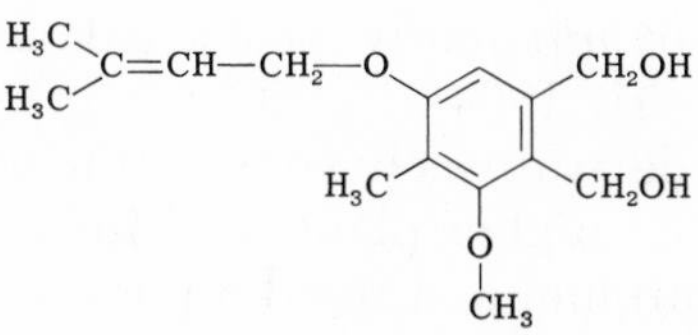

Zinniol

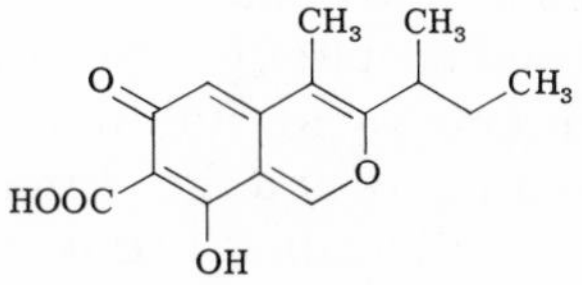

Ascochitine

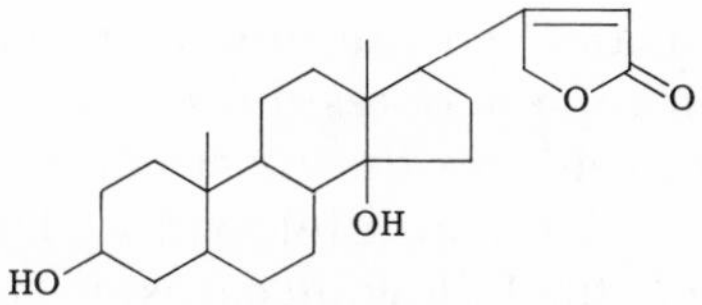

Digitoxigenin

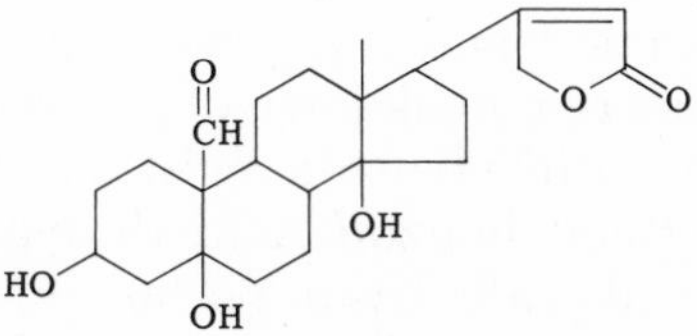

Strophanthidin

Fig. 38. *(continued)*

blight disease of various species of the Solanaceae caused by *Alternaria solani* (Owens, 1969). Ascochitine (Fig. 38) is a sesquiterpenoid-like compound, which was isolated from culture filtrates of *Ascochyta fabae,* the causal fungus of brown spot disease of broad bean (Owens, 1969). Application of small amounts of the toxin to coleoptiles of broad bean causes the brown necrotic spots characteristic of the disease.

The basic steroid nucleus is the same as that of tetracyclic triterpenoids, but only two methyl groups are attached to the ring system (Robinson, 1963). As far as I have been able to ascertain, very few steroids have ever been linked to allelopathy. Digitoxigenin and strophanthidin (Fig. 38) are two well-known examples that have strong antimicrobial activity (Evenari, 1949). Both are aglycones of cardiac glycosides. Digitoxigenin is the aglycone of the digilanides A, B, and C produced by foxglove, *Digitalis pupurea,* and strophanthidin is the aglycone of convallatoxin produced by *Convallaria majalis* (Robinson, 1963).

F. Simple Phenols, Benzoic Acid, and Derivatives

The compounds listed in this category have somewhat of a mixed origin. Some compounds, such as gallic (Fig. 42) and protocatechuic acids, originate directly from dehydroshikimic acid (Neish, 1964), and some compunds, such as phloroglucinol, apparently are formed directly from acetate (Robinson, 1963), but apparently most are derived from cinnamic acid (Robinson, 1963; Neish, 1964).

This category and the cinnamic acid derivatives have been the most commonly identified toxins produced by higher plants and involved in allelopathy. As long ago as 1908, Schreiner and Reed reported that vanillin, vanillic acid, and hydroquinone (Fig. 39) are among phenolic compounds commonly produced by plants that are inhibitory to seedling growth. Hydroquinone is the aglycone of arbutin. Gray and Bonner (1948b) identified 3-acetyl-6-methoxybenzaldehyde as the toxin produced in leaves of *Encelia farinosa*. Börner (1959) found that phloroglucinol and *p*-hydroxybenzoic acid are two inhibitors produced during the breakdown of phlorizin from apple root residues.

p-Hydroxybenzoic acid and vanillic acid are the most commonly identified benzoic acid derivatives involved in allelopathy. These were identified as important inhibitors in the following cases: in *Camelina alyssum* (Grümmer and Beyer, 1960); in soil (Whitehead, 1964); in residues of corn, wheat, sorghum, and oats (Guenzi and McCalla, 1966a); in cropped soil (Guenzi and McCalla, 1966b); in many soils in France (Hennequin and Juste, 1967); in soils in Taiwan (Wang *et al.*, 1967); and in sugar beet flower clusters (Battle and Whittington, 1969). Guenzi and McCalla (1966a,b) found syringic acid (Fig. 39) in the same residues and in soils also.

Arbutin was found to be the inhibitor in *Arctostaphylos uva-ursi* (Winter, 1961) and to be one inhibitor in the leachate of foliaceous branches of *Arctostaphylos glandulosa* along with hydroquinone, gallic, protocatechuic, vanillic, and *p*-hydroxybenzoic acids (Chou and Muller, 1972). The latter authors also found *p*-hydroxybenzoic and syringic acids in soil under the shrub. Gallic acid is one inhibitor produced by *Euphorbia corollata* (Rice, 1965a), *Euphorbia supina* (Rice, 1969), and *Eucalyptus camaldulensis* (del Moral and Muller, 1970). Gentisic acid (2,5-dihydroxybenzoic acid) is one of the toxins produced by *Celtis laevigata* (Lodhi and Rice, 1971) and *Eucalyptus globulus* (del Moral and Muller, 1969). Hattingh and Louw (1969b) isolated a strain of *Pseudomonas* from the rhizoplane of *Trifolium*

II. Chemical Compounds Identified as Inhibitors

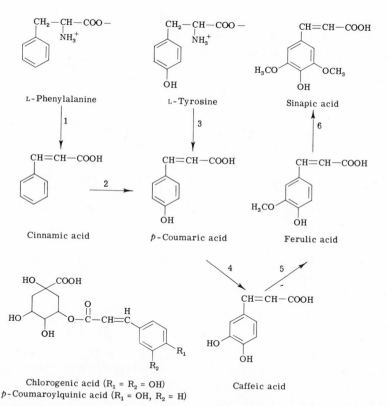

Fig. 39. Some benzoic and cinnamic acid derivatives and related compounds that have been identified as allelopathic agents. The proposed pathway of biosynthesis of cinnamic acid and its derivatives is shown. (After Neish, 1964.)

repens which inhibited development of clover seedlings. They suspected on the basis of previous work that the inhibitor involved was 2,4-diacetyl -phloroglucinol, but did not confirm it. Sulfosalicylic acid (2-hydroxy-5-sulfonicbenzoic acid) is one of the inhibitors produced by crabgrass (Parenti and Rice, 1969), and phenolcarbonic acid is a potent inhibitor apparently exuded from the roots of tomatoes (Gaidamak, 1971).

G. Cinnamic Acid and Derivatives

These compounds are clearly derived from phenylalanine or tyrosine (Fig. 39) through the shikimic acid pathway (Neish, 1964), and they are widespread in higher plants.

These substances have been implicated in many cases of allelopathy since Schreiner and Reed (1908) demonstrated that cinnamic acid (Fig. 39), *o*-coumaric acid and *o*-hydrocoumaric acid are among several organic compounds known to be produced by plants that are inhibitory to seedling growth. Bonner and Galston (1944) identified *trans*-cinnamic acid (the common isomer) as the toxin produced by roots of guayule. Other examples in which cinnamic acid derivatives have been implicated as the toxins involved in allelopathic actions are caffeic and ferulic acids in tomato juice (Evenari, 1949); chlorogenic and caffeic acids (Fig. 39), which are fungistatic agents produced by potatoes in response to inoculation with *Helminthosporium carbonum* (Kúc *et al.*, 1956); and *p*-hydroxyhydrocinnamic acid, which is an inhibitor produced in the breakdown of phlorizin from apple residues (Börner, 1959). Several cinnamic acid derivatives were identified as germination inhibitors in many species and families (Van Sumere and Massart, 1959). Several cinnamic acid derivatives, including chlorogenic acid, were identified as growth and germination inhibitors in many dry fruits (Varga and Köves, 1959). Ferulic acid is one inhibitor produced by *Camelina alyssum* (Grümmer and Beyer, 1960). *p*-Coumarylquinic (Fig. 39) and chlorogenic acids were identified in apple leaves (Williams, 1960) and may be involved in the apple replant problem. Whitehead (1964) identified *p*-coumaric and ferulic acids in several soils. Chlorogenic acid is one inhibitor in *Galium mollugo* (Kohlmuenzer, 1965a). Chlorogenic and isochlorogenic acids are the chief inhibitors in *Helianthus annuus* (Rice, 1965a). Chlorogenic acid, isochlorogenic acid, and a glucose ester of caffeic acid are toxins produced by *Ambrosia psilostachya* and *A. elatior* (=*A. artemisiifolia*, Rice 1965c). Ferulic and *p*-coumaric acids are among the inhibitors present in residues of corn, wheat, sorghum, and oats and in soil under these crops (Guenzi and McCalla, 1966a,b). Chlorogenic and p-coumaric acids are inhibitors in *Sorghum hale-pense* (Abdul-Wahab and Rice, 1967). p-Coumaric and ferulic acids were found in many cultivated soils (Hennequin and Juste, 1967). A glucose ester of ferulic acid is one of six phenolic inhibitors produced by *Bromus japonicus* (Rice and Parenti, 1967). p-Coumaric and ferulic acid were found in soils in Taiwan (Wang *et al.*, 1967). p-Coumarylqui-nic and chlorogenic acids are inhibitors in fog drip from *Eucalyptus globulus* (del Moral and Muller, 1969). Ferulic and p-coumaric acids are two of the inhibitors present in flower clusters of sugar beet (Battle and Whittington, 1969). Chlorogenic and isochlorogenic acids are in-hibitors in *Digitaria sanguinalis* (Parenti and Rice, 1969). Caffeic, chlorogenic, p-coumaric, and ferulic acids are among the toxins in the leaf leachate of *Eucalyptus camaldulensis* (del Moral and Muller, 1970). Chlorogenic acid, isochlorogenic acid, neochlorogenic acid, band-510, and o-coumaric acid are toxins produced by *Platanus occi-dentalis* (Al-Naib and Rice, 1971). Ferulic, caffeic, and p-coumaric acids are toxins in *Celtis laevigata* leaves (Lodhi and Rice, 1971). Hydrocinnamic and ferulic acids are toxins produced during decompo-sition of rye residues (Patrick, 1971). p-Coumaric and ferulic acids are inhibitors in *Sporobolus pyramidatus* (Rasmussen and Rice, 1971). Chlorogenic acid was found in the leachate of leaves of *Arcto-staphylos glandulosa* and p-coumaric, ferulic, and o-coumaric acids were found in soil under the plant (Chou and Muller, 1972). Isochloro-genic acid is actually a mixture of 4,5-, 3,4-, and 3,5-dicaffeoylquinic acids (Corse *et al.*, 1965). It apparently sometimes contains a small amount of a monoferuloyl monocaffeoylquinic acid also.

H. Coumarins

The coumarins are lactones of o-hydroxycinnamic acid (Robinson, 1963). Various kinds of side chains may be present, with isoprenoids being especially common. They occur in all parts of plants and are widely distributed in the plant kingdom.

Schreiner and Reed (1908) reported that coumarin (Fig. 40) and esculin (6-glucoside of esculetin, Fig. 40) are very inhibitory to the growth of wheat seedlings. Evenari (1949) also listed coumarin as a very potent inhibitor of seed germination. Esculin is a toxin produced by *Aesculus hippocastanum,* and coumarin is one produced by *Meli-lotus alba* (Winter, 1961). A glycoside of esculetin, probably esculin,

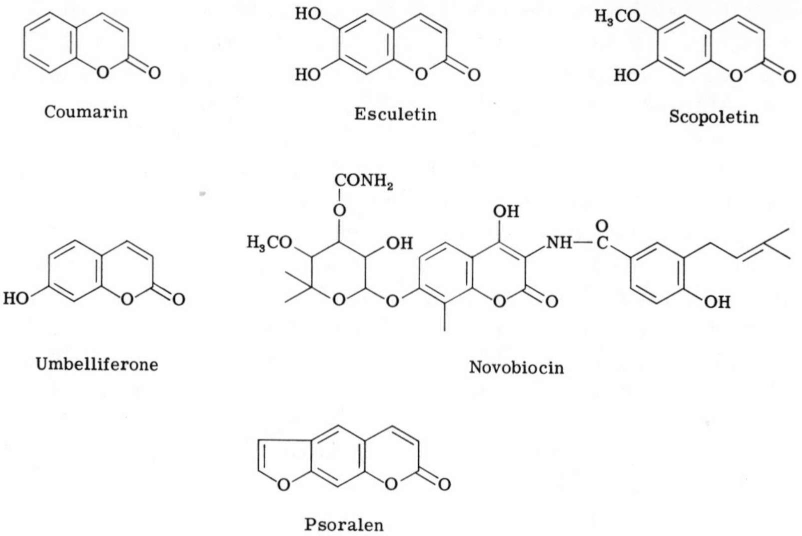

Coumarin   Esculetin   Scopoletin

Umbelliferone   Novobiocin

Psoralen

Fig. 40.   Some coumarins that have been implicated in allelopathy.

is produced prominently in *Phleum pratense* roots (Avers and Goodwin, 1956). Scopoletin (Fig. 40) and/or its 7-glucoside, scopolin, have been reported as inhibitors in oat roots (Goodwin and Kavanagh, 1949; Martin, 1957), in *Galium mollugo* (Kohlmuenzer, 1965a), in *Platanus occidentalis* (Al-Naib and Rice, 1971), and in *Celtis laevigata* (Lodhi and Rice, 1971). Van Sumere and Massart (1959) listed several coumarins as inhibitors of seed germination in many species and families of plants.

The antibiotic, novobiocin (Fig. 40), is a coumarin with some rather complex side chains (Neish, 1964). It is produced by *Streptomyces niveus* according to Neish.

There are a few examples of furanocoumarins that have been identified as plant inhibitors. These are compounds with a furan ring fused with the benzene ring of coumarin (Robinson, 1963). Psoralen (Fig. 40) is produced by some species of *Psoralea* (Robinson, 1963; Baskin *et al.*, 1967), and byakangelicin, isopimpinellin, and another unidentified furanocoumarin are produced by *Thamnosma montana* (Bennett and Bonner, 1953).

I. Flavonoids

The flavonoids have a basic C_6–C_3–C_6 skeleton (Fig. 41) in which the A ring is of acetate origin and the B ring of shikimic acid origin (Neish,

1964). The largest group of flavonoids is characterized by having a pyran ring linking the 3-carbon chain with one of the benzene rings (Robinson, 1963). There is a huge variety of flavonoids, and they are very widespread in seed plants (Harborne and Simmonds, 1964). In spite of the large numbers and wide distribution, only a relatively small number have been reported as toxins implicated in allelopathy. I feel this may be due in part to the difficulties involved in identifying many of the flavonoids and their numerous glycosides. Work in progress in my laboratory indicates that many of them, both aglycones and glycosides, are extremely potent toxins to seed germination and to at least some bacteria.

Börner (1959) found that phlorizin in apple root residues is very inhibitory to growth of apple seedlings. This compound is the 6-glucoside of phloretin (Fig. 41), and Börner found that phloretin, phloroglucinol, p-hydroxyhydrocinnamic acid, and p-hydroxybenzoic acid are all produced from phlorizin during the decomposition of apple root residues; all are inhibitory to apple seedlings. Börner (1959) also

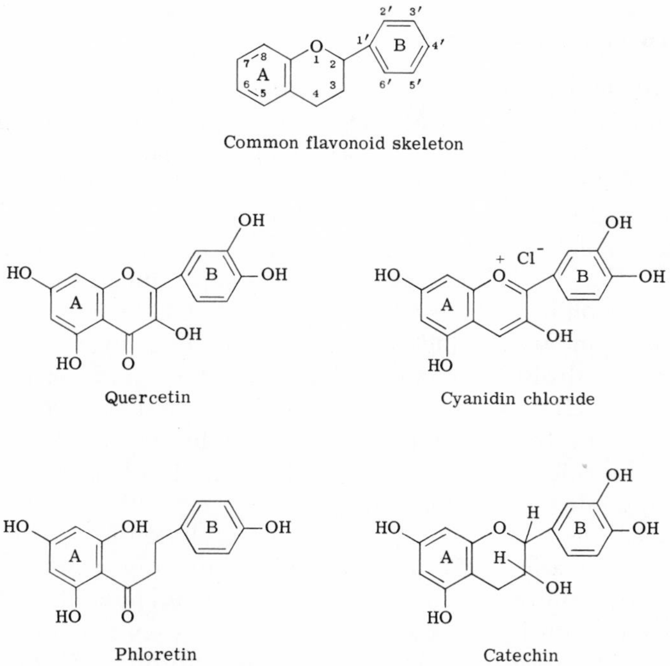

Common flavonoid skeleton

Quercetin

Cyanidin chloride

Phloretin

Catechin

Fig. 41. Some flavonoids (after Neish, 1964) that are important in allelopathy, either directly or indirectly. Catechin is thought to be involved along with flavan-3,4-diols in the synthesis of condensed tannins, and cyanidin chloride is formed in the hydrolysis of condensed tannins by concentrated HCl (Brown, 1964).

found quercitrin, a glycoside of quercetin (Fig. 41), in apple bark, but he did not test it for possible inhibitory activity. Williams (1960) reported that numerous glycosides of quercetin and kaempferol, and epicatechin and catechin are all present in apple residues, and possibly these compounds may play roles in the apple replant problem in addition to those played by phlorizin and its breakdown products.

Kohlmuenzer (1965a) identified the flavonoid, diosmetin trioside, as one of the inhibitors produced by *Galium mollugo*; and Grümmer (1961) listed quercitrin as an inhibitor in leaves of *Artemisia absinthium*. Fottrell *et al.* (1964) found that the flavonol, myricetin, which is present in some legume seeds, is inhibitory to *Rhizobium*. E. L. Rice and S. K. Pancholy (unpublished) have found several flavonoids and their glycosides in several herbaceous species from the tall-grass prairie and the post oak–blackjack oak forest and have found them to be very inhibitory to nitrifying bacteria and to seed germination.

J. Tannins

1. HYDROLYZABLE TANNINS

The only logical reason for including the hydrolyzable and condensed tannins in one category is that both types possess an astringent taste and can tan leather. The former contains ester linkages that can be hydrolyzed by boiling with dilute mineral acid, which is not true of the condensed tannins. The most common hydrolyzable tannins are sugar esters of gallic acid or of gallic and hexaoxydiphenic acid (Robinson, 1963) (Fig. 42). Ellagic acid (Fig. 42) is produced from hexaoxydiphenic acid on hydrolysis (Robinson, 1963). Chebulic acid (Fig. 42) is another secondary product formed from the hydrolysis of some tannins. Some hydrolyzable tannins are complex mixtures of several phenolic acids (Robinson, 1963). Digallic (Fig. 42) and trigallic acids sometimes result from the mild hydrolysis of hydrolyzable tannins, as well as gallic acid. There are obviously many kinds of hydrolyzable tannin molecules possible, and they are very difficult to identify specifically. They are widespread in dicotyledonous plants (Bate-Smith and Metcalfe, 1957; Swain, 1965), but only a relatively few workers have reported them as inhibitors involved in allelopathy.

They have been identified to be among the toxins involved in the following cases: as growth and germination inhibitors in several dry fruits (Varga and Köves, 1959); as inhibitors of nitrogen-fixing and

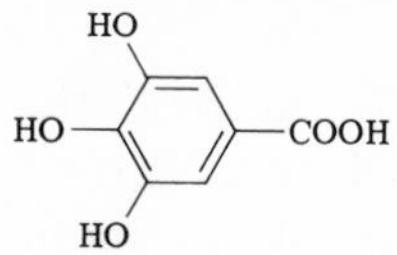

Gallic acid

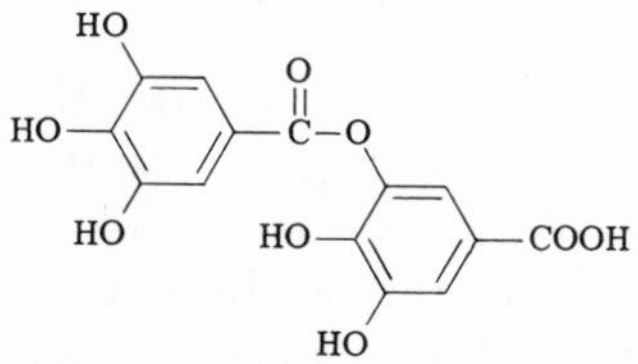

m-Digallic acid

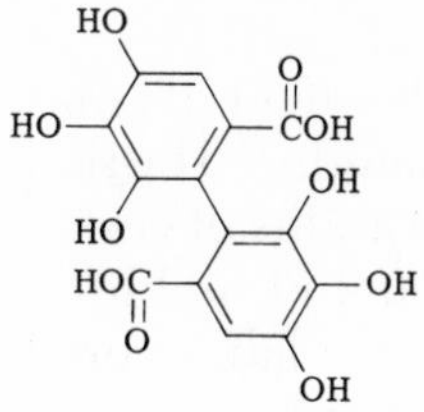

Hexaoxydiphenic acid

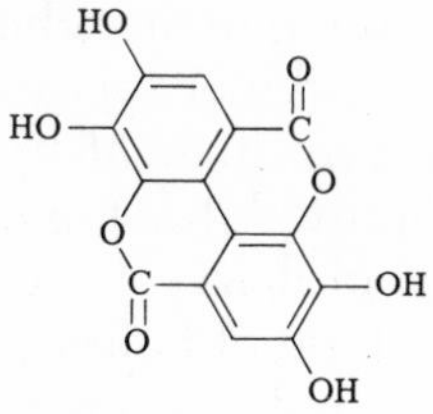

Ellagic acid

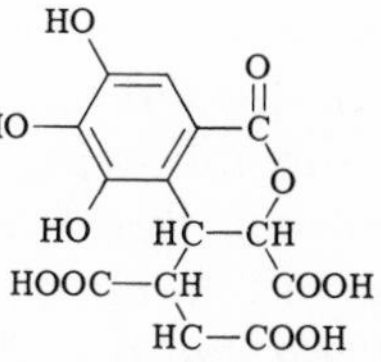

Chebulic acid

Fig. 42. Some acid components of hydrolyzable tannins. (After Robinson, 1963.)

nitrifying bacteria in *Euphorbia corollata, E. supina,* and *E. marginata* (Rice, 1965a,b, 1969); as inhibitors of *Rhizobium* in *Rhus copallina* (Blum and Rice, 1969); as inhibitors of seedling growth in *Carpinus betulus* (Mitin, 1970); as inhibitors of seed germination and seedling growth in *Arctostaphylos glandulosa* (Chou and Muller, 1972); and as inhibitors of nitrification in *Quercus marilandica, Q. stellata,* and *Q. velutina* (Rice and Pancholy, 1973). Plant residues that contain hydrolyzable tannins often contain either gallic or ellagic acid or both, and sometimes digallic acid. All of these are potent inhibitors of nitrification in soil and occur naturally in some forest soils in concentrations above those required to inhibit nitrification in those soils (Rice and Pancholy, 1973).

2. CONDENSED TANNINS

Condensed tannins apparently arise by the oxidative polymerization of catechins (Fig. 41) and flavan-3,4-diols (Brown, 1964). The latter have OH groups at the 3 and 4 positions in the pyran ring. Condensed tannins can be only partially broken down by rather drastic heating with concentrated acid to release cyanidin chloride (Fig. 41), which has a bright red color, and some red-brown polymers that are often termed phlobaphenes (Robinson, 1963). Obviously, there can be huge numbers of kinds of condensed tannins just on the basis of the length of the polymer chain alone.

There are even fewer reports of the involvement of condensed tannins in allelopathy than of hydrolyzable tannins. Harris and Burns (1970, 1972) reported that the tannins in the grains of certain sorghum hybrids inhibit preharvest seed germination and molding. They did not specify the type of tannins, but work in my laboratory has shown that the grasses analyzed for tannins contain only condensed tannins (Rice and Pancholy, 1973). I have found nothing else in the literature on the chemistry of grass tannins.

Mitin (1970) identified the seedling growth inhibitors in dead leaves of the beech, *Fagus silvatica,* as condensed tannins. We have found in my laboratory that condensed tannins are important inhibitors of nitrifying bacteria in the following species of the tall-grass prairie, the post oak–blackjack oak forest, and the oak–pine forest: *Andropogon gerardi, A. scoparius, A. virginicus, Aristida oligantha, Panicum virgatum, Sorghastrum nutans, Pinus echinata, Quercus marilandica, Q. stellata,* and *Q. velutina* (Rice and Pancholy, 1973).

As we mentioned in a previous chapter, Starkey and his colleagues demonstrated that condensed tannins markedly inhibit the rate of decomposition of organic matter in soil (Benoit and Starkey, 1968a,b; Benoit *et al.,* 1968).

Somers and Harrison (1967) isolated condensed and hydrolyzable tannins from wood shavings and found that all tannin fractions inhibited germination and hyphal growth of spores of *Verticillium albo-atrum,* which causes the *Verticillium* wilt disease. The main condensed tannin of highest molecular weight was most inhibitory.

Basaraba (1964) reported that both hydrolyzable and condensed tannins inhibited nitrification when added to soil.

K. Amino Acids and Polypeptides

Amino acids and peptides are among the best-known constituents of living matter and are well described in most general biochemistry textbooks. Suffice it to say here that amino acids are carboxylic acids having at least one amino group (Robinson, 1963). Peptides are polymers of two or more amino acid molecules connected by peptide (C–N) linkages. The amino acids can be divided arbitrarily into two major groups: one group is found in all living systems either in the free state or condensed as peptides, whereas representatives of the second group occur in a limited number of organisms and do not occur in proteins.

There are only a few instances in which amino acids have been identified as inhibitors in allelopathy, and in most cases the specific amino acids have not been identified. Thus, it is impossible to say at this time whether both groups of amino acids described above may be involved as inhibitors. In the case of rhizobitoxine, which is produced by certain strains of *Rhizobium japonicum* and causes chlorosis in new leaf growth of the soybean host plant, it is an amino acid of the noncommon category (Owens, 1969; Owens *et al.*, 1972). Owens *et al.* (1972) identified it as 2-amino-4(2-amino-3-hydroxypropoxy)-*trans*-but-3-enoic acid. This compound irreversibly inactivates β-cystathionase and inhibits the conversion of methionine into ethylene.

Gressel and Holm (1964) found that several free amino acids were the compounds present in seeds of *Abutilon theophrasti*, which were inhibitory to germination of seeds of several crop plants. They did not identify the amino acids, however. Prutenskaya *et al.* (1970) reported that amino acids are among the inhibitory compounds produced during the decomposition of soybean plant residue, but they did not identify the specific amino acids. Gaidamak (1971) found that unspecified amino acids are among the phytotoxins exuded by roots of cucumbers and tomatoes. It would be interesting to know if the inhibitory amino acids involved in these last three cases are unusual amino acids acting as antimetabolites in amino acid or protein synthesis.

Several of the known marasmins produced by pathogenic microorganisms are polypeptides and related glycopeptides (Owens, 1969). One of these whose structure has been identified is lycomarasmin (Fig. 46) (Owens, 1969). This toxin is produced by *Fusarium oxysporum f. lycopersicum,* and it causes wilting of tomato cuttings.

Other marasmins that have been identified as polypeptides according to Owens (1969) are victorin produced by *Helminthosporium victoriae,* which causes blight in Victoria oats and its derivative cultivars, *Helminthosporium carbonum* toxin; carbtoxinine produced by *H. carbonum* also; and toxin A and toxin B produced by *Periconia circinata,* which causes milo disease in certain grain sorghums. *Helminthosporium carbonum* is pathogenic to certain corn hybrids.

Some marasmins that have been identified as glycopeptides according to Owens (1969) are *Corynebacterium sepidonicum* toxin; *C. michiganense* toxins, I, II, III; and colletotin produced by *Colletotrichum fuscum*, which infects *Digitalis*. *Corynebacterium sepidonicum* infects potato plants, and *C. michiganense* infects tomato plants.

L. Alkaloids and Cyanohydrins

The logic for including these types of compounds together is that they are derived from amino acids and contain nitrogen (Neish, 1964).

1. ALKALOIDS

The nitrogen of the alkaloids may be in heterocyclic rings or in side chains, but, in any event, the simple aliphatic amines are not included in this category. The alkaloids as a group are distinguished generally from most other plant components by being basic, and they usually occur in plants as the salts of various organic acids (Robinson, 1963). Caffeine (Fig. 46) is often included as an alkaloid, but I am including it with the purines because of its obvious purine ring structure (Robinson, 1963). The alkaloids are best known for their physiological effects on man and their use in pharmacy.

There has been virtually no recent work on the role of alkaloids in allelopathy. Evenari (1949) emphasized strongly, however, the importance of these compounds as seed germination inhibitors. He stated, in fact, that all seeds and fruits known for their high alkaloid content are strong inhibitors of seed germination and that the alkaloids are the main, if not the only, cause of inhibition. He listed the following as strong inhibitors of seed germination: cocaine, physostigmine, caffeine, quinine, strychnine, berberine, codeine (see Fig. 43 for structures of these compounds), cinchonin, cinchonidin, and tropa acid. He listed narkotine, scopolamine, emetine (Fig. 43), papaverine (Fig. 43), ephedrine (Fig. 43), piperine, and atropine (Fig. 43) as weak inhibitors of seed germination.

Fusaric acid (Fig. 43) is a marasmin produced by many species of *Fusarium* and has been detected in infected tomato plants and wilted cotton (Owens, 1969). α-Picolinic acid (Fig. 43) acts as a marasmin in some cases also (Owens, 1969), and salts or esters of fusaric acid and α-picolinic acid are alkaloids.

2. CYANOHYDRINS

Tyrosine appears to be the precursor of the aglycone of dhurrin (Fig. 44), and phenylalanine appears to be the precursor of the aglycone of amygdalin and prunasin (Fig. 44) (Neish, 1964).

Dhurrin was reported by Conn and Akazawa (1958) to be present in sorghum (*Sorghum vulgare*) seedlings, and they found that the seedlings also contain enzymes that hydrolyze dhurrin to an equimolar mixture of glucose, HCN, and p-hydroxybenzaldehyde (Fig. 44). Later, Abdul-Wahab and Rice (1967) found that HCN and p-hydroxybenzaldehyde are among the phytotoxins produced by Johnson grass (*Sorghum halepense*), and they demonstrated that dhurrin is the source of these inhibitors in Johnson grass.

Proebsting and Gilmore (1941) and Patrick (1955) pointed out that HCN and benzaldehyde (Fig. 44) are produced by the breakdown of amygdalin that is present in peach root residues. They found that HCN and benzaldehyde are inhibitory to the growth of peach seedlings, but amygdalin is not.

Evenari (1949) reported that seeds of many species of the Prunaceae and Pomaceae contain large amounts of cyanogenic glucosides and that the HCN, which is released slowly from these glucosides, inhibits germination. He further pointed out that large quantities of HCN are released from *Crataegus* seeds just before germination and suggested that this may be the culmination of the period of after-ripening. The HCN could thus be liberated from the tissues, and germination processes could proceed.

M. Sulfides and Mustard Oil Glycosides

The sulfur or sulfur- and nitrogen-containing compounds included in this category have considerable diversity, but are thought to be derived from amino acids (Robinson, 1963). The sulfides are volatile and have an offensive odor. Robinson (1963) stated that there is no conclusive evidence for the occurrence of di- and polysulfides in plants and that they probably arise through secondary transformations brought about by plant enzymes. Allicin (Fig. 45) is an example of a disulfide known to be produced enzymatically from alliin (Fig. 45) when garlic, *Allium sativum*, is crushed (Robinson, 1963).

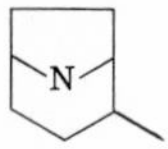

Cocaine 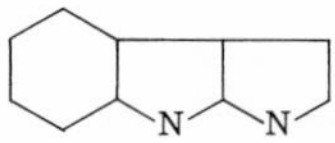   Physostigmine 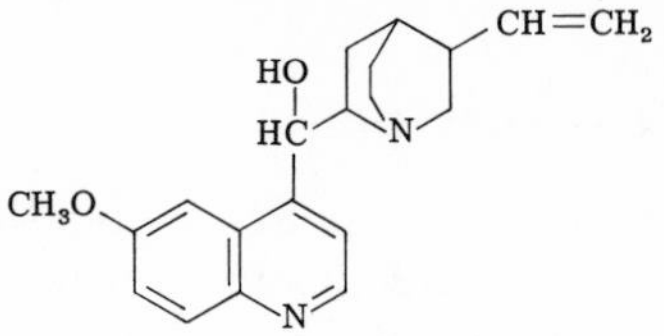   Quinine

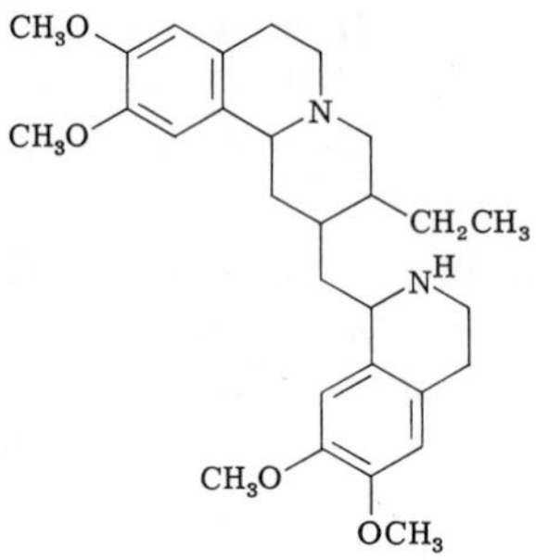

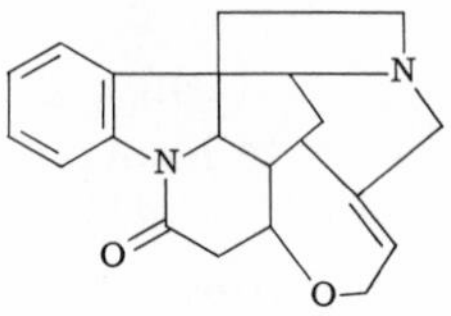

Strychnine

Emetine

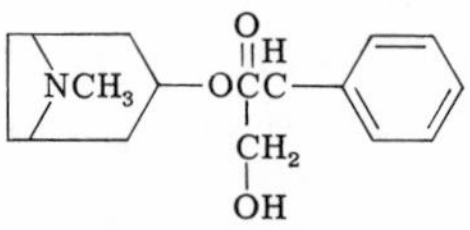

Atropine 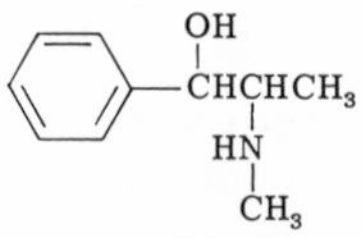   Ephedrine

Fig. 43. Alkaloids and related compounds that have been identified as allelopathic agents. Salts and esters of fusaric and picolinic acids are alkaloids.

As early as 1936, McKnight and Lindegren reported that vapors from crushed garlic are bactericidal to *Mycobacterium cepae*. Cavallito *et al.* (1944) identified allicin as the antibacterial substance.

Mustard oils, such as allyl isothiocyanate and allyl thiocyanate (Fig. 45), are hydrolysis products of mustard oil glycosides such as sinigrin (Fig. 45) (Robinson, 1963). The aglycones undergo rearrangement on hydrolysis and therefore often bear little resemblance to the aglycones that exist in the glycosides.

According to Evenari (1949), mustard oils are produced by all organs of plants belonging to the Cruciferae and are produced in espe-

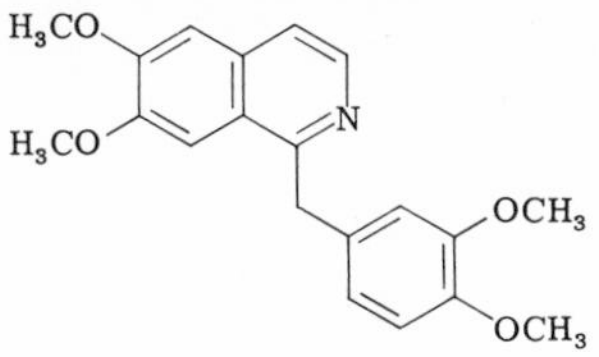

Papaverine

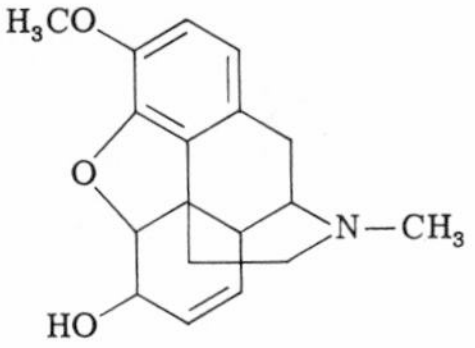

Codeine

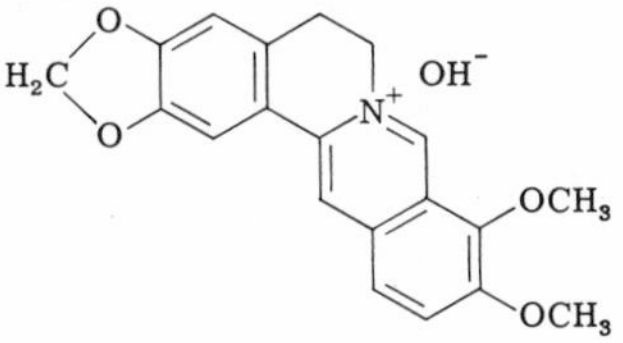

Berberine

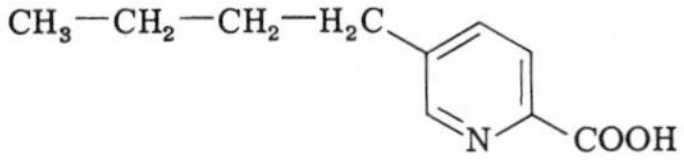

Fusaric acid

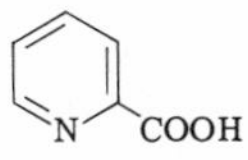

α-Picolinic acid

Fig. 43. *(continued)*

cially large amounts in the genera *Brassica* and *Sinapis*. He pointed out that mustard oils are potent inhibitors of seed germination and of microorganisms.

As I pointed out in Chapter 7, Bell and Muller (1973) found that large quantities of allyl isothiocyanate are liberated when leaves of *Brassica nigra* are macerated. They also found that this mustard oil is very inhibitory to seed germination in laboratory tests, but could not demonstrate any appreciable activity under field conditions.

N. Purines and Nucleosides

The purines are best known, of course, as constituents of nucleic acids, and the specific ones involved in both ribonucleic acid (RNA) and deoxyribonucleic acid (DNA) are adenine and guanine. When a sugar molecule is attached by a β-glycosidic bond to nitrogen in position 9 of a purine, the resulting compound is called a nucleoside

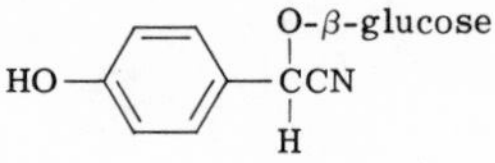

Dhurrin

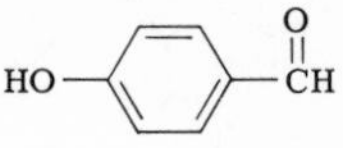

p-Hydroxybenzaldehyde

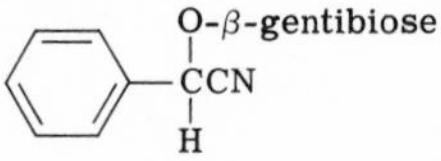

Amygdalin

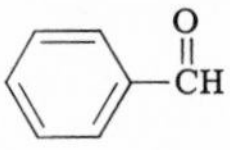

Benzaldehyde

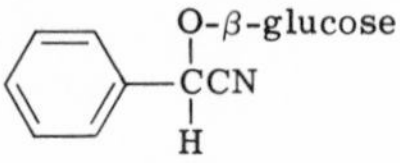

Prunasin

Fig. 44. Representative cyanogenic glycosides and their hydrolysis products. (After Robinson, 1963.)

(Robinson, 1963). The sugar involved in DNA is deoxyribose, and the one involved in RNA is ribose.

There are several known naturally occurring purines and nucleosides in plants in addition to those involved in nucleic acids (Robin-

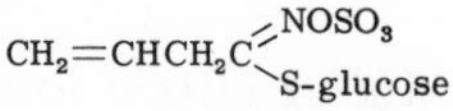

Sinigrin

$CH_2{=}CHCH_2NCS$

Allyl isothiocyanate

$CH_2{=}CHCH_2SCN$

Allyl thiocyanate

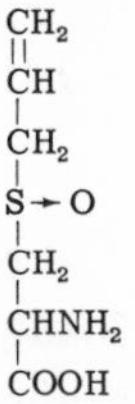

Alliin

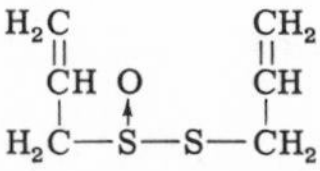

Allicin

Fig. 45. Sulfides, a mustard oil glycoside, and mustard oils implicated in allelopathy. (After Robinson, 1963.)

son, 1963). The only one I know of in higher plants that has been shown to be involved in allelopathy is caffeine (Fig. 46), which is a purine. Evenari (1949) included this as an alkaloid and pointed out that it is one of the most potent alkaloids in the inhibition of seed germination.

Several antibiotics produced by various microorganisms have been shown to be nucleosides. Among these are nebularine, cordycepin, and nucleocidin (Fig. 46). Cordycepin is produced by *Cordyceps militaris*, and the sugar involved is cordycepose, which is attached to an adenine base (Bentley *et al.*, 1951). Nucleocidin is a glycoside of adenine in which sulfamic acid is bound to the sugar moiety by an ester linkage (Waller *et al.*, 1957), and nebularine has a rather unusual 6-carbon sugar attached to the 9 position of purine (Löfgren *et al.*, 1954).

O. Miscellaneous

There are several toxins, which have been implicated in allelopathy, that do not fit clearly into any of the specific categories I have discussed, although they usually have relationships to one or more categories. Phenylacetic and 4-phenylbutyric acids are among the phytotoxins produced during the decomposition of rye residues (Patrick, 1971), and these compounds are apparently produced directly from either shikimic acid or cinnamic acid (Robinson, 1963). Phenethyl alcohol is one of the autoantibiotics produced by the fungus *Candida albicans*, and it probably fits into the same category as the compounds just mentioned (Lingappa *et al.*, 1969). Tryptophol is another autoantibiotic produced by *C. albicans* (Lingappa *et al.*, 1969), and this compound possibly is produced from the amino acid, tryptophan, as has been suggested in higher plants (Leopold, 1955).

Ethylene ($CH_2=CH_2$) is the volatile inhibitor produced by various fruits, such as apples and pears (Molisch, 1937), and it is derived from the amino acid, methionine (Owens *et al.*, 1971). Abscisic acid is one of the inhibitors of seed germination present in leaves of *Fagus silvatica* (Mitin, 1971) and in flower clusters of sugar beet (Battle and Whittington, 1969). This is a rather unusual compound, and apparently nothing definite is known as to its derivation.

Agropyrene is a compound produced by *Agropyron repens*, which is known to be antimicrobial, but nothing is known concerning its effect on higher plants (Grümmer, 1961). It has the following side chain ($-CH_2-C\equiv C-C\equiv C-CH_3$) attached to a benzene ring, and apparently nothing is known of its derivation.

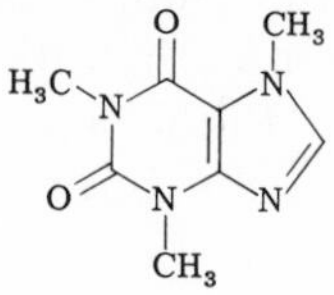

Caffeine

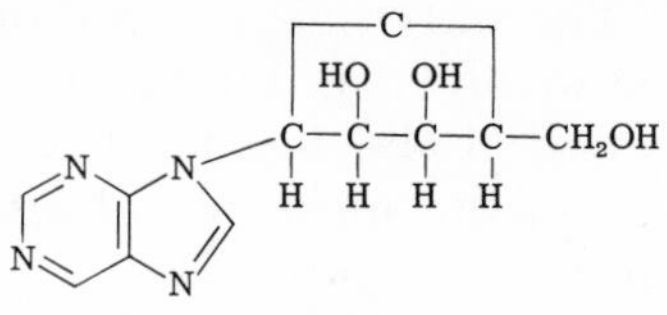

Nebularine

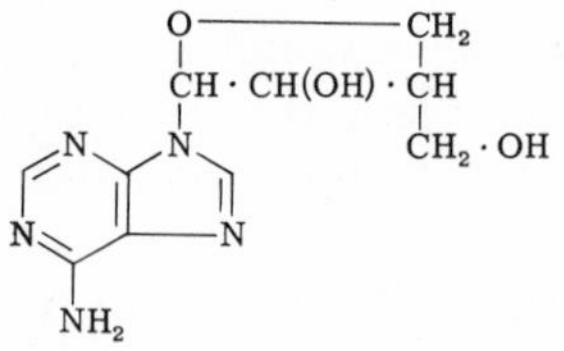

Cordycepin

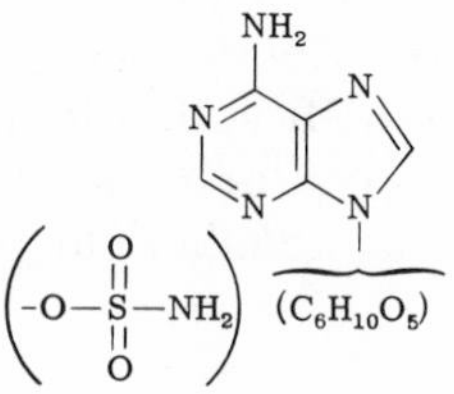

Nucleocidin

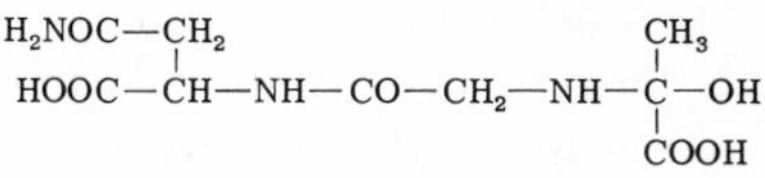

Lycomarasmin

Fig. 46. A representative polypeptide (lycomarasmin—Owens, 1969), purine (caffeine), and some nucleosides (cordycepin—Bentley *et al.*, 1951; nucleocidin—Walter *et al.*, 1957; nebularine—Löfgren *et al.*, 1954) known to be involved in allelopathy.

III. UNIDENTIFIED INHIBITORS

There are a great many cases in which significant allelopathic mechanisms are known to be operative and in which nothing is known of the toxins involved. There are no doubt important unidentified inhibitors in numerous cases in which some inhibitors have been identified. Much work remains to be done in this area because the inhibitors need to be known before significant advances can be made in determining mechanisms of action, amounts present in the environment, and methods and rates of decomposition.

13

Mechanisms of Action of Inhibitors

I. INTRODUCTION

Unfortunately, the surface has only been scratched in determining the mechanisms by which the different kinds of toxins exert their inhibitory actions. One reason is that it is very difficult to separate secondary effects from primary causes. Moreover, if one works with enzyme systems, he cannot be certain that observed effects of inhibitors on them will occur in the same way in intact plants. If one is measuring effects of certain inhibitors on whole-plant photosynthesis, he cannot be sure that observed effects are due to direct action on the process of photosynthesis. Changes in stomatal opening, membrane permeability, water content, or rates of many other processes could affect the overall rate of photosynthesis. In spite of the pitfalls, it is extremely important that work be done in this area. All information may be important in helping put the various pieces of the many puzzles together.

More information is available on the mechanisms of action of some of the antibiotics important in medicine than on inhibitors important at other levels. As has been my practice throughout this book, however, I will not discuss such antibiotics to any appreciable extent.

II. MECHANISMS OF ACTION

A. Inhibition of Cell Division and Elongation

The chief criteria used in determining the presence or relative effectiveness of allelopathic agents are increases in size and weight of test organisms. Appreciable increases in either of these require cell division and enlargement. A discussion of the effects of known toxins on these processes seems to be a logical starting point in a consideration of mechanisms of action.

A saturated aqueous solution of coumarin blocks all mitoses in onion and lily roots within 2–3 hours (Cornman, 1946). The initial effect is similar to that resulting from colchicine treatment: destruction of the spindle with the resultant interruption of anaphases and accumulation of metaphases. These interrupted mitoses form tetraploid nuclei or binucleate cells (Cornman, 1946). Coumarin also prevents the entry of cells into mitosis. Parasorbic acid in a saturated aqueous solution causes an accumulation of metaphases in onion roots, but apparently only by slowing mitosis because the retarded metaphases eventually continue in normal anaphases and telophases (Cornman, 1946). Parasorbic acid also prevents the inception of mitosis.

Jensen and Welbourne (1962) found a marked decrease in numbers of root cells of *Pisum sativum* in mitosis 4 and 8 hours after treatment with an aqueous extract of *Juglans nigra* hulls, or *trans*-cinnamic acid. Moreover, during treatment with the walnut hull extract, sizable numbers of cells were found in metaphase at 8 and 12 hours after beginning the treatment, whereas no metaphases were found in the controls at those times. They concluded, therefore, that the walnut hull extract probably slows mitosis and also prevents inception of the process. They made no additional comments on *trans*-cinnamic acid, but their results suggest that perhaps it prevents inception of mitosis only.

Volatile terpenes from macerated leaves of *Salvia leucophylla* completely prevent mitosis in roots of *Cucumis sativus* seedlings (W. H. Muller, 1965). In addition, they prevent the cells present from elongating in both the roots and hypocotyls. The cells do become wider than control cells so they have a considerably different appearance. The terpenes found in the air near *S. leucophylla* plants in the field are cineole and camphor.

W. H. Muller (1965) found that volatiles from leaves of *Salvia leucophylla* inhibited growth (cell division) of 32 of 44 bacterial isolates obtained from soil in and around *Salvia* stands. Five were stimulated, and seven were not affected. He found that a relatively small concentration of cineole inhibited growth of all 36 isolates tested.

Avers and Goodwin (1956) reported that scopoletin and coumarin decrease mitosis in *Phleum pratense* roots and that scopoletin is most effective in doing so.

Bukolova (1971) found that toxins from three weedy species, *Son-*

chus arvensis, Chenopodium album, and *Cirsium arvense,* reduce mitotic activity in roots of wheat, rye, and garden cress.

B. Inhibition of Gibberellin- or Indoleacetic Acid-Induced Growth

It seems logical to me to consider next the effects of allelopathic agents on plant growth hormones. Considerable work has been done on this subject since Andreae (1952) reported that scopoletin inhibits oxidation of indoleacetic acid (IAA). Sondheimer and Griffin (1960) found that indoleacetic acid oxidase from etiolated pea epicotyls is inhibited by chlorogenic acid, isochlorogenic acid, neochlorogenic acid, band 510, and dihydrochlorogenic acid, all of which are polyphenols. They found that dihydro-*p*-coumaric and *p*-coumaric acids were strong activators of the enzyme.

Lee and Skoog (1965) found that the monohydroxybenzoic acids are stimulatory to the inactivation of IAA by a crude enzyme extract of tobacco callus, and that the order of increasing effectiveness is 2-, 3-, and 4-hydroxybenzoic acid. 2,4-Dihydroxybenzoic acid is very stimulatory to IAA inactivation, but 3,4-dihydroxybenzoic acid is inhibitory. In fact, at equimolar concentrations, 3,4-dihydroxybenzoic acid completely prevents the stimulatory effect of 4-hydroxybenzoic acid on IAA inactivation. They found also that *p*-coumaric acid strongly accelerates IAA inactivation, whereas ferulic acid strongly inhibits it. 2-Hydroxyphenylacetic and 2-methoxyphenylacetic acids are moderate inhibitors if IAA inactivation. The same relative activities were found in the case of horseradish peroxidase breakdown of IAA.

Tomaszewski and Thimann (1966) supported the previous work and suggested that polyphenols synergize IAA-induced growth by counteracting IAA decarboxylation. They pointed out that ferulic acid and sinapic acid act like polyphenols. They suggested also that monophenols stimulate the decarboxylation of IAA under conditions where they depress growth, and that this action is enhanced by Mn^{2+}. They hypothesized further that the major role of polyphenolase may be the control of hormone balance, since changing monophenols to polyphenols changes their action from auxin destroying to auxin preserving.

Stenlid (1968) reported that phlorizin and some related flavonoid glycosides, as well as naringenin and 2',4,4'-trihydroxychalcone, are strong stimulators of IAA oxidase. This could certainly help explain the potent growth-inhibitory effects of many flavonoids.

Kefeli and Turetskaya (1967) reported that the natural phenolic growth inhibitors from *Salix rubra* and apple trees suppress the activity of IAA and gibberellin. Wurzburger and Leshem (1969) reported that the germination inhibitor contained in the glumes and hull of the grass species, *Aegilops kotschyi,* appears to inhibit gibberellin-induced growth. Corcoran (1970) found that the inhibitors from carob, *Ceratonia siliqua,* also inhibit gibberellin-induced growth, but not IAA-induced growth.

Six chemically defined tannins were found to inhibit hypocotyl growth induced by gibberellic acid in cucumber seedlings (Geissman and Phinney, 1972), but growth induced by IAA was not inhibited. In addition, 14 chemically defined hydrolyzable tannins and six impure mixtures of either condensed or hydrolyzable tannins were found to inhibit the gibberellin-induced growth of light-grown dwarf pea seedlings. Eight compounds related to tannins, including coumarin, cinnamic acid, and a number of phenolic compounds were tested and showed some inhibition of gibberellin-induced growth in dwarf pea seedlings, but not as much as tannins.

C. Effect on Mineral Uptake

Growing sugar beets alters the zinc status of the soil to the extent that zinc-sensitive crops such as corn and beans are severely zinc deficient when they follow beets in the cropping sequence (Boawn, 1965). This has been observed in all parts of the United States where sugar beets are grown. Boawn found in field experiments that beets did not remove as much zinc as sorghum, which does not cause zinc deficiency in subsequent crops. Moreover, he found that sugar beets did not change the acid-extractable zinc, titratable alkalinity, or pH any more than did sorghum. His only conclusion was that excessive removal of zinc by sugar beets cannot be considered a factor contributing to zinc deficiency in subsequent crops. It seems to me, therefore, that sugar beets must be adding some toxin to the soil which interferes with the uptake of zinc by some crops.

Chambers and Holm (1965) measured the uptake of phosphorus-32 (^{32}P) by bean plants (*Phaseolus vulgaris*) growing alone or in association with other bean plants, pigweed (*Amaranthus retroflexus*), or green foxtail (*Setaria viridis*). They found that one associated bean plant reduced the ^{32}P uptake by the test bean plant as much as two, three, or four associated bean plants. Moreover, the weed species caused less reduction of phosphorus uptake than did associated bean plants even though these particular weed species are noted for absorbing large quantities of the major elements. In fact, they found that the pigweed absorbed seven times as much total phosphorus as the bean and still had less effect on absorption of ^{32}P by the test bean plant than other bean plants did. All these facts indicate that competition for limited phosphorus was not the causal factor in reduced phosphorus uptake by the bean plants. Consequently, the authors concluded that an allelopathic interrelationship was involved.

Tillberg (1970) found that salicylic acid at concentrations of 10^{-6}–10^{-3} M decreased phosphorus uptake by the alga, *Scenedesmus*, but *trans*-cinnamic and abscisic acids had no effect.

Lastuvka and Minarz (1970) reported that when maize and peas are grown together in solution culture, the removal of nitrogen, phosphorus, and potassium is almost always greater than when each crop is grown alone. Under the mixed condition, the migration of nutrients into the aboveground parts of maize is better and of peas is worse than in pure culture. This suggested that root exudates were affecting mineral uptake, and in subsequent experiments, Lastuvka (1970) used differentially permeable membranes to separate macromolecular root secretions and found that the substances secreted affected ion absorption and accumulation by test plants.

Buchholtz (1971) observed that corn plants growing in areas infested with quackgrass, *Agropyron repens*, appear to be suffering from a severe deficiency of mineral elements, particularly nitrogen and potassium. Analysis of corn stover from such areas demonstrated that it is very low in nitrogen and potassium compared with controls from nonquackgrass areas. Heavy fertilization with nitrogen and potassium in quackgrass areas did not improve the yield of corn greatly, even though it was found that only a small part of the added elements was absorbed by the quackgrass.

In a subsequent experiment, a container was buried flush with the soil surface and filled with full-strength Hoagland's solution. Two seminal roots of a corn seedling were placed in the solution, and the remainder of the root system of the corn was allowed to grow outside the container in quackgrass-infested soil. In this type of experiment, the corn plants grew almost as well as controls without quackgrass, even though most of the roots of the test corn plants were in the quackgrass-infested soil. He concluded, therefore, that the allelopathic effect of quackgrass is predominantly localized and not systemic and that the reduced growth of corn plants associated with quackgrass is definitely due to a deficiency of minerals within the corn-shoot tissue. Buchholtz suggested four possible reasons for the failure of shoots of corn plants growing in quackgrass-infested soil to obtain sufficient potassium and nitrogen for normal growth: (1) nutrients in the soil are made unavailable in some way other than by depletion, (2) the corn root system may be reduced, (3) the absorptive capacity of the corn roots may be impaired, and (4) the nitrogen and potassium may be absorbed but are not transported to the shoots. From various bits of evidence, Buchholtz felt that reasons (2) and (4) are not very likely reasons. The problem is still unsolved and waiting for someone to pursue it further.

Croak (1972) studied the effects of ferulic acid on the rate of depletion of four macronutrients and three micronutrients from a defined medium by suspension cultures of Paul's scarlet rose cells. The macronutrients involved were potassium, magnesium, calcium, and phosphorus; the micronutrients were iron, molybdenum, and manganese. A 10^{-4} M concentration of ferulic acid decreased the depletion of macronutrients per flask, but the total depletion on a fresh weight basis (μmoles per gm of cells) was greater in cells treated with ferulic acid than in control cells, with the exception of phosphorus. The reason for this marked difference depending on the criterion used was that the ferulic acid inhibited the growth of the cells in test flasks. Obviously, there was no reduction in ion uptake. Similar results were reported for the effects of chlorogenic and tannic acids on uptake of K^+ and Ca^{2+} by *Amaranthus retroflexus* seedlings (Olmsted and Rice, 1970).

A 10^{-4} M concentration of ferulic acid increased the rate of depletion of the micronutrients from the medium also when calculated on the basis of μmoles per gram fresh weight of rose cells per day. Again, therefore, a slight increase in ion uptake occurred rather than a decrease. Actually, the concentrations of the elements involved in the defined medium were considerably higher than available amounts of the same elements under field conditions so such uptake studies probably do not have much ecological significance.

In order to try to get more realistic data on ion uptake at low levels of available ions, Croak (1972) studied the effect of ferulic acid on rubidium-86 (^{86}Rb) uptake by rose cell suspension cultures. Incubation of 5-day rose cells in 10^{-4} M ferulic acid during a 10-minute absorption period resulted in a subsequent inhibition of uptake of ^{86}Rb from both 0.2 and 5.0 mM solutions (Figs. 47 and 48). Inhibition of uptake was consistently greater at high external salt concentrations (5.0 mM RbCl). Incubation of 10-day cells in the same concentration of inhibitor had very little effect, however, on the rate of ^{86}Rb absorption at either high or low external salt concentrations. Apparently, as the cells age they become less susceptible to the effects of ferulic acid, at least insofar as it

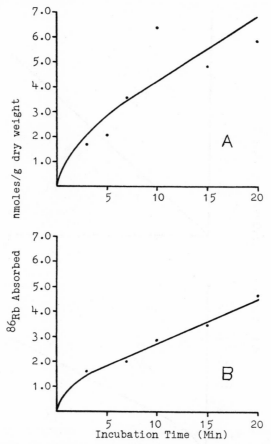

Fig. 47. (A) Rate of uptake of ^{86}Rb from 0.2 mM RbCl by normal 5-day cells. Control rate, 14.17 nmoles/gm dry weight/hour. (B) Effect of $10^{-4}M$ ferulic acid on rate of uptake of ^{86}Rb from 0.2 mM RbCl by 5-day cells. Test rate, 10.81 nmoles/gm dry weight/hour. (From Croak, 1972.)

affects ion uptake. Hodges *et al.* (1971) reported a similar differential sensitivity with age to Rb uptake in oat root sections treated with the antibiotics gramicidin and nigericin.

Two systems of ion uptake (Welch and Epstein, 1969) operate in the ion accumulation process in rose-cell suspension cultures according to Croak (1972). Young cells incubated in a ferulic acid solution showed inhibition of ^{86}Rb uptake in both systems, with inhibition being greater in system 2 operating at high concentrations.

Ion uptake is certainly of basic importance in the growth and reproduction of organisms of all levels of complexity, and evidence is

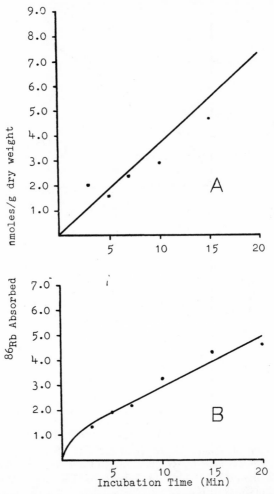

Fig. 48. (A) Rate of uptake of ^{86}Rb from 5.0 mM RbCl by normal 5-day cells. Control rate, 224.32 nmoles/gm dry weight/hour. (B) Effect of 10^{-4} M ferulic acid on rate of uptake of ^{86}Rb from 5.0 mM RbCl by 5-day cells. Test rate, 122.82 nmoles/gm dry weight/hour. (From Croak, 1972.)

accumulating that many types of allelopathic agents affect the rate of ion uptake. I feel, therefore, that this is a very important mechanism of action of many such agents, and much more work needs to be done in this area at all levels, from one-celled organisms to intact higher plants.

D. Retardation of Photosynthesis

In spite of the basic importance of this process to all autotrophic organisms, very little work has been done concerning the effects on photosynthesis of inhibitors implicated in allelopathy. Einhellig *et al.* (1970) found that scopoletin markedly inhibited the photosynthetic rate of intact plants of Russian Mammoth sunflower, tobacco (var. One Sucker), and pigweed (*Amaranthus retroflexus*). There was a large reduction in net photosynthesis in tobacco the second day after treatment in $10^{-3} M$ and $5 \times 10^{-4} M$ concentrations (Fig. 49). This reduction reached a low point by the fourth day (34% of the control rate) and was followed by a gradual recovery phase. The degree of reduction correlated well with the concentration of scopoletin used in treatment, and leaf area expansion also correlated well with the concentration of scopoletin. Moreover, a calculation of CO_2 fixed per hour of illumination in the daily photosynthesis of tobacco showed a striking relationship with reduced CO_2 fixation in the treated plants (Fig. 50). By the end of the experiment, the $10^{-3} M$ scopoletin-treated tobacco plants fixed only 51% as much CO_2 as the controls. The dark respira-

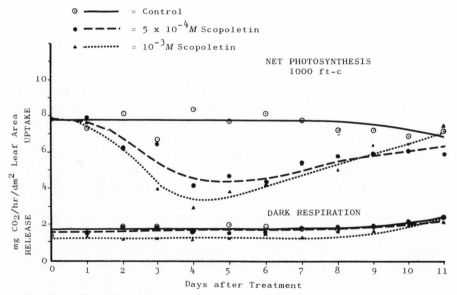

Fig. 49.   Effects of scopoletin treatment on net photosynthesis and dark respiration in tobacco seedlings. Each point is mean of four plants (From Einhellig *et al.*, 1970.)

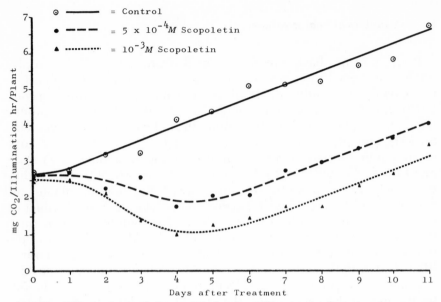

Fig. 50.   Effects of scopoletin on CO_2 fixed per illumination hour in tobacco seedlings. Each point is computed from mean leaf area and net photosynthesis of four plants.
(From Einhellig *et al.*, 1970.)

tion rate was not significantly affected by scopoletin treatment (Fig.
49). The results with sunflower were very similar to those with tobacco; the photosynthetic and dark respiration rates in pigweed were
measured only on the fifth day after treatment, and results were similar on that day to the results obtained with sunflower and tobacco.

Einhellig *et al.* (1970) found that the inhibitory activity of scopoletin on total plant growth correlated well with decreases in net photosynthesis, but, as previously stated, no respiration differences were
found. They felt that the overall evidence indicated that the effect of
scopoletin on net photosynthesis was the cause of growth reduction,
but pointed out that the evidence did not eliminate other possible
causes of growth reduction.

Sikka *et al.* (1972) found that three quinones tested inhibited CO_2
fixation by isolated chloroplasts. The quinones were 2,3-dichloro-1,4-
naphthoquinone (Dichlone); 2-amino-3-chloro-1,4-naphthoquinone
(06K-Quinone); and 2,3,5,6-tetrachloro-1,4-benzoquinone (Chloranil).
Dichlone was a strong inhibitor of both photosystems I and II;
photosystem I was more sensitive to 06K-Quinone than was photosystem II, but the reverse was true in the case of Chloranil. These

quinones are obviously commercially produced ones and, to my knowledge, have not been shown to be produced by plants. Nevertheless, they do indicate that quinones can inhibit photosynthesis and suggest that tests should be run using quinones that have been identified as allelopathic agents.

E. Inhibition or Stimulation of Respiration

1. OXYGEN UPTAKE BY ROOTS, SEEDS, AND YEAST CELLS

Patrick (1955) found that water extracts of soil in which peach root residues were decomposing were very inhibitory to respiration in excised peach roots. Patrick and his colleagues demonstrated later that water extracts of soils in which several different crop residues were decomposing were inhibitory to respiration in excised tobacco roots (Patrick and Koch, 1958; Patrick et al., 1964).

Koeppe (1972) found that 500 μM concentrations of juglone (5-hydroxynaphthoquinone) inhibited oxygen uptake by excised corn roots by more than 90% after a 1-hour treatment. Lesser inhibitions occurred with 50 μM and 250 μM concentrations of juglone.

Van Sumere et al. (1971) reported that several quinones, aldehydes, benzoic acid and cinnamic acid derivatives, and coumarins affect the rate of oxygen uptake by yeast (Saccharomyces cerevisiae) cells (Table 55). Most of the compounds stimulated uptake of oxygen, but a few inhibited it, notably the quinones. This is in agreement with the results of Koeppe (1972) on effects of juglone on corn roots.

Van Sumere et al. (1971) found that the same compounds have effects on oxygen uptake by lettuce seeds that are very similar to those on uptake by yeast cells. Oxygen uptake by barley seeds was affected by these compounds, but there were many more cases of reduction in uptake, particularly on a short-term test basis (10 minutes).

2. RESPIRATION BY SUSPENSION OF ISOLATED MITOCHONDRIA

Muller et al. (1969) found that two volatile terpenes, cineole and dipentene, which emanate from leaves of Salvia leucophylla, markedly reduce oxygen uptake by suspensions of mitochondria from Avena fatua or Cucumis sativus. The inhibition appeared to be localized in that part of the Kreb's cycle where succinate is converted to fumarate or fumarate to malate. Koeppe (1972) demonstrated that, in the absence of inorganic phosphate (P_i), juglone stimulated the rate of

TABLE 55

Effects of Phenolics and Coumarins on the Respiration of Yeast [a,b]

Compound [c]	$10^{-4}M$		$5 \times 10^{-4} M$		$10^{-3} M$	
	5.6	7.0	5.6	7.0	5.6	7.0
2-Methylnaphthoquinone	+30	+100	+20	−10	−15	−25
Benzaldehyde	0	0	0	0	+10	+10
Salicylaldehyde	+15	+15	+30	+65	+45	+100
p-Hydroxybenzaldehyde	0	+10	+10	+15	+25	+25
β-Resorcylaldehyde	+10	+10	+35	+25	+50	+80
Vanillin	0	+15	+15	+35	+25	+60
Cinnamaldehyde	+10	+10	+25	+30	+35	+40
Benzoic acid	0	0	0	0	0	0
Cinnamic acid	+20	+10	+25	+20	+30	+25
o-Coumaric acid	0	0	0	0	+10	+10
p-Coumaric acid	0	+10	0	+15	+10	+25
Ferulic acid	0	0	+10	+10	+15	+15
Coumarin	0	+10	+10	+20	+20	+25
Umbelliferone	0	0	0	+10	+10	+20
Scopoletin	0	0	0	0	+10	+10

[a] Modified from Van Sumere et al. (1971).
[b] Results are expressed as percent change from the respiration of the blank, after 300 minutes.
[c] Flasks contained 2.5 ml of 1.2% yeast suspension in 0.05 M phthalate-NaCH buffer (5.6) or 0.05 M tris-HCl buffer (pH 7.0). Test substances were added in 0.5 ml solution containing 1 mg D-glucose and 0.66 mg KH_2PO_4.

oxygen uptake by isolated corn mitochondria oxidizing reduced nicotinamide adenine dinucleotide (NADH), succinate, or malate + pyruvate. However, in the presence of P_i, juglone concentrations of 3 μM or greater inhibited the state 3 oxidation rates of succinate and malate + pyruvate; lowered respiratory control and ADP/O ratios obtained from the oxidation of NADH, malate + pyruvate, or succinate; and reduced the coupled deposition of calcium phosphate within isolated mitochondria driven by the oxidation of malate + pyruvate. Koeppe concluded that this uncoupling of ATP (adenosine triphosphate) production correlates well with the inhibition that results when tissues or organisms are treated with juglone.

Van Sumere et al. (1971) found that several of the compounds that stimulate oxygen uptake by yeast cells (Table 55) lower the ADP/O ratio resulting from the oxidation of NADH by suspensions of isolated yeast mitochondria. Of those compounds listed in Table 55, 2-methyl-1,4-naphthoquinone, salicylaldehyde, β-resorcylaldehyde, cinnamaldehyde, cinnamic acid, o-coumaric acid, and scopoletin lowered the ADP/O ratio and thus proved to be uncouplers of oxidative phosphorylation (prevent ATP formation). An additional compound tested, caffeic acid, also is an uncoupler of oxidative phosphorylation in yeast respiration.

Hulme and Jones (1963) tested a large number of simple phenols, derivatives of benzoic acid, digallic and ellagic acids, tannic acid, cinnamic acid derivatives, esculetin, and flavonoids against oxidation of succinate by succinoxidase in suspensions of isolated apple peel mitochondria. Most of the compounds tested were found to inhibit succinoxidase to at least some degree and many were very inhibitory. Two flavonoid compounds and tannic acid and chlorogenic acid were tested against decarboxylation of malate by the malic enzyme in apple peel mitochondria, and all were found to be inhibitory to the malic enzyme except chlorogenic acid, which had a stimulatory effect after the first hour.

4-Hydroxybenzoic acid is very stimulatory to the oxidation of NADH by enzymes from tobacco leaves (Lee, 1966), but a shift of the hydroxyl group from the 4- to the 3-position and from the 3- to the 2-position decreases the activity. In the presence of 4-hydroxybenzoic, 2,4-dihydroxybenzoic and 2,5-dihydroxybenzoic acids further stimulate oxidation of NADH. On the other hand, 3,4-dihydroxybenzoic, 2,3-dihydroxybenzoic, and 2,6-dihydroxybenzoic acids inhibit oxidation of NADH by the same enzymes.

Stenlid (1968) found that the flavonoids, naringenin, and 2',4,4'-trihydroxychalcone inhibit oxidative phosphorylation in higher plants and give a distinct uncoupling effect. He found, however, that phlorizin and related glycosides are less active in this respect.

The fact that respiratory activity by isolated respiratory enzymes, isolated mitochondria, one-celled organisms, and organs of plants has been shown to be adversely affected by many identified allelopathic agents indicates that respiratory effects probably represent an important mechanism of action of at least some inhibitors.

F. Inhibition or Stimulation of Stomatal Opening

Einhellig *et al.* (1970) found a loss in turgor pressure in tobacco plants treated with 10^{-3} *M* scopoletin in addition to the pronounced reduction in photosynthesis previously discussed. They suggested, therefore, that scopoletin may operate through effects on the stomata. This was a logical suggestion, since stomata are the portals through which carbon dioxide enters the interior of the leaf during photosynthesis and through which large quantities of water vapor diffuse in transpiration. Moreover, Shimshi (1963a) found that spraying phenylmercuric acetate on tobacco and sunflower plants reduced stomatal apertures, affected transpiration, and reduced growth. Similar treatment reduced photosynthesis in maize (Shimshi, 1963b). In addition, Zelitch (1967) reported that leaf disks of tobacco floated on a $10^{-3} M$ chlorogenic acid solution had 50% stomatal closure.

Einhellig and Kuan (1971) followed up on the suggestion of Einhellig *et al.* (1970) and found that whole plants of tobacco and sunflower treated with $10^{-3} M$ and $5 \times 10^{-4} M$ scopoletin and chlorogenic acid (root immersion) showed stomatal closure for several days after treatment. They found that $10^{-4} M$ concentrations of both inhibitors stimulated opening of the stomates of both test species. They concluded that inhibition of stomatal opening by scopoletin correlates well with growth inhibition under similar conditions. They pointed out also that a comparison of the photosynthetic curves of Einhellig *et al.* (1970) with the curves of the effects of scopoletin on stomatal aperture indicates that the closing and partial closing of stomata are closely related to photosynthetic reductions. They cautioned, however, that it is not clear whether stomatal closure induced by scopoletin causes a reduction in photosynthesis or the latter induces the former. They pointed out that photosynthesis is one of the processes implicated in light-induced stomatal opening.

A $10^{-3} M$ tannic acid solution causes significant reductions in stomatal apertures of tobacco plants for about 5 days after treatment, but a $10^{-4} M$ tannic acid solution does not affect stomatal opening of tobacco, even though it significantly reduces plant growth (Einhellig, 1971). Surprisingly, the stomata of the $10^{-3} M$ tannic acid-treated plants return to normal aperture at a time when the plants appear to be in a deteriorative condition. Thus, stomatal aperture changes cannot account for the pronounced growth effects of tannic acid on tobacco plants.

Vikherkova (1970) reported that extracts of fresh rhizomes of *Agropyron repens* added to soil in which *Linum usitatissimum* is growing causes decreased transpiration, water content, and osmotic pressure of the cell sap and reduces opening of the stomates. However, he felt that these changes are secondary and are caused by a water deficit that could be due to limitation of water inflow into the roots of the plant.

Turner (1972) found that oat plants treated with the marasmin, victorin (see Chapter 12), have a reduced stomatal aperture and a decreased rate of transpiration. On the other hand, fusicoccin, which is also a marasmin, stimulates opening of stomata and increases transpiration (Turner, 1972). A great many of the marasmins produced by pathogenic microorganisms cause plants to wilt. Thus, it would be interesting to determine if a great many of them act like fusicoccin and increase transpiration.

The overall evidence on the effects of allelopathic agents on stomatal opening is confusing at this point in time. It appears to me that the effects may generally be secondary ones, but much more research needs to be done before anything definite can be concluded.

G. Inhibition of Protein Synthesis and Changes in Lipid and Organic Acid Metabolism

Krylov (1970) reported that potatoes produce toxic substances when cultivated in the space between rows of young apple trees which inhibit tree growth, decrease the total nitrogen content in the branches and roots, change the composition of proteins in the bark of the branches, increase the amount of soluble albumins, and decrease the amount of residual proteins.

Other persons, working with much simpler one-celled organisms or cell suspensions, have also noted effects of allelopathic agents on protein synthesis and other synthetic processes (Van Sumere *et al.*, 1971; Croak, 1972; Zweig *et al.*, 1972). Zweig *et al.* (1972) investigated the effects of certain quinones on the photosynthetic incorporation of $^{14}CO_2$ by the alga, *Chlorella*. They found that the quinones caused an increase in the proportion of ^{14}C in sucrose and glycine accompanied by a reduction in ^{14}C in lipids and glutamic acid. They suggested, therefore, that the quinones inactivate coenzyme A and cause a shortage of NADPH.

Croak (1972) studied the effects of cinnamic and ferulic acids on the metabolism of L-[U-^{14}C]glucose by Paul's scarlet rose cell suspension cultures. Treatment of the cells with $10^{-5} M$ cinnamic acid during the 210-minute incubation period in labeled glucose resulted in a significant decrease in incorporation of ^{14}C into the alcohol-insoluble residue (primarily protein) (Fig. 51). On the other hand, ^{14}C incorporation into soluble amino acids was significantly increased. There was also a decrease in ^{14}C incorporation into protein amino acids, which was additional evidence for decreased incorporation into protein. An analysis of the percent distribution of ^{14}C in soluble amino acids was made in the control and treated cells to determine whether the inhibition of protein synthesis might be the result of a reduced

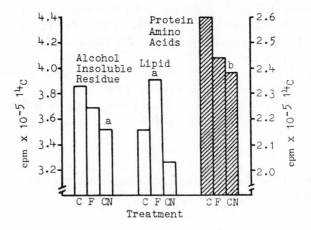

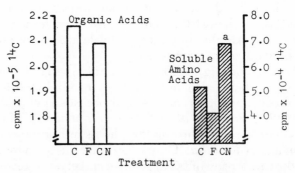

Fig. 51. Distribution of ^{14}C in various cell fractions following 210 minutes of incubation of cells in [L-U-^{14}C] glucose medium containing $10^{-4} M$ ferulic acid or $10^{-5} M$ cinnamic acid. Data, mean of three replicates; C, control; F, ferulic acid; CN, cinnamic acid; a, significantly different from control at 5% level; b, significantly different from control at 10% level. (From Croak, 1972.)

synthesis of a particular amino acid. No significant increase or reduction of incorporation of ^{14}C into a particular amino acid was found.

Cinnamic acid reduced the total incorporation of ^{14}C from glucose into the organic acid fraction also (Fig. 51). Detailed analyses indicated that a significantly greater amount of the ^{14}C appeared in succinate in treated cells, and reduced amounts appeared in malate and citrate. Incorporation of ^{14}C into soluble lipids was also reduced in cells treated with cinnamic acid (Fig. 51).

Ferulic acid also reduced the incorporation of ^{14}C into the alcohol-insoluble residue, protein, amino acids, and organic acids, but the rest of the labeling pattern was considerably different from that resulting from the cinnamic acid treatment (Fig. 51). A significantly greater portion of the label appeared in the soluble lipid fraction of the ferulic acid-treated cells, but the amount in the soluble amino acid fraction was greatly reduced.

Although ^{14}C incorporation into total protein and soluble amino acids was reduced, no significant alteration in the percentage distribution of ^{14}C into the constituent amino acids was noted. Again, as with cinnamic acid-treated cells, changes did occur in the distribution of ^{14}C in organic acids compared with control cells. Incorporation of the label into succinate was slightly increased, and incorporation into malate slightly reduced.

Croak (1972) concluded that the reduction in protein synthesis resulting from ferulic or cinnamic acid treatment, if maintained through the normal 14-day growth cycle of the rose-cell suspensions, would certainly lead to a reduction in growth of the cultures. She concluded also that ferulic and cinnamic acids affect protein synthesis in different ways. In cells treated with cinnamic acid, incorporation of ^{14}C into all soluble amino acids was enhanced, indicating that the reduction in protein synthesis was not due to a lack of supply of a particular amino acid but apparently to inhibition of the mechanism of protein synthesis. In contrast, in cells treated with ferulic acid, there was a reduction of incorporation of ^{14}C into soluble amino acids, protein, and organic acids with a concomitant increase of incorporation into lipids. Thus, it appears that ferulic acid causes a diversion of [^{14}C]acetate into lipid synthesis rather than into Kreb's cycle and subsequent pathways leading to amino acids and proteins. Croak suggested that these alterations in the flow of carbon into cellular constituents because of cinnamic and ferulic acid may be particularly significant during seed germination and seedling development when storage reserves are being mobilized and resynthesized into other compounds necessary for growth.

Van Sumere et al. (1971) investigated the effects of a large number of known inhibitors on incorporation of [1-^{14}C]phenylalanine into protein in yeast cells. They found that most of the inhibitors reduced the incorporation of the labeled phenylalanine into protein in yeast cells (Table 56). In other experiments, they tested the effects of ferulic acid and coumarin on the incorporation of [1-^{14}C]phenylalanine into protein in lettuce seeds and in barley seeds and embryos. They found that both inhibitors markedly reduced the incorporation of labeled phenylalanine in all cases. These workers found that the uptake of labeled phenylalanine was also generally reduced in yeast and in the

TABLE 56

Effect of Different Phenolics and Related Substances (25 μmoles) on the Uptake, Oxidation, and Incorporation of [1-^{14}C]DL-Phenylalanine (0.75 μmoles) by Yeast (3.2 gm Wet Weight in 25 ml 0.1 M Phosphate Buffer pH 7.2) [a,b,c]

Activity in DPM × 10⁶ after 10 hours	Control	A	B	C	D	E	F	G	H	I	J	K	L	M
Remaining in the medium	4.1 (100%)	103	114	124	115	101	117	147	123	96	97	96	125	164
$^{14}CO_2$ respired	0.4 (100%)	94	97	78	68	108	85	50	67	110	119	120	75	11
Intact cells	1.8 (100%)	87	74	64	80	88	74	33	61	93	87	87	45	10
Pool	1.1 (100%)	103	70	67	64	109	56	49	64	108	111	117	81	51
Balance	98	97	95	97	95	97	95	98	95	96	96	97	95	98
Protein fraction	0.5 (100%)	74	83	65	101	98	86	33	78	108	97	82	62	11

[a] Modified from Van Sumere *et al.* (1971).

[b] Results are expressed as percent of the controls. (Apparent K_m of [1-^{14}C]DL-phenylalanine uptake:1.68 × 10^{-5} M or 0.9 × 10^{-5} M for [1-^{14}C]DL-phenylalanine.) Activity in the medium at the start of the experiment was 7.5 × 10⁶ dpm. Analogous results were obtained when a [1-^{14}C]DL-phenylalanine concentration of 25 μmoles was employed.

[c] A, benzaldehyde; B, salicylaldehyde; C, β-resorcylaldehyde; D,benzoic acid; E, *p*-hydroxybenzoic acid; F, vanillic acid; G, cinnamaldehyde (125 μmoles); H, cinnamic acid (125 μmoles); I, *p*-coumaric acid; J, caffeic acid; K, ferulic acid; L, coumarin (125 μmoles); M, menadione (2-methyl-1,4-naphthoquinone).

seeds by the inhibitors. They concluded, therefore, that the allelopathic agents studied may reduce growth by inhibiting the transport of amino acids and the formation of proteins.

It is significant that Croak (1972) and Van Sumere *et al.* (1971) concluded that cinnamic and ferulic acids inhibit protein formation, because very different cells and organs were used in the investigations. Furthermore, the results of Zweig *et al.* (1972), using still a different organism (see above), support the same conclusion in the case of quinones. I feel, therefore, that this is one of the important mechanisms of action of many inhibitors. Einhellig (1971) stated that unpublished work in his laboratory suggested that tannic acid may affect RNA synthesis or release. It is evident that this is a fruitful area for future research on mechanisms of action of allelopathic agents.

H. Inhibition of Hemoglobin Synthesis

There is much evidence that several plants found to inhibit *Rhizo-bium* reduce nodule numbers on heavily inoculated legumes and he-moglobin content of the nodules (Rice, 1964, 1968, 1971a, 1972; Blum and Rice, 1969). As I pointed out in Chapter 4, legume nodules have to contain hemoglobin in order to be effective in nitrogen-fixation. It is obvious, therefore, that reduction of nodulation and of hemoglobin formation could certainly reduce the growth of legumes in areas low in nitrogen.

I have observed many times (E. L. Rice, unpublished) that heavily inoculated bean plants growing in soil in pots with plants known to produce inhibitors of *Rhizobium* have unusual patterns of chlorosis. In addition to a general appearance of nitrogen deficiency, the pri-mary leaves are often completely devoid of chlorophyll in certain sections. Often the entire blade on one side of the midvein will be apparently completely devoid of chlorophyll. When one considers this in relation to the inhibition of hemoglobin synthesis, it appears that some allelopathic agents interfere with porphyrin synthesis. This appears to be another fertile area for future research.

I. Changes in Permeability of Membranes

Muller *et al.* (1969) stated that two volatile terpenes, cineole and dipentene, from leaves of *Salvia leucophylla* appear to decrease the permeability of cell membranes. They did not, however, furnish any actual evidence for such a change. Levitan and Barker (1972) presented definite evidence, on the other hand, that several known allelopathic agents do change membrane permeability. They found that salicylate, benzoate, cinnamate, 2-naphthoate, and derivatives in-creased the permeability of neuronal membranes of the marine mol-lusk, *Navanax inermis,* to potassium and decreased permeability of the membranes to chloride. Moreover, they found that the relative effectiveness in changing membrane permeability is closely corre-lated (positively) with the octanol–water partition coefficient and pK_a value. The effect, in other words, is related to the solubility of the compound in the membrane and the concentration of aromatic anions available.

Owens (1969) pointed out that several of the polypeptide antibiot-ics, polypeptide marasmins, and animal polypeptide toxins are postulated to exert their biological influence primarily by altering the permeability of certain membranes. The primary effect of victorin is thought to be a change in membrane permeability. When victorin-treated tissue from a susceptible oat variety is placed in a bathing solution, the tissue begins to lose electrolytes into the solution within 5 minutes from the time of treatment (Owens, 1969). Tissues from resistant oat varieties are not affected, which shows that the effect is host specific.

Four glycopeptide wilt toxins produced by *Corynebacterium* have been shown also to change membrane permeability (Owens, 1969). Another marasmin, fusaric acid, produced by several species of *Fusarium* causes changes in membrane permeability, as do α-picolinic and dehydrofusaric acids (Owens, 1969). Owens stated, in fact, that, with few exceptions, the most common early sign of marasmin damage to cells is an alteration in water or ion permeability of the cytoplasmic membrane. He pointed out further, however, that it is not known in many cases whether this is the primary effect of the toxins.

The evidence is clear that changes in permeability of membranes represent an important mechanism of action of at least some allelopathic substances. This field is wide open for further research, however.

J. Inhibition of Specific Enzymes

1. PECTOLYTIC ENZYMES

The ability of pathogens to penetrate host cells depends strongly on the effectiveness of the pectolytic enzymes produced by the pathogens. Knowledge of effects of plant-produced substances on pectolytic enzymes is of considerable importance, therefore, in an understanding of resistance of plants to diseases. According to Williams (1963), Cole demonstrated in 1958 that apple juice inhibits pectolytic enzymes of *Sclerotinia fructigena*, which causes the fungal brown rot of fruit. Williams and a colleague subsequently investigated the effects of known simple phenols, chlorogenic acid, and flavonoids (unoxidized and enzymatically oxidized) present in the apple against tissue-macerating and polygalacturonase activity of culture filtrates of *S. fructigena* (Williams, 1963). None of the unoxidized compounds had an appreciable effect on either the macerating or polygalacturonase activity. All the oxidized compounds were effective against both types of activity, with oxidized chlorogenic acid being least effective. In other experiments, they found tannic acid to be an extremely effective inhibitor of both types of activity and the larger molecules of the gallotannins to be even more effective. They concluded that the minimum molecular size for inhibitory activity at concentrations up to 0.2% is about 500. Benoit and Starkey (1968b) found the wattle tannin, a condensed tannin, also markedly inhibited the activity of a purified commercial polygalacturonase.

It is evident, therefore, that some well-known allelopathic agents inhibit activity of pectolytic enzymes, at least after oxidation of the compounds. This effect of some phytoncides produced by higher plants on the activity of pathogenic microorganisms probably has very significant ecological importance.

2. CELLULASE

Cellulase is extremely important ecologically because of its role in decomposition and the large amount of cellulose in plants. Benoit and Starkey (1968b) demonstrated that wattle tannin strongly inhibits the action of cellulase. They previously demonstrated that wattle tannin slows the decomposition of hemicellulose and cellulose by cultures of microorganisms obtained from fresh barnyard soil (Benoit and Starkey, 1968a). Thus, although they did not specifically study the effect of tannin on hemicellulase, it appears that tannin also inhibits the action of that enzyme.

I feel that the role of allelopathic substances in decomposition is very important ecologically and that this area of research has not had the attention it merits.

3. CATALASE AND PEROXIDASE

The information is very limited concerning effects of inhibitors on these enzymes. Dzubenko and Petrenko (1971) reported that root secretions of *Lupinus albus* and *Zea mays* inhibited growth and catalase and peroxidase activity of two weed species, *Chenopodium album* and *Amaranthus retroflexus*.

In Section II,B above, I discussed the evidence of Lee and Skoog (1965) concerning the effects of several phytotoxins on horseradish peroxidase breakdown of IAA. Possibly many more types of inhibitors can affect plant growth through their effects on peroxidase and thus on IAA inactivation.

Benoit and Starkey (1968b) stated that tannins inactivate peroxidase and catalase.

4. PHOSPHORYLASES

Schwimmer (1958) found that potato tubers contain polyphenols which inhibit the activity of potato phosphorylase. He tested the activity of chlorogenic acid, caffeic acid, and catechol individually against activity of the enzyme and found that all were very inhibitory. He decided that chlorogenic acid is the most important inhibitor of phosphorylase in the potato peel, however. Sondheimer (1962) stated that the concentration of polyphenols in the peel is probably sufficiently high to inhibit the phosphorylase completely.

5. OTHER ENZYMES

There is a great deal of published information on factors and substances that regulate the activity of many enzymes, but most of the evidence does not relate to the role of established allelopathic agents.

According to Benoit and Starkey (1968b), other workers have demonstrated that tannins inactivate the following enzymes not mentioned previously: amylase, myrosinase, pepsin, proteinase, dehydrogenases, decarboxylases, invertase, phosphatases, β-glucosidase, aldolase, polyphenoloxidase, lipase, urease, trypsin, and chymotrypsin. References can be found in their paper.

6. MISCELLANEOUS MECHANISMS

Hauschka *et al.* (1945) found that cysteine and glutathione have a pronounced effect in inactivating parasorbic acid, but this is not true of cystine, glycine, or glutamic acid. They suggested, therefore, that this phytotoxin and related unsaturated lactones such as patulin, penicillic acid, etc., may interfere with cellular proliferation because of their reactivity with SH groups essential to enzyme function. Cavallito and Haskell (1945) reported the same phenomenon about the same time. They found that the antibiotic properties of penicillin and several widely different bacteriostatic substances, all of which were unsaturated lactones, were inactivated by compounds having SH groups. They determined the details of how the compounds combine, and also the end products in most cases. They concluded that unsaturated lactone antibiotics may inhibit enzyme activity by uniting with SH and possibly amino groups of enzyme proteins. This could apparently be a basic mechanism of action of all the unsaturated lactone inhibitors including the coumarins, protoanemonin, strophanthidin, digitoxigenin, etc., in addition to others named above.

Ilag and Curtis (1968) examined 228 species of fungi belonging to all classes for production of ethylene, and they found that 58, or 25.6%, definitely produce this potent growth regulator. They suggested that it is probably produced regularly by fungi. They also were able to verify ethylene production by one culture of a streptomycete. They concluded that the production of ethylene should be considered in studies of growth disturbance in healthy and diseased plants.

Morgan and Powell (1970) investigated the effect of coumarin on the hypocotyl hook of etiolated bean plants and found that coumarin stimulated ethylene production. About the same time, Fuchs (1970) discovered that various phenol derivatives stimulate ethylene production by citrus fruit peel. In addition, Riov et al. (1969) reported that the induction of phenylalanine ammonia-lyase (PAL) in citrus fruit peel is controlled by ethylene. PAL is the enzyme involved in the formation of cinnamic acid from phenylalanine and, thus, there is a demonstrated connection between ethylene and possible allelopathic effect in this case. It is interesting that Owens et al. (1971) found that rhizobitoxine inhibited ethylene production in light-grown sorghum and senescent apple tissue by 75%. It appears to inhibit the production of ethylene from methionine and not the synthesis of methionine.

As was pointed out in Chapter 9, allelopathic substances sometimes promote the infection of plants by pathogens (Patrick and Koch, 1963; Toussoun and Patrick, 1963). In fact, they sometimes make species susceptible to certain diseases to which they are normally resistant (Patrick and Koch, 1963).

Sandfaer (1968) made the interesting observation that when two barley varieties were grown in mixtures, the resulting percentage of sterile flowers increased in one variety and decreased in the other compared with results in pure stands. Subsequent work indicated that this happened even when the roots were kept in separate containers and no competition of any kind was allowed. He suggested, therefore, that some volatile compounds might be involved, but pointed out that all other possibilities had not been ruled out completely.

Adams et al. (1970) reported that water-repellant soils are present under several shrub species in southeastern California and that these are particularly pronounced under Larrea divaricata, Prosopis juliflora, and Cercidium floridum. The outward extension generally coincides with the extension of the crown, indicating that substances leached from the aboveground parts of the plants are responsible. Fire increases the thickness of the hydrophobic layer of soil, and no annual plants start for several years after a fire even if the crowns are removed. Hummocks under the shrubs are nearly devoid of annual vegetation even without fire, whereas the surrounding soil is densely populated with annuals. This is clearly a case of allelopathy, because the effect is due to substances added to the environment by the shrubs, but it certainly represents an apparently unusual mechanism of action. In this case, available soil moisture is simply decreased under the shrubs.

As I stated at the beginning of this chapter, the mechanisms of action of allelopathic agents have not been adequately researched. The future will no doubt reveal many important mechanisms that we know nothing about at present. I hope this brief coverage may stimulate much more research in this important area of allelopathic studies.

14

Factors Affecting Quantities of Inhibitors Produced by Plants

I. INTRODUCTION

There is a growing interest on the part of biochemists, physiologists, ecologists, and others concerning the roles of phenolics and related compounds in living organisms. Consequently, considerable research has been carried out to determine factors that affect the amounts of such compounds in organisms, particularly in higher plants.

Early in my own research in allelopathy, I found that inhibitor plants growing in glass houses do not produce as large quantities of inhibitors as the same kinds of plants growing out-of-doors. This suggested an important effect of light quality on the production of inhibitors. My students, colleagues, and I also became interested in the possible roles of mineral deficiency in the production of inhibitors, because we were interested in old-field succession, and the old fields with which we were working were abandoned from cultivation because of low fertility (see Chapter 4). Our early work led to the study of the effects of other stress factors on the content of various phenolic inhibitors in plants. Many other persons have investigated effects of various factors on the phenolic content of plants because of an interest in the possible physiological roles of such compounds.

There has been a great deal of research done also on the effects of various factors on the production of commercially important antibiotics by microorganisms, but I will not review that work here.

II. EFFECTS OF RADIATION

A. Light quality

1. IONIZING RADIATION

Ionizing radiation markedly increases the amounts of various phenolic inhibitors in tobacco and sunflower plants (Fomenko, 1968; Koeppe *et al.*, 1970a). Fomenko (1968) found that exposure of sunflower plants to 20,000 R of ionizing radiation greatly increases the concentrations of caffeic acid and quercetin. Koeppe *et al.* (1970a) investigated the effects of 1000, 2500, and 4400 R of X irradiation on the concentrations of chlorogenic acid and scopolin (SCP) in tobacco plants (*Nicotiana tabacum* var. One Sucker). Amounts of chlorogenic acid (3-0-caffeoylquinic acid), neochlorogenic acid (5-0-caffeoylquinic acid), and band 510 (4-0-caffeoylquinic acid) were determined separately in this project and most others presented later, but I will add these values together and report the sum as total chlorogenic acids in my discussions here. Plants were harvested and analyzed at 12, 21, and 29 days after irradiation.

Substantial increases in scopolin because of irradiation were found at first harvest in roots, stems, and leaves, and the amounts were dose dependent. The concentrations remained higher in leaves and stems of plants exposed to the two highest doses throughout the test period. Total chlorogenic acids were decreased by all doses except for a temporary increase in leaves at first harvest owing to the highest dose.

2. ULTRAVIOLET RADIATION

Many workers have investigated the effects of UV treatment on the phenolic content of plants since Frey-Wyssling and Babler (1957) reported that greenhouse tobacco (*Nicotiana tabacum* var. Mont Calme brun) does not produce any rutin and only about one-seventh of the normal amount of chlorogenic acid (Lott, 1960; Koeppe *et al.*, 1969; del Moral, 1972; Hadwiger, 1972). Frey-Wyssling and Babler (1957) found that supplementation of greenhouse light with UV light improved the growth of greenhouse tobacco and increased the chlorogenic acid content from 0.41 to 2.52%. This approached the concentration present in control plants grown out-of doors, 2.72%.

Lott (1960), working with the same variety of tobacco as Frey-Wyssling and Babler (1957), found that the maximum increase in concentration of chlorogenic acid he could achieve in open air by supplementing natural radiation with UV light was 79%. On the other hand, he achieved a maximum increase of 550% in the greenhouse by supplementing the radiation with UV light. When he removed the short UV rays (below 350nm) from the supplemental irradiation, the maximum increase attained in the greenhouse was 287%. He found also that supplementation of normal radiation with short-wavelength UV light gave a maximum increase in concentration of rutin of 27% in open air plants and 28.5% in greenhouse plants.

Koeppe *et al.* (1969) conducted a thorough investigation of the effects of different levels of supplemental UV irradiation on concentrations of chlorogenic acids and scopolin in tobacco (*Nicotiana tabacum* var. One Sucker) and Russian mammoth sunflower plants. All levels of UV increased concentrations of scopolin in old leaves, young leaves, and stems of tobacco (Table 57), but only the low UV dose increased the concentration of this compound in the roots. All doses increased the concentrations of total chlorogenic acids in young leaves and stems of tobacco (Table 57), and the low dose increased the concentration in old leaves and roots. The medium dose increased the concentration of chlorogenic acids in old leaves also. All doses markedly increased the scopolin concentration in sunflower leaves, and the two highest doses increased the concentration of chlorogenic acids in sunflower leaves.

Del Moral (1972) found that supplemental UV light markedly increased concentrations of total chlorogenic and isochlorogenic acids in sunflower (*Helianthus annuus* var. not given) leaves, stems, and roots.

Hadwiger (1972) reported that psoralen plus 4 minutes of 366 nm UV light caused twice as much phenylalanine ammonia lyase (PAL) activity to be present in pea plants 3 hours after irradiation as in controls and 12 times as much PAL activity 20 hours after irradiation. Psoralen alone did not have this effect. PAL is the enzyme responsible for the formation of cinnamic acid from phenylalanine, and cinnamic acid derivatives and coumarins are produced from cinnamic acid (see Chapter 12, Sections II,G and H).

3. RED AND FAR-RED LIGHT

Jaffe and Isenberg (1969) demonstrated that concentrations of several phenolic compounds were increased at a faster rate in potato

TABLE 57

Effects of Varying Supplemental UV Intensities on Concentrations of Chlorogenic Acids and Scopolin in Tobacco Plants [a]

	μg/gm fresh weight	
Treatment [b]	Total chlorogenic acids	Scopolin
Older leaves		
Control	657	2.1
Low UV	910	3.1
Medium UV	675	11.3
High UV	464	59.3
Younger leaves		
Control	1290	4.5
Low UV	2076	7.6
Medium UV	1615	28.1
High UV	1797	38.6
Stems		
Control	143	11.0
Low UV	290	15.9
Medium UV	229	38.7
High UV	323	34.1
Roots		
Control	222	39.4
Low UV	234	46.2
Medium UV	187	37.4
High UV	89	19.5

[a] Data from Koeppe et al. (1969). Reproduced by permission of Microforms International Marketing Corporation.

[b] UV in mW/ft^2: Low, 1–1.5; medium, 4–5; high, 5–8.

tuber disks irradiated with red light than in disks irradiated with an equivalent dose of far-red light. The only phenolics identified were ferulic and p-coumaric acids.

In connection with a study on the effect of photoperiod on concentrations of alkaloids and phenolic compounds in tobacco plants, Tso et al. (1970) gave some plants on each photoperiod 5 minutes of red light at the end of each day (light period) and others 5 minutes of far-red light. Within each photoperiod, the plants receiving the red light every day had significantly higher concentrations of total alkaloids than those receiving far red. On the other hand, plants that received far red last each day had higher concentrations of soluble phenols, particularly of chlorogenic acid. The results concerning phenolics appear to be just the opposite from those of Jaffe and Isenberg (1969). This probably is not true, however, because the experiments were different in so many ways: (1) Jaffe and Isenberg worked with potato tuber disks, (2) the disks were irradiated with the given light quality for 24 hours each day, (3) Tso *et al.* used whole tobacco plants, and (4) the plants received only 5 minutes of red or far-red light at the end of each light cycle. Thus, the question concerning the relative effects of these two light qualities on the phenolic content of intact plants is still unanswered.

B. Intensity of Visible Light

Zucker (1963) found that visible light stimulates the synthesis of chlorogenic acid in potato tuber disks in water and it stimulates synthesis of *p*-coumaryl esters in similar disks in phenylalanine culture. A brief exposure to light of low intensity doubles the rate of synthesis of chlorogenic acid over that in darkness. Later, Zucker (1969) found that some photosynthetic product is necessary in apparently very small amounts for the synthesis of phenylalanine ammonia-lyase in *Xanthium* leaf disks. A very weak light for a short period suffices to produce the required material, however.

Jaffe and Isenberg (1969) found that white light at an intensity of 244 μW cm^{-2} sec^{-1} was not quite as effective in stimulating the formation of lignin in peeled potato tubers as red light at an intensity of 73 μW cm^{-2} sec^{-1}. They did not test other intensities of white light, so it is possible that a lower-intensity white light would be more effective than the intensity used. The relationship to the question being discussed is that cinnamic acid derivatives are precursors of lignin.

C. Daylength

It appears that long days generally increase phenolic acids and terpenes in plants regardless of the daylengths required for flowering (Taylor, 1965; Burbott and Loomis, 1967; Zucker, 1969). However, Zucker *et al.* (1965) discovered that concentrations of the chlorogenic acids increase markedly in the leaves of Maryland mammoth tobacco (short-day plant) and *Nicotiana sylvestris* (long-day plant) just prior to the change of the meristem from the vegetative to the flowering shape. This increase occurs under short days in Maryland mammoth tobacco and under long days in *N. sylvestris*. Taylor (1965) stated in his review of the literature that the biosynthesis of anthocyanins in *Kalanchoe blossfeldiana* is regulated also by the same photoperiodic conditions that regulate flowering.

Xanthium pennsylvanicum is a striking short-day plant because it will flower if given a single, long dark period. Nevertheless, much higher concentrations of chlorogenic acid, isochlorogenic acid, flavonoid aglycones, and quercetin glycosides are produced in the leaves on very long days (Taylor, 1965).

Burbott and Loomis (1967) found that *Mentha piperita* grows better and produces considerably greater concentrations of monoterpenes on long days. Under 8-hour days, temperature affects the composition of the terpenes produced, with warm nights producing oxidized terpenes, such as pulegone and menthofuran, while cold nights favor production of the more reduced compound, menthone. In long days, temperature does not affect the composition, with menthone predominating whatever the temperature.

Zucker (1969) reported that the induction of phenylalanine ammonia lyase increases in leaf disks of *Xanthium pennsylvanicum* with increases in daylength. This correlates well, of course, with the report of Taylor (1965) that many phenolics increase in leaves of *Xanthium pennsylvanicum* with increases in daylength, including several cinnamic acid derivatives.

III. MINERAL DEFICIENCIES

A. Boron

Watanabe *et al.* (1961) discovered a 20-fold increase in scopolin in leaves of tobacco plants that grew in a boron-free solution for 38 days. A few years later, Dear and Aronoff (1965) found a pronounced increase in caffeic and chlorogenic acids in leaves and growing points of boron-deficient sunflower plants. They found, also, that the ratio of caffeic acid to chlorogenic acid increased tenfold in the leaves and fourfold in the growing points of boron-deficient plants.

B. Calcium

Loche and Chouteau (1963) reported that concentrations of scopolin increase and those of chlorogenic acid decrease in leaves of tobacco plants deficient in calcium. This is the only report I have seen on the subject and much more needs to be done because calcium deficiency is very common in areas with high precipitation.

C. Magnesium

Loche and Chouteau (1963) found increases in concentrations of scopolin and decreases in chlorogenic acid in magnesium-deficient tobacco leaves just as they did in the case of calcium. Their results were supported by Armstrong *et al.* (1971) who found exactly the same effects in magnesium-deficient tobacco leaves. The scopolin concentration did not change, however, in Mg-deficient stems, but decreased in the deficient roots. The total chlorogenic acids decreased in concentration in Mg-deficient stems and roots, just as in the leaves.

D. Nitrogen

Chouteau and Loche (1965) again did some of the early research on effects of nitrogen deficiency on concentrations of phenolics in plants. They reported an increase in concentration of chlorogenic acid in nitrogen-deficient tobacco leaves, but did not analyze roots and stems. Shortly thereafter, Tso *et al.* (1967) reported a direct relationship between amounts of applied nitrogen and concentrations of chlorogenic acid and scopolin in three varieties of tobacco, with an inverse relationship in the fourth. For some strange reason, only the results with the fourth variety agree with the results of Chouteau and Loche (1965) and other workers (Armstrong *et al.*, 1970; del Moral, 1972; Lehman and Rice, 1972).

Armstrong *et al.* (1970) found very large increases in concentrations of total chlorogenic acids and scopolin in roots, stems, and leaves of nitrogen-deficient tobacco plants (*N. tabacum* var. One Sucker) (Table 58). There was almost a fivefold increase in concentration of total chlorogenic acids in leaves and stems and of scopolin in stems. Lehman and Rice (1972) found similar large increases in concentration of total chlorogenic acids in old leaves, stems, and roots of nitrogen-deficient Russian mammoth sunflower plants (Table 59). There was a very slight decrease, however, in concentration of scopolin in old leaves and stems of nitrogen-deficient sunflower plants. This last point is not of much significance, however, because the concentra-

TABLE 58

Concentrations of Chlorogenic Acids and Scopolin in Nitrogen-Deficient and Control Tobacco Plants 5 Weeks from Start of Treatment [a]

	μg/gm fresh weight	
Plant organ and treatment	Total chlorogenic acids	Scopolin
Leaves		
Control	1325	7.2
Deficient	6410	13.6
Stems		
Control	192	14.8
Deficient	932	70.8
Roots		
Control	479	140.6
Deficient	923	289.9

[a] Data from Armstrong *et al.* (1970). Reproduced by permission of Microforms International Marketing Corporation.

TABLE 59

Concentrations of Chlorogenic Acids and Scopolin in Nitrogen-Deficient and Control Sunflower Plants 5 Weeks from Start of Treatment [a]

	μg/gm fresh weight	
Plant organ and treatment	Total chlorogenic	Scopolin
Older leaves		
Control	1139	7.2
Deficient	8884	6.4
Younger leaves		
Control	1737	—[b]
Deficient	873	—[b]
Stems		
Control	383	1.8
Deficient	3275	—[b]
Roots		
Control	303	—[b]
Deficient	490	—[b]

[a] Data from Lehmen and Rice (1972).
[b] Below amounts determinable by procedure used.

tions of scopolin are low in various parts of sunflower plants. The increase in concentration of total chlorogenic acids in nitrogen-deficient old leaves was about eightfold, and it was about 8½-fold in N-deficient stems.

Del Moral (1972) reported very large increases in concentrations of total chlorogenic and isochlorogenic acids in roots, stems, and leaves of nitrogen-deficient sunflower plants. There was about a 10½-fold increase in concentration of total chlorogenic acids in N-deficient plants, based on his weighted mean data, and approximately an eightfold increase in concentration of isochlorogenic acids.

The very great increases in concentrations of inhibitors in plants that result from nitrogen deficiency are probably of great significance in allelopathy, because there are large areas of land deficient in nitrogen. I feel this is extremely important in connection with allelopathic mechanisms operating in revegetation of infertile old fields (see Chapter 4).

E. Phosphorus

Loche and Chouteau (1963) reported increases in scopolin concentration and decreases in chlorogenic acid in tobacco leaves deficient in phosphorus.

D. E. Koeppe (personal communication) grew Russian mammoth sunflower plants in three different levels of phosphorus: complete, one-tenth of the phosphorus in the complete solution, and no phosphorus. He analyzed the plants for concentrations of chlorogenic acids 22 days after the start of the treatments and found substantial increases in concentrations of total chlorogenic acids in leaves and stems treated with one-tenth phosphorus. There were very large increases in concentrations of total chlorogenic acids in the minus-phosphorus plants.

There is a widespread deficiency of easily soluble phosphorus in many soils (Rice et al., 1960). Over half the soils tested in eastern Oklahoma have been found to be deficient in phosphorus, with the subsurface soils having even lower amounts than the surface soils. Available phosphorus is particularly low in old fields that have been abandoned because of low fertility (Rice et al., 1960). Thus, the pronounced increases in inhibitors in plants resulting from phosphorus deficiency are probably very important in the allelopathic mechanisms operating during old-field succession (see Chapter 4).

F. Potassium

Chouteau and Loche (1965) reported decreased concentrations of chlorogenic acid in leaves of potassium-deficient tobacco plants. The results of Armstong *et al.* (1971) supported this report, because Armstrong *et al.* found decreases in concentrations of total chlorogenic acids in roots, stems, and leaves of tobacco plants (One Sucker) maintained on a potassium-free solution for 3–5 weeks. Concentrations of scopolin almost doubled in leaves of potassium-deficient tobacco plants, and they were slightly higher in roots and stems.

Lehman and Rice (1972) found that maintenance of Russian mammoth sunflower plants on a potassium-free solution for 5 weeks caused marked increases in concentrations of total chlorogenic acids in young leaves and stems (Table 60). Concentrations were increased in old leaves during the period from 1 to 4 weeks after start of treatment also. Concentrations of scopolin were increased in old leaves, young leaves, and stems of potassium-deficient sunflower plants (Table 60). In fact, the concentration in potassium-deficient old leaves was more than doubled 5 weeks after the start of treatment.

TABLE 60

Concentrations of Chlorogenic Acids and Scopolin in Potassium-Deficient and Control Sunflower Plants 5 Weeks after Start of Treatment [a]

Plant organ and treatment	μg/gm fresh weight	
	Total chlorogenic acids	Scopolin
Older leaves		
Control	1139	7.2
Deficient	832	16.5
Younger leaves		
Control	1737	—[b]
Deficient	2001	1.1
Stems		
Control	383	1.8
Deficient	1458	2.1
Roots		
Control	303	—[b]
Deficient	178	—[b]

[a] Data from Lehmen and Rice (1972).
[b] Below amounts determinable by procedure used.

TABLE 61

Concentrations of Chlorogenic Acids and Scopolin in Sulfur-Deficient and Control Sunflower Plants 5 Weeks after Start of Treatment [a]

Plant organ and treatment	μg/gm fresh weight	
	Total chlorogenic acids	Scopolin
Older leaves		
Control	1139	7.2
Deficient	4399	7.7
Younger leaves		
Control	1737	—[b]
Deficient	4272	—[b]
Stems		
Control	383	1.8
Deficient	1192	0.6
Roots		
Control	303	—[b]
Deficient	464	1.8

[a] Data from Lehmen and Rice (1972).
[b] Below amounts determinable by procedure used.

G. Sulfur

Lehman and Rice (1972) reported that the concentrations of total chlorogenic acids were substantially increased in old leaves, young leaves, stems, and roots of Russian mammoth sunflower plants grown in a sulfur-free solution for 5 weeks (Table 61). The concentrations of scopolin were slightly increased also in old leaves and roots of the sulfur-deficient plants, but slightly decreased in stems.

The increases in concentrations of total chlorogenic acids resulting from sulfur deficiency were surprisingly great, ranking second in amount only to the extremely large increases resulting from nitrogen deficiency.

IV. WATER STRESS

It has no doubt become obvious that all the factors discussed so far in this chapter which result in increased concentrations of inhibitors represent stress conditions to the plants. Water stress is certainly a very obvious stress condition, but very little has been done to determine its effect on the inhibitor content of plants.

Del Moral (1972) used NaCl in the culture solution to cause water stress of sunflower (*Helianthus annuus*) plants. The osmotic potential of the solution in the drought stress vessels ranged from −4.0 to −4.3 atmospheres during a 24-hour test period. After 31 days of treatment, the drought stress resulted in substantial increases in concentrations of total chlorogenic and isochlorogenic acids in roots, stems, and leaves over amounts in control plants.

Del Moral (1972) also tested effects of combinations of stress factors, and he found that a combination of water stress and exposure to supplemental UV light increased concentrations of total chlorogenic and isochlorogenic acids more than either factor alone, with normal nitrogen (Table 62). With nitrogen deficiency, however, the stimulatory effects of drought plus UV light were less than with drought alone. The greatest increases in concentrations of total chlorogenic and isochlorogenic acids, on a whole-plant basis, resulted from a combination of drought stress and nitrogen deficiency. This combination resulted in a 15-fold increase in concentration of total chlorogenic acids and a 16-fold increase in concentration of total isochlorogenic acids.

The synergistic effects of stress factors are particularly important because they generally occur in combinations under field conditions.

TABLE 62

Effects of Stress Factors on Concentrations of Total chlorogenic Acids and Total Isochlorogenic Acids in Sunflower Plants [a]

	μg/gm dry weight [b]	
Stress applied	Total chlorogenic acids	Total isochlorogenic acids
None—control	43	135
UV light	113	203
−H$_2$O	258	320
UV; −H$_2$O	455	512
−Nitrogen	458	1065
−Nitrogen; UV	310	375
−Nitrogen; −H$_2$O	645	2185
−Nitrogen; −H$_2$O; UV	546	979

[a] Data from del Moral (1972).
[b] Weighted mean of leaf, stem, and root tissues.

TABLE 63

Effect of Chilling Temperatures on Concentrations of Chlorogenic Acids
and Scopolin in Tobacco Plants 24 Days after Start of Treatment [a]

| Organ and treatment | μg/gm fresh weight [b] | |
	Total chlorogenic acids	Scopolin
Older leaves		
Control	1204	9.4
Chilled	3812	12.2
Younger leaves		
Control	1714	4.0
Chilled	4387	1.1
Stems		
Control	205	109.0
Chilled	965	96.5
Roots		
Control	2460	555.0
Chilled	860	178.0

[a] Data from Koeppe et al. (1970b).

Conditions that cause low fertility in soils, such as excessive erosion, often result in soils with lower infiltration rates and thus in soils that are often deficient in available water. These combinations would increase, therefore, the allelopathic potentials of inhibitory species.

V. TEMPERATURE

Martin (1957) found that about 7½ times as much scopoletin exuded from roots of oat plants in 72 hours at 30°C than in 135 hours at 19°C. Obviously, this does not necessarily relate directly to the amount of scopoletin produced, but it does relate to the intensity of any allelopathic effect resulting from the scopoletin.

Koeppe et al. (1970b) maintained tobacco plants (One Sucker) on temperatures of either 32°C (control) or 8°–9°C (chilled) during a 16-hour light period each day, and all plants were subjected to a dark period temperature of 15°–16°C each day. Chilling increased the concentrations of total chlorogenic acids markedly in old leaves, young leaves, and stems, but decreased the concentration in the roots (Table 63). Chilling also increased the concentration of scopolin slightly in old leaves, but decreased the concentrations substantially in young

VII. AGE OF PLANT ORGANS

Koeppe *et al.* (1969) found that the concentrations of scopolin and chlorogenic acids in leaves of tobacco plants varied with the ages of the leaves, even in control plants. Because of these results, Koeppe *et al.* (1970c) decided to determine the effect of tissue age on concentrations of chlorogenic and isochlorogenic acids in native sunflower plants (*Helianthus annuus*) collected in old fields near Norman, Oklahoma. Concentrations of total chlorogenic acids increased with increase in age of leaves to node 6 (Table 64), after which they declined. On the other hand, concentrations of total isochlorogenic acids decreased with increasing age of leaves from the apex. Concentrations of both total chlorogenic acids and total isochlorogenic acids in stems decreased with increasing age from the apex to node 5 or node 6, after which the concentrations began to increase again very slowly with age.

Koeppe *et al.* (1970b) discovered that the concentrations of scopolin

TABLE 64

Effect of Age on Concentrations of Chlorogenic and Isochlorogenic Acids in Leaves of Native Sunflower, *Helianthus annuus,* in Field [a]

	μg/gm fresh weight	
Harvest time and leaf position	Total chlorogenic acids	Relative isochlorogenic acids
May 2[b]		
Apex	2465	157.3
Nodes 3,4	3094	109.2
Nodes 5,6	3894	66.4
May 24 [b]		
Apex	1892	182.5
Nodes 3,4	1960	146.0
Node 6	2603	159.2
Node 8	2445	100.8
Node 10	2082	88.2
Node 12	925	30.6
Node 14	863	28.4

Data from Koeppe *et al.* (1970c). Reproduced by permission of Microforms International Marketing Corporation.

[b] May 2, plants 16–24 cm tall; May 24, plants 48–64 cm tall.

and total chlorogenic acids decreased with age of leaves in tobacco but, owing to the increase in size with age, the total amounts of these compounds increased with age in the leaves.

VIII. GENETICS

Unfortunately, I know of no published work that presents data relating the relative allelopathic effect of any plants to their genetic make-up. There has been considerable research done concerning the kinds of phenolic compounds present in many species of plants (Harborne, 1964; Harborne and Simmonds, 1964) and on the genetic variation of anthocyanin pigments in flowers and other plant parts (Harborne, 1960; Pecket, 1960). Feenstra (1960) worked out the genetics concerning the formation of phenolic compounds in the seedcoat of the French bean (*Phaseolus vulgaris*), but this was just in relation to seed-coat color.

All persons who have worked in the field of allelopathy become aware very quickly that plants of the same species growing close together vary greatly in their allelopathic effects. Obviously, this could be due in part to differences in the microhabitats and thus to differences in stress conditions. It is logical to assume that genetics must play an important role also in determining amounts of inhibitors produced by a given plant and the sensitivity of the plant to the stress factors discussed above.

I suspect that a species such as *Ambrosia psilostachya* [which invades old fields in Oklahoma in the pioneer weed stage, almost entirely disappears before the *Aristida oligantha* stage (second stage) becomes prominent, reappears in the perennial bunchgrass stage, and remains in the climax prairie] may vary greatly genetically in the different stages. The plants of this species which appear in the pioneer weed stage are very inhibitory to several species of that stage and probably help to eliminate the pioneer weed stage rapidly (Neill and Rice, 1971). I feel it is doubtful that the plants of this species which persist into the climax exert the same allelopathic impact, but only additional research can determine whether this suggestion is correct.

I feel there is a great need for research on the genetics of allelopathy. It seems to me that individuals interested in both genetics and allelopathy could make important contributions to both areas by combining them.

15

Interrelations of Allelopathy with Other Types of Chemical Interactions

I. INTRODUCTION

Molisch (1937), the originator of the term allelopathy, was very much aware of the biochemical interactions between plants and animals, and between one animal and another, in addition to the interaction between plants. Early in his book on allelopathy, he pointed out that he was confining himself to the mutual influence of plants and was omitting animals from consideration. As research has progressed, it has become increasingly obvious that there are many close relationships between the various types of chemical interactions. Many of the same, or related, compounds are involved in all the types of interaction listed above, as has been so admirably pointed out by Whittaker (1971) and Whittaker and Feeny (1971). In recognition of this fact, Whittaker (1971) suggested that all interspecies chemical agents significant for chemical effects other than use as food be called allelochemics.

The question may arise in the minds of some readers as to why I have not included all types of interspecies interactions in this monograph under the title of "allelochemics," and the answer is primarily a lack of space. I feel it is very important, however, that the reader be left with a better appreciation of relationships between the various types of biochemical interactions than these brief remarks can accomplish. The rest of this chapter is devoted, therefore, to a rather brief discussion of selected examples of plant–animal interactions.

II. CHEMICAL INTERACTIONS BETWEEN PLANTS AND INSECTS

One obvious example of this type of chemical interaction is that between plants and gall-forming insects in which the insects produce chemicals that stimulate the plant tissue to proliferate (Grümmer, 1955). Conversely, plants produce compounds that are of special significance to insects. Here belong the chemicals that determine the feeding behavior of insects, the growth and molting of insects (the ecdysones), the juvenile hormones, and the lures or attractants directing parasitic insects to their host plants (the pheromones).

One of the fundamental relationships between insects and plants involves the feeding behavior of phytophagous insects (Fraenkel, 1959). In lepidopterous larvae, both olfaction and taste are important in food–plant preference and in the initiation of feeding in general (Dethier, 1969). An important aspect of plant survival involves the production by plants of chemicals that prevent feeding by various insects. Klun (1969) reported that 2,4-dihydroxy-7-methoxy-1,4($2H$) benzoxazin-3-one is an important chemical factor in the resistance of dent corn to the European corn borer. Wahlroos and Virtanen (1959) had previously isolated this compound from maize. Quantitative analysis of dried whorl corn tissue for the benzoxazolinone degradation product of the inhibitor can be used as a chemical indicator of level of host plant resistance in single cross strains and inbred strains of corn (Klun, 1969). The extrafloral nectaries of one species of cotton (*Gossypium hirsutum*) are an important food source for various cotton-attacking insects of the genus *Heliothis* (Lukefahr *et al.*, 1969). These investigators transferred the nectariless character from *Gossypium tomentosum* to certain strains of *G. hirsutum*, making these strains more resistant to feeding by *Heliothis* spp. Todd *et al.* (1971) reported that resistance in barley to the greenbug, *Schizaphis graminum*, is apparently related to the presence in the barley of numerous phenolic and flavonoid compounds and related substances.

Lukefahr *et al.* (1969) found that gossypol and related compounds in cotton plants inhibit larval growth of these insects. Thorsteinson (1969) showed that adult female diamondback moths lay eggs much more densely on rugose plastic surfaces coated with allyl isothiocyanate (mustard oil), a characteristic constituent of their food plants. He found that the mustard oil also stimulates ovarian development in adult moths that are in a prereproductive state.

Many ecdysones (molting hormones) have been isolated from plants and identified (Nakanishi, 1969). A massive screening of plant species for these compounds has been carried on in Japan because of the obvious practical role the ecdysones could play in insect control. By 1967, 186 of the 188 families of higher plants in Japan, including 738 genera and 1056 species had already been assayed for ecdysone activity (Nakanishi, 1969). Forty species provided active extracts.

A female polyphemus moth (*Polyphemus*) will not release her sex pheromone except in the presence of oak leaves which emit *trans*-2-hexenal (Riddiford and Williams, 1967; Riddiford, 1969). In rather low concentrations, this compound promotes the release of the attractant pheromone, but in high concentrations it elicits ovipositional behavior even from virgin female moths. Rudinsky (1966, 1969) found that the Douglas fir beetle, *Dendroctonus pseudotsugae*, first aggregates in response to host substances (i.e., oleoresin and terpenes: camphene, limonene, and α-pinene). Female beetles are attracted to physiologically weakened trees characterized by low oleoresin pressure and high internal water stress. After tunneling into the phloem, these beetles signal their presence by secreting a pheromone that attracts additional males and females. Rudinsky found that similar primary and secondary attraction exists in *Pseudohylesinus nebulosus* and *Scolytus unispinosus*, and that terpenes are also the substances aggregating the predators of these beetles. Among ambrosia beetles, *Trypodendron lineatum* produces its pheromone only after mating and feeding on wood particles. According to Rudinsky (1969), most of the terpenes found in the Douglas fir act as repellents at concentrations above 1%, but are attractants at 0.1% and below to most of the insect species associated with Douglas fir.

Another scolytid beetle, *Ips confusus*, also uses an assembly pheromone in its attack on the ponderosa pine, *Pinus ponderosa* (Silverstein *et al.*, 1966; Silverstein, 1969). The tree is first attacked by a few male beetles, and, as they tunnel into the bark, they produce frass containing an extremely potent attractant for both male and female *Ips confusus*.

III. CHEMICAL INTERACTIONS BETWEEN PLANTS AND ANIMALS OTHER THAN INSECTS

There is much less organized material of a basic ecological nature on this subject than the previous one concerning chemical interactions between plants and insects. Nevertheless, there are many kinds of biochemical interactions between plants (including micro-organisms) and animals other than insects. One obvious and significant area is that of production of toxins by bacteria and fungi which are pathogenic to man and other mammals (Grümmer, 1955). Several of the fleshy fungi, such as some species of *Amanita*, are very poisonous to man and some other animals.

Several species of *Ranunculus,* buttercup, produce chemicals that make them very distasteful to grazing animals, and some species pro-duce protoanemonin, which can lead to fatal convulsions in livestock (Kingsbury, 1964). According to Kingsbury (1964), *Digitalis purpurea* and some other plants produce steroid cardiac glycosides that cause convulsive heart attacks in vertebrates that eat them. He points out that there are other numerous higher plant species poisonous to man and other animals. Virtually everyone is aware of certain plants, such as *Rhus radicans,* poison ivy, and others which cause a dermatitis in man.

Man has made use of many biochemicals produced by plants in his treatment of ailments of humans and other animals, certainly since the beginning of recorded history and probably before. A great many ani-mals use carotin produced by green plants to manufacture vitamin A in their own bodies. According to Boutwell (1967), some materials of plant origin such as croton oil, certain euphorbia latices, citrus oils, and extracts of unburned tobacco promote the development of skin cancers in mice. He pointed out also that tannic acid administered parenterally to rats caused benign multiple liver tumors to develop in 56% of those that survived treatment for 300 days.

According to Lucas (1947), Pearcey, in 1885, reported a scarcity of herring in waters where the diatoms *Rhizosolenia shrubsolei* and *Tha-lassiosira nordenskioldii* were abundant as well as the scarcity of zoo-plankton under such conditions. Kofoid (1911) suggested that the wholesale death of fish off the California coast might be due to the products of the dense masses of dinoflagellates that were associated with the fish. Numerous later workers confirmed Pearcey's observa-tions concerning the scarcity of herring in places where various dia-toms were present in large numbers (Lucas, 1947). Much evidence has accumulated also indicating that Kofoid may have been correct in his suggestion. *Gonyaulax catenella* synthesizes a toxin that is about ten times as potent as strychnine when tested on mice (Saunders, 1957). The toxin has little effect on fish, but humans have been killed by eating shellfish that collect *Gonyaulax* in their guts. *Gonyaulax tamerensis* poisonings have been reported from Novia Scotia. Accord-ing to Davis (1948), *Gymnodinium brevis* has caused the mass death of marine organisms off the west coast of Florida. Shilo and Aschner (1953) reported that *Prymnesium parvum,* a phytoflagellate of the Chrysophyceae, produces an extracellular toxin that kills fish or other organisms which obtain oxygen by means of gills.

Prescott (1948) and Scott (1952) reported that several blue-green algae produce intracellular toxins that are released only on death and decay or ingestion by animals. Sheep, horses, dogs, pigs, cattle, chickens, turkeys, ducks, geese, and rabbits have been reported to be killed by drinking water that contains large numbers of these algae. Injections of the algae into test animals killed the animals, but injection of pond water from which the algae were filtered did not affect the test animals. The genera of the Cyanophyta which have been reported to contain toxic species are *Anabaena, Aphanizomenon, Coelosphaerium, Microcystis,* and *Nodularia* (Saunders, 1957).

It is obvious that plant–animal and plant–plant biochemical interactions have many similar important ecological implications. It is noteworthy that many of the same terpenes, phenols, flavonoids, and other types of compounds are involved in both major types of chemical interactions (Muller and Muller, 1964; Rice, 1965a, 1969; Rudinsky, 1966, 1969; Boutwell, 1967; Wilson and Rice, 1968; Lukefahr *et al.,* 1969; Parenti and Rice, 1969; Silverstein, 1969; Al-Naib and Rice, 1971; Lodhi and Rice, 1971; Todd *et al.,* 1971; Whittaker, 1971; Whittaker and Feeny, 1971; Chou and Muller, 1972).

Bibliography

Abdul-Wahab, A. S. (1964). The toxicity of Johnson grass excretions: A mechanism of root competition. Master's Thesis, Louisiana State University, Baton Rouge.

Abdul-Wahab, A. S., and Rice, E. L. (1967). Plant inhibition by Johnson grass and its possible significance in old-field succession. *Bull. Torrey Bot. Club* **94**, 486–497.

Adams, S., Strain, B. R., and Adams, M. S. (1970). Water-repellent soils, fire, and annual plant cover in desert scrub community of southeastern California. *Ecology* **51**, 696–700.

Addoms, R. M. (1937). Nutritional studies of loblolly pine. *Plant Physiol.* **12**, 199–205.

Agnihothrudu, B. (1955). Incidence of fungistatic organisms in the rhizosphere of pigeon pea (*Cajanus cajan*) in relation to resistance and susceptibility to wilt caused by *Fusarium udum* Butler. *Naturwissenschaften* **42**, 373.

Agnihotri, V. P., and Vaartaja, O. (1968). Seed exudates from *Pinus resinosa* and their effects on growth and zoospore germination of *Pythium afertile*. *Can. J. Bot.* **46**, 1135.

Ahshapanek, D. C. (1962). Ecological studies on plant inhibition by *Solanum rostratum*. Ph.D. Dissertation, University of Oklahoma, Norman.

Akehurst, S.C. (1931). Observations on pond life, with special reference to the possible causation of swarming of phytoplankton. *J. Roy. Microsc. Soc.* [3]**51**, 237–265.

Alexander, M. (1961). "Introduction to Soil Microbiology." Wiley, New York.

Alexander, M., and Clark, F. E. (1965). Nitrifying bacteria. *In* "Methods of Soil Analysis" (C. A. Black *et al.*, eds.), Vol. 2, pp. 1477–1483. Amer. Soc. Agron., Madison, Wisconsin.

Allison, F. E. (1931). Forms of nitrogen assimilated by plants. *Quart. Rev. Biol.* **6**, 313–321.

Al-Naib, F. A. (1968). Allelopathic effects of *Platanus occidentalis* L. Master's Thesis, University of Oklahoma, Norman.

Al-Naib, F. A., and Rice, E. L. (1971). Allelopathic effects of *Platanus occidentalis*. *Bull. Torrey Bot. Club* **98**, 75–82.

Andreae, W. A. (1952). Effects of scopoletin on indoleacetic acid metabolism. *Nature (London)* **170**, 83–84.

Anonymous. (1962). Dutch elm disease fungus makes anti-ATP. *Chem. & Eng. News* **40**, 55.

Anonymous. (1969). Natural weed killer. *Sci. Amer.* **221**, 54.

317

Armstrong, G. M., Rohrbaugh, L. M., Rice, E. L., and Wender, S. H. (1970). The effect of nitrogen deficiency on the concentration of caffeoylquinic acids and scopolin in tobacco. *Phytochemistry* **9**, 945–948.

Armstrong; G. M., Rohrbaugh, L. M., Rice, E. L., and Wender, S. H. (1971). Preliminary studies on the effect of deficiency in potassium or magnesium on concentration of chlorogenic acid and scopolin in tobacco. *Proc. Okla. Acad. Sci.* **51**, 41–43.

Arnold, J. F. (1964). Zonation of understory vegetation around a juniper tree. *J. Range Manage.* **17**, 41–42.

Asplund, R. O. (1968). Monoterpenes: Relationship between structure and inhibition of germination. *Phytochemistry* **7**, 1995–1997.

Asplund, R. O. (1969). The phytotoxicity of essential oils of different species of sage-brush. *Wyo. Range Manage.* **270**, 40–43.

Avers, C. J., and Goodwin, R. H. (1956). Studies on roots. IV. Effects of coumarin and scopoletin on the standard root growth pattern of *Phleum pratense. Amer. J. Bot.* **43**, 612–620.

Baer, H., Holden, M., and Seegal, B. C. (1946). The nature of the antibacterial agent from *Anemone pulsatilla. J. Biol. Chem.* **162**, 65–68.

Baker, H. G. (1966). Volatile growth inhibitors produced by *Eucalyptus globulus. Madrono, S. Francisco* **18**, 207–210.

Ballester, A., and Vieitez, E. (1971). Estudio de sustancias de crecimiento aisladas de *Erica cinerea* L. *Acta Cient. Compostelana* **8**, 79–84.

Basaraba, J. (1964). Influence of vegetable tannins on nitrification in soil. *Plant Soil* **21**, 8–16.

Baskin, J. M., Ludlow, C. J., Harris, T. M., and Wolf, F. T. (1967). Psoralen, an inhibitor in the seeds of *Psoralea subacaulis* (Leguminosae). *Phytochemistry* **6**, 1209–1213.

Bate-Smith, E. C., and Metcalfe, C. R. (1957). The nature and systematic distribution of tannins in dicotyledonous plants. *J. Linn. Soc. London, Bot.* **55**, 669–705.

Battle, J. P., and Whittington, W. J. (1969). The relation between inhibitory substances and variability in time to germination of sugar beet clusters. *J. Agr. Sci.* **73**, 337–346.

Bauchop, T. (1971). Stomach microbiology of primates. *Annu. Rev. Microbiol.* **25**, 429–436.

Becker, Y., Guillemat, J., Guyot, L., and Lelievre, D. (1951). Sur un aspect phytopathologique du probleme des substances racinaires toxiques. *C. R. Acad. Sci.* **233**, 198–199.

Becking, J. H. (1961). A requirement of molybdenum for the symbiotic nitrogen fixation in alder (*Alnus glutinosa* Gaertn.). *Plant Soil* **15**, 217–227.

Beggs, J. P. (1964). Spectacular clover establishment with formalin treatment suggests growth inhibitor in soil. *N. Z. J. Agr.* **108**, 529–535.

Bell, D. T., and Koeppe, D. E. (1972). Noncompetitive effects of giant foxtail on the growth of corn. *Agron. J.* **64**, 321–325.

Bell, D. T., and Muller, C. H. (1973). Dominance of California annual grasslands by *Brassica nigra. Amer. Mid. Natur.* **90**, 277–299.

Benedict, H. M. (1941). The inhibitory effect of dead roots on the growth of bromegrass. *J. Amer. Soc. Agron.* **33**, 1108–1109.

Bennett, E., and Bonner, J. (1953). Isolation of plant growth inhibitors from *Thamnosma montana. Amer. J. Bot.* **40**, 29–33.

Benoit, R. E., and Starkey, R. L. (1968a). Enzyme inactivation as a factor in the inhibition of decomposition of organic matter by tannins. *Soil Sci.* **105**, 203–208.

Benoit, R. E., and Starkey, R. L. (1968b). Inhibition of decomposition of cellulose and some other carbohydrates by tannin. *Soil Sci.* **105**, 291–296.

Benoit, R. E., Starkey, R. L., and Basaraba, J. (1968). Effect of purified plant tannin on decomposition of some organic compounds and plant materials. *Soil Sci.* **105**, 153–158.

Bentley, H. R., Cunningham, K. G., and Spring, F. S. (1951). Cordycepin, a metabolic product from cultures of *Cordyceps militaris* (Linn.) Link. Part II. The structure of cordycepin. *J. Chem. Soc., London*, pp. 2301–2305.

Berestetsky, O. A. (1970). On the role of decomposition products of root residue for garden soil toxicity. *In* "Physiological–Biochemical Basis of Plant Interactions in Phytocenoses" (A. M. Grodzinsky, ed.), Vol. 1, pp. 113–118. Naukova Dumka, Kiev. (In Russian)

Berestetsky, O. A. (1972). Formation of phytotoxic substances by soil microorganisms on root residues of fruit trees. *In* "Physiological-Biochemical Basis of Plant Interactions in Phytocenoses" (A. M. Grodzinsky, ed.), Vol. 3, pp. 121–124. Naukova Dumka, Kiev. (In Russian)

Berlier, Y., Dabin, B., and Leneuf, N. (1956). Comparaison physique, chimique et microbiologique entre les sols de foret et de savane sur les sables tertiaires de la Basse Côte d'Ivoire. *Trans. Int. Congr. Soil Sci., 6th, 1956* E. pp. 499–502.

Bevage, D. I. (1968). Inhibition of seedling hoop pine (*Araucaria cunninghamii* Aiz.) on forest soils by phytotoxic substances from the root zone of *Pinus*, *Araucaria*, and *Flindersia*. *Plant Soil* **29**, 263–273.

Bieber, G. L., and Hoveland, C. S. (1968). Phytotoxicity of plant materials on seed germination of crownvetch, *Coronilla varia* L. *Agron. J.* **60**, 185–188.

Blum, U., and Rice, E. L. (1969). Inhibition of symbiotic nitrogen-fixation by gallic and tannic acid, and possible roles in old-field succession. *Bull. Torrey Bot. Club* **96**, 531–544.

Boawn, L. C. (1965). Sugar beet induced zinc deficiency. *Agron. J.* **57**, 509.

Bode, H. R. (1940). Über die Blattausscheidungen des Wermuts und ihre Werkung auf andere Pflanzen. *Planta* **30**, 567–589.

Bode, H. R. (1958). Beiträge zur Kenntnis Allelopathischer Erscheinungen bei einigen Juglandaceen. *Planta* **51**, 440–480.

Bold, H. C. (1949). The morphology of *Chlamydomonas chlamydogama* sp. nov. *Bull. Torrey Bot. Club* **76**, 108.

Bonner, J. (1946). Further investigation of toxic substances which arise from guayule plants: Relation of toxic substances to the growth of guayule in soil. *Bot. Gaz. (Chicago)* **107**, 343–351.

Bonner, J. (1950). The role of toxic substances in the interactions of higher plants. *Bot. Rev.* **16**, 51–65.

Bonner, J., and Galston, A. W. (1944). Toxic substances from the culture media of guayule which may inhibit growth. *Bot. Gaz. (Chicago)* **106**, 185–198.

Booth, W. E. (1941a). Revegetation of abandoned fields in Kansas and Oklahoma. *Amer. J. Bot.* **28**, 415–422.

Booth, W. E. (1941b). Algae as pioneers in plant succession and their importance in erosion control. *Ecology* **22**, 38–46.

Börner, H. (1959). The apple replant problem. I. The excretion of phlorizin from apple root residues. *Contrib. Boyce Thompson Inst.* **20**, 39–56.

Börner, H. (1960). Liberation of organic substances from higher plants and their role in the soil sickness problem. *Bot. Rev.* **26**, 393–424.

Börner, H. (1963a). Untersuchungen über die Bildung antiphytotischer und antimikrobieller Substanzen durch Mikroorganismen im Boden und ihre mogliche Bedeutung für die Bodenmudigkeit beim Apfel (*Pirus malus* L.) I. Bildung von Patulin und einer phenolischen Verbindung durch *Penicillium expansum* auf Wurzel-und Blattrückstanden des Apfel. *Phytopathol. Z.* **48**, 370–396.

Börner, H. (1963b). Untersuchungen über die Bildung antiphytotischer und antimikrobieller Substanzen durch Mikroorganismen im Boden und ihre mogliche Bedeutung für die Bodenmudigkeit beim Apfel (*Pirus malus* L.). II. Der Einflutz verschiedener Factoren auf die Bildung von Patulin und einer phenolischen Verbindung durch *Penicillium expansum* auf Blatt-und Wurzelrückstanden des Apfels. *Phytopathol. Z.* **49**, 1–28.

Boughey, A. S., Munro, P. E., Meiklejohn, J., Strang, R. M., and Swift, M. J. (1964). Antibiotic reactions between African savanna species. *Nature (London)* **203**, 1302–1303.

Bould, C., and Hewitt, E. J. (1963). Mineral nutrition of plants in soils and in culture media. *In* "Plant Physiology" (F. C. Steward, ed.), Vol. 3, pp. 15–133. Academic Press, New York.

Boutwell, R. K. (1967). Phenolic compounds as tumor-promoting agents. *In* "Phenolic Compounds and Metabolic Regulation" (B. J. Finkle and V. C. Runeckles, eds.), pp. 121–141. Appleton, New York.

Bowen, G. D. (1961). The toxicity of legume seed diffusates toward Rhizobia and other bacteria. *Plant Soil* **15**, 155–165.

Bremner, J. M. (1965). Inorganic forms of nitrogen. *In* "Methods of Soil Analysis" (C. A. Black *et al.*, eds.), Vol. 2, pp. 1179–1237. Amer. Soc. Agron., Madison, Wisconsin.

Brown, D. D. (1968). The possible ecological significance of inhibition by *Euphorbia supina*. Master's Thesis, University of Oklahoma, Norman.

Brown, R. T. (1967). Influence of naturally occurring compounds on germination and growth of jack pine. *Ecology* **48**, 542–546.

Brown, S. A. (1964). Lignin and tannin biosynthesis. *In* "Biochemistry of Phenolic Compounds" (J. B. Harborne, ed.), pp. 361–398. Academic Press, New York.

Buchholtz, K. P. (1971). The influence of allelopathy on mineral nutrition. *In* "Biochemical Interactions among Plants" (U. S. Nat. Comm. for IBP, eds.), pp. 86–89. Nat. Acad. Sci., Washington, D. C.

Bukolova, T. P. (1971). A study of the mechanism of action of water-soluble substances of weeds on cultivated plants. *In* "Physiological-Biochemical Basis of Plant Interactions in Phytocenoses" (A. M. Grodzinsky, ed.), Vol. 2, pp. 66–69. Naukova Dumka, Kiev. (In Russian)

Burbott, A. J., and Loomis, W. D. (1967). Effects of light and temperature on the monoterpenes of peppermint. *Plant Physiol.* **42**, 20–28.

Burkholder, P. R., Burkholder, L. M., and Almdóvar, L. R. (1960). Antibiotic activity of some marine algae of Puerto Rico. *Bot. Mar.* **2**, 149–156.

Buxton, E. W. (1960). Effects of pea root exudate on the antagonism of some rhizosphere microorganisms toward *Fusarium oxysporum f. pisi. J. Gen. Microbiol.* **22**, 678–689.

Byrde, R. J. W., Fielding, A. H., and Williams, A. H. (1960). The roles of oxidized polyphenols in the varietal resistance of apples to brown rot. *In* "Phenolics in Plants in Health and Disease" (J. B. Pridham, ed.), pp. 95–99. Pergamon, Oxford.

Cadman, C. H. (1959). Some properties of an inhibitor of virus infection from leaves of raspberry. *J. Gen. Microbiol.* **20**, 113–128.

Cain, J. C. (1952). A comparison of ammonium and nitrate nitrogen for blueberries. *Proc. Amer. Soc. Hort. Sci.* **59**, 161.

Campbell, H. (1964). Notes on viability of honey locust seeds in relation to age. *Turtox News* **42**, 134–135.

Cavallito, C. J., and Bailey, J. H. (1944). Allicin, the antibacterial principle of *Allium sativum*. I. Isolation, physical properties and anti-bacterial action. *J. Amer. Chem. Soc.* **66**, 1950–1951.

Cavallito, C. J. and Haskell, T. H. (1945). The mechanism of antibiotics. The reaction of unsaturated lactones with cysteine and related compounds. *J. Amer. Chem. Soc.* **67**, 1991–1994.

Cavallito, C. J., Buck, J. S., and Suter, C. M. (1944). Allicin, the antibacterial principle of *Allium sativum*. II. Determination of the chemical structure. *J. Amer. Chem. Soc.* **66**, 1952–1954.

Cavallito, C. J., Bailey, J. H., and Buck, J. S. (1945). The antibacterial principle of *Allium sativum*. III. Its precursor and "essential oil" of garlic. *J. Amer. Chem. Soc.* **67**, 1032–1033.

Chaffin, W. A. (no date). Soil improvement program for Oklahoma, *Okla., Agr. Exp. Sta., Extension Ser., Cir.* **412**.

Chambers, E. E., and Holm, L. G. (1965). Phosphorus uptake as influenced by associated plants. *Weeds* **13**, 312–314.

Chesters, C. G. C., and Stott, J. A. (1956). The production of antibiotic substances by seaweeds. *Proc. Int. Seaweed Symp., 2nd, 1956*, pp. 49–54.

Chou, C-H., and Muller, C. H. (1972). Allelopathic mechanisms of *Arctostaphylos glandulosa* var. *zacaensis*. *Amer. Midl. Natur.* **88**, 324–347.

Chouteau, J., and Loche, J. (1965). Incidence de la nutrition azotée de la plante de tabac sur l'accumulation des composés phenoliques dans les feuilles. *C. R. Acad. Sci.* **260**, 4568–4588.

Christersson, L. (1972). The influence of urea and other nitrogen sources on growth rate of Scots pine seedlings. *Physiol. Plant.* **27**, 83–88.

Clark, R. S., Kúc, J., Henze, R. E., and Quackenbush, F. W. (1959). The nature and fungitoxicity of an amino-acid addition product of chlorogenic acid. *Phytopathology* **49**, 594–597.

Cobb, E. W. J., Krstic, M., Zavarin, E., and Barbe, H. W., Jr. (1968). Inhibitory effects of volatile oleoresin component on *Fomes annosus* and four *Ceratocystis* species (disease resistance). *Phytopathology* **58**, 1327–1335.

Cochrane, V. W. (1948). The role of plant residues in the etiology of root rot. *Phytopathology* **38**, 185–196.

Condon, P., and Kúc, J. (1960). Isolation of a fungitoxic compound from carrot root tissue inoculated with *Ceratocystis fimbriata*. *Phytopathology* **50**, 267–270.

Conn, E. E., and Akazawa, T. (1958). Biosynthesis of p-hydroxybenzaldehyde. *Fed. Proc., Fed. Amer. Soc. Exp. Biol.* **17**, 205.

Conn, H. J., and Bright, J. W. (1919). Ammonification of manure in soil. *J. Agr. Res.* **16**, 313–350.

Cook, M. T. (1921). Wilting caused by walnut trees. *Phytopathology* **11**, 346.

Cook, M. T., and Taubenhaus, J. J. (1911). The relation of parasitic fungi to the contents of the cells of the host plants. I. The toxicity of tannin. *Del., Agr. Exp. Sta., Bull.* **91**, 3–77.

Cooper, W. E., and Chilton, S. J. P. (1950). Studies on antibiotic soil organisms. I. Actinomycetes antibiotic to *Pythium arrhenomanes* in sugar-cane soils in Louisiana. *Phytopathology* **40**, 544–552.

Cooper, W. S., and Stoesz, A. D. (1931). The subterranean organs of *Helianthus scaberrimus*. *Bull. Torrey Bot. Club* **58**, 67–72.

Corcoran, M. R. (1970). Inhibitors from Carob (*Ceratonia siliqua* L.) II. Effect on growth induced by indoleacetic acid or gibberellins A_1, A_4, A_5, and A_7. *Plant Physiol.* **46**, 531–534.

Cornelius, D. R. (1969). Influence of temperature and leachate on germination of *Atriplex polycarpa. Agron. J.* **61**, 209–211.

Cornman, I. (1946). Alteration of mitosis by coumarin and parasorbic acid. *Amer. J. Bot.* **33**, 217.

Corse, J., Lundin, R. E., and Waiss, A. C., Jr. (1965). Identification of several components of isochlorogenic acid. *Phytochemistry* **4**, 527–529.

Cowles, H. C. (1911). The causes of vegetative cycles. *Bot. Gaz. (Chicago)* **51**, 161–183.

Craigie, J. S., and McLachlan, J. (1964). Excretion of colored ultraviolet absorbing substances by marine algae. *Can. J. Bot.* **42**, 23–33.

Cramer, M., and Myers, J. (1948). Nitrate reduction and assimilation in *Chlorella. J. Gen. Physiol.* **32**, 92–102.

Croak, M. (1972). Effects of phenolic inhibitors on growth, metabolism, mineral depletion, and ion uptake in Paul's scarlet rose cell suspension cultures. Ph.D. Dissertation, University of Oklahoma, Norman.

Cruickshank, I. A. M., and Perrin, D. R. (1960). Isolation of a phytoalexin from *Pisum sativum. Nature (London)* **187**, 799–800.

Cruickshank, I. A. M., and Perrin, D. R. (1964). Pathological function of phenolic compounds in plants. *In* "Biochemistry of Phenolic Compounds" (J. B. Harborne, ed.), pp. 511–544. Academic Press, New York.

Cummins, D. G. (1971). Relationship between tannin content and forage digestibility in sorghum. *Agron. J.* **63**, 500–502.

Curtis, J. T., and Cottam, G. (1950). Antibiotic and autotoxic effects in prairie sunflower. *Bull. Torrey Bot. Club* **77**, 187–191.

Dadykin, V. P., Stepanov, L. N., and Ryzhkova, B. E. (1970). On importance of volatile plant secretions under the development of closed systems. *In* "Physiological-Biochemical Basis of Plant Interactions in Phytocenoses" (A. M. Grodzinsky, ed.), Vol. 1, pp. 118–124. Naukova Dumka, Kiev. (In Russian)

Daniel, H. A., and Langham, W. H. (1936). The effect of wind erosion and cultivation on the total nitrogen and organic matter content of soil in the southern high plains. *J. Amer. Soc. Agron.* **28**, 587–596.

Davis, C. C. (1948). *Gymnodinium brevis.* A cause of discolored water and animal mortality in the Gulf of Mexico. *Bot. Gaz. (Chicago)* **109**, 358–360.

Davis, R. F. (1928). The toxic principle of *Juglans nigra* as identified with synthetic juglone and its toxic effects on tomato and alfalfa plants. *Amer. J. Bot.* **15**, 620.

Dear, J., and Aronoff, S. (1965). Relative kinetics of chlorogenic and caffeic acids during the onset of boron deficiency in sunflower. *Plant Physiol.* **40**, 458–459.

DeCandolle, M. A-P. (1832). "Physiologie Vegetale," Vol. III. Bechet Jeune, Lib. Fac. Med., Paris.

Deleuil, M. G. (1950). Mise en évidence de substances toxiques pour les thérophytes dans les associations du Rosmarino-Ericion. *C .R. Acad. Sci.* **230**, 1362–1364.

Deleuil, M. G. (1951a). Origine des substances toxiques du sol des associations sans thérophytes du Rosmarino-Ericion. *C. R. Acad. Sci.* **232**, 2038–2039.

Deleuil, M. G. (1951b). Explication de la présence de certains thérophytes recontrés parfois dans les associations du Rosmarino-Ericion. *C. R. Acad. Sci.* **232**, 2476–2477.

del Moral, R. (1972). On the variability of chlorogenic acid concentration. *Oecologia* **9**, 289–300.

del Moral, R., and Cates, R. G. (1971). Allelopathic potential of the dominant vegetation of western Washington. *Ecology* **52**, 1030–1037.

del Moral, R., and Muller, C. H. (1969). Fog drip: A mechanism of toxin transport from *Eucalyptus globulus*. *Bull. Torrey Bot. Club*. **96**, 467–475.

del Moral, R., and Muller, C. H. (1970). The allelopathic effects of *Eucalyptus camaldulensis*. *Amer. Midl. Natur.* **83**, 254–282.

Dethier, V. G. (1969). Electrophysiological studies of food-plant relationships of lepidopterous larvae. *In* "Insect-Plant Interactions" (U.S. Nat. Comm. for IBP, eds.), p. 20. Nat. Acad. Sci., Washington, D.C.

Dieterman, L. J., Lin, C-Y., Rohrbaugh, L. M., Thiesfeld, V., and Wender, S. H. (1964a). Identification and quantitative determination of scopolin and scopoletin in tobacco plants treated with 2,4-dichlorophenoxyacetic acid. *Anal. Biochem.* **9**, 139–145.

Dieterman, L. J., Lin, C.-Y., Rohrbaugh, L. M. and Wender, S. H. (1964b). Accumulation of ayapin and scopolin in sunflower plants treated with 2,4-dichlorophenoxyacetic acid. *Arch. Biochem. Biophys.* **106**, 275–279.

Dobbs, C. G., and Hinson, W. H. (1953). A wide-spread fungistasis in soil. *Nature (London)* **172**, 197–199.

Dominguez, X. A., Franco, R., Rojas, P., Elizondo, A., Valenzuela, J., and Martinez, E. G. (1964). Determinación de la acción antibiótica de noventa y dos plantas mejicanos tóxicas al ganado o utilizadas con propósitos medicinales. *Ciencia (Mexico City)* **23**, 99–103.

Dommergues, Y. (1952). Influence du défrichement de forêt suivi d'incendie sur l'activité biologique du sol. *Mem. Inst. Sci. Madrid, Ser. D* **4**, pp. 273–296.

Dommergues, Y. (1954). Biology of forest soils of central and eastern Madagascar. *Trans. Int. Congr. Soil Sci., 5th, 1954* Vol. 3, pp. 24–28.

Dommergues, Y. (1956). Study of the biology of soils of dry tropical forests and their evolution after clearing. *Trans. Int. Congr. Soil Sci., 6th, 1956* E, pp. 605–610.

Drew, W. B. (1942). The revegetation of abandoned cropland in the Cedar Creek area, Boone and Callaway counties, Missouri. *Mo., Agr. Exp. Sta., Bull.* **344**.

Dzubenko, N. N., and Petrenko, N. I. (1971). On biochemical interaction of cultivated plants and weeds. *In* "Physiological-Biochemical Basis of Plant Interactions in Phytocenoses" (A. M. Grodzinsky, ed.), Vol. 2, pp. 60–66. Naukova Dumka, Kiev. (In Russian)

Eberhardt, F. (1954). Ausscheidung einer organischen Verbindung aus den Wurzeln des Hafers (*Avena sativa* L.). *Naturwissenshaften* **41**, 259.

Eden, T. (1951). Some agricultural properties of Ceylon montane tea soils. *J. Soil Sci.* **2**, 43–49.

Einhellig, F. A. (1971) Effects of tannic acid on growth and stomatal aperture in tobacco. *Proc. S. Dak. Acad. Sci.* **50**, 205–209.

Einhellig, F. A., and Kuan, L. (1971). Effects of scopoletin and chlorogenic acid on stomatal aperture in tobacco and sunflower. *Bull. Torrey Bot. Club* **98**, 155–162.

Einhellig, F. A., Rice, E. L., Risser, P. G., and Wender, S. H. (1970). Effects of scopoletin on growth, CO_2 exchange rates, and concentration of scopoletin, scopolin, and chlorogenic acids in tobacco, sunflower, and pigweed. *Bull. Torrey Bot. Club* **97**, 22–33.

Elkan, G. H. (1961). A nodulation-inhibiting root excretion from a non-nodulating soybean strain. *Can. J. Microbiol.* **7**, 851–856.

Elmer, O. H. (1932). Growth inhibition of potato sprouts by the volatile products of apples. *Science* **75**, 193.

Grodzinsky, A. M. (1965). "Allelopathy in the Life of Plants." Naukova Dumka, Kiev. (In Russian)

Grodzinsky, A. M. (1967). Ein Keimungshemmstoff in den Fruchten des tatarischen Meerkohls (*Crambe tataria* Sebeok) and seine ökologischphysiologische Bedeutung. *In* "Physiology, Ecology, and Biochemistry of Germination" (H. Borriss, ed.), pp. 789–793. Ernst-Moritz-Arndt-Univ., Greifswald.

Grodzinsky, A. M. (1969). Über den Metabolitenaustauch zwischen benachbarten Pflanzen. *Qual. Plant. Mater. Veg.* **17**, 93–100.

Grodzinsky, A. M., and Gaidamak, V. M. (1971). Allelopathic influence of woody plants on herbaceous ones in the Ukrainian forest-steppe region. *In* "Physiological-Biochemical Basis of Plant Interactions in Phytocenoses" (A. M. Grodzinsky, ed.), Vol. 2, pp. 3–11. Naukova Dumka, Kiev. (In Russian)

Grümmer, G. (1955). "Die gegenseitige Beeinflussung hoherer Pflanzen-Allelopathie." Fischer, Jena.

Grümmer, G. (1961). The role of toxic substances in the interrelationships between higher plants. *Symp. Soc. Exp. Biol.* **15**, 219–228.

Grümmer, G., and Beyer, H. (1960). The influence exerted by species of *Camelina* on flax by means of toxic substances. *In* "The Biology of Weeds" (J. L. Harper, ed.), pp. 153–157. Blackwell, Oxford.

Guenzi, W. D., and McCalla, T. M. (1962). Inhibition of germination and seedling development by crop residues. *Soil Sci. Soc. Amer., Proc.* **26**, 456–458.

Guenzi, W. D., and McCalla, T. M. (1966a). Phenolic acids in oats, wheat, sorghum, and corn residues and their phytotoxicity. *Agron. J.* **58**, 303–304.

Guenzi, W. D., and McCalla, T. M. (1966b). Phytotoxic substances extracted from soil. *Soil Sci. Soc. Amer., Proc.* **30**, 214–216.

Guenzi, W. D., McCalla, T. M., and Norstadt, F. A. (1967). Presence and persistence of phytotoxic substances in wheat, oat, corn and sorghum residues. *Agron. J.* **59**, 163–165.

Guyot, A. L. (1957). Les microassociations végétales au sein du Brometrum Erecti. *Vegetatio, Haag* **7**, 321–354.

Guyot, A. L., Becker, Y., Guillemat, J., Lelievre, D., Massenot, M., and Montegut, J. (1951). Sur un aspect du déterminisme biologique de l'évolution floristique de quelques groupements végétaux. *C. R. Acad. Sci.* **239**, 3–14.

Hadwiger, L. A. (1972). Induction of phenylalanine ammonia lyase and pisatin by photosensitive psoralen compounds. *Plant Physiol.* **49**, 779–782.

Harborne, J. B. (1960). The genetic variation of anthocyanin pigments in plant tissues. *In* "Phenolics in Plants in Health and Disease" (J. B. Pridham, ed.), pp. 109–117. Pergamon, Oxford.

Harborne, J. B. (1964). Phenolic glycosides and their natural distribution. *In* "Biochemistry of Phenolic Compounds" (J. B. Harborne, ed.), pp. 129–169. Academic Press, New York.

Harborne, J. B., and Simmonds, N. W. (1964). The natural distribution of the phenolic aglycones. *In* "Biochemistry of Phenolic Compounds" (J. B. Harborne, ed.), pp. 77–127. Academic Press, New York.

Harper, H. J. (1932). Easily soluble phosphorus in Oklahoma soils. *Okla., Agr. Exp. Sta., Bull.* **205**.

Harris, H. B., and Burns, R. E. (1970). Influence of tannin content on preharvest seed germination in sorghum. *Agron. J.* **62**, 835–836.

Harris, H. B., and Burns, R. E. (1972). "Inhibiting Effects of Tannin in Sorghum Grain on Preharvest Seed Molding," Agron. abstr., 1972 Annu. Meet. Amer. Soc. Agron., Madison, Wisconsin.

Harris, H. B., Cummins, D. G., and Burns, R. E. (1970). Tannin content and digestibility of sorghum grain as influenced by bagging. *Agron. J.* **62,** 633–635.

Hattingh, M. J., and Louw, H. A. (1969a). Clover rhizoplane bacteria antagonistic to *Rhizobium trifolii. Can. J. Bot.* **15,** 361–364.

Hattingh, M. J., and Louw, H. A. (1969b). The influence of antagonistic rhizoplane bacteria on the clover-*Rhizobium* symbiosis. *Phytophylactica* **1,** 205–208.

Hauschka, T., Toennies, G., and Swain, A. P. (1945). The mechanism of growth inhibition by hexenolactone. *Science* **101,** 383–385.

Havis, L., and Gilkeson, A. L. (1947). Toxicity of peach roots. *Proc. Amer. Soc. Hort. Sci.* **50,** 203–205.

Hayes, L. E. (1947). Survey of higher plants for presence of antibacterial substances. *Bot. Gaz. (Chicago)* **108,** 408–414.

Heilman, A. S., and Sharp, A. J. (1963). A probable antibiotic effect of some lichens on bryophytes. *Rev. Bryolog. Lichenol.* **32,** 215.

Henis, Y., Tagari, H., and Volcani, R. (1964). Effect of water extract of carob pods, tannic acid, and their derivatives on the morphology and growth of microorganisms. *Appl. Microbiol.* **12,** 204–209.

Hennequin, J. R., and Juste, C. (1967). Présence d'acides phénols libres dans le sol. Etude de leur influence sur la germination et la croissance des végétaux. *Ann. Agron.* **18,** 545–569.

Hoagland, D. R., and Arnon, D. I. (1950). The water-culture method of growing plants without soil. *Calif., Agr. Exp. Sta., Circ.* **347.**

Hodges, T. K., Darding, R. L., and Weidner, T. (1971). Gramicidin-D-stimulated influx of monovalent cations into plant roots. *Planta* **97,** 245–256.

Holowczak, J., Kúc, J., and Williams, E. G. (1960). Metabolism in vitro of phloridzin and other host compounds by *Venturia inaequalis. Phytopathology* **50,** 640.

Horton, J. S., and Kraebel, C. J. (1955). Development of vegetation after fire in the chamise chaparral of southern California. *Ecology* **36,** 244–262.

Hughes, J. C., and Swain, T. (1960). Scopolin production in potato tubers infected with *Phytophthora infestans. Phytopathology* **50,** 398–400.

Hulme, A. C., and Jones, J. D. (1963). Tannin inhibition of plant mitochondria. *In* "Enzyme Chemistry of Phenolic Compounds" (J. B. Pridham, ed.), pp. 97–120. Macmillan, New York.

Hungate, R. E. (1966). "The Rumen and its Microbes." Academic Press, New York.

Ilag, L., and Curtis, R. W. (1968). Production of ethylene by fungi. *Science* **159,** 1357–1358.

Iuzhina, Z. I. (1958). Relationship between toxic properties of soil of Kola Peninsula and number of bacterial antagonists of *Azotobacter. Microbiology (USSR)* **27,** 452–456.

Ivanov, V. P., and Yakobson, G. A. (1970). Biochemical role of root secretions in interrelations of plants in cenosis. *In* "Physiological-Biochemical Basis of Plant Interactions in Phytocenoses." (A. M. Grodzinsky, ed.), Vol. 1, pp. 40–49. Naukova Dumka, Kiev. (In Russian)

Jackson, R. M. (1965). Antibiosis and fungistasis of soil microorganisms. *In* "Ecology of Soil-Borne Plant Pathogens" (K. F. Baker and W. C. Snyder, eds.), pp. 363–369. Univ. of California Press, Berkeley.

Jacquemin, H., and Berlier, Y. (1956). Evolution du pouvoir nitrifiant d'un sol de bosse

Côte d'Ivoire sous l'action du climat et de la végétation. *Trans. Int. Congr. Soil Sci.*, *6th 1956* C, pp. 343–347.

Jaffe, M. J., and Isenberg, F. M. R. (1969). Red light photoenhancement of the synthesis of phenolic compounds and lignin in potato tuber tissue. *Фуton* **26**, 51–67.

Jameson, D. A. (1961). Growth inhibitors in native plants of northern Arizona. *U.S., Forest Serv., Rocky Mt. Forest Range Exp. Sta. Res. Notes* No. 61.

Jameson, D. A. (1963). Plant extracts retard growth of grass seedlings. *In* "Annual Report for 1963" (Rocky Mt. Forest and Range Exp. Sta., ed.), p. 57. USDA, Fort Collins, Colorado.

Jameson, D. A. (1966). Pinyon-juniper litter reduces growth of blue grama. *J. Range Manage.* **19**, 214–217.

Jensen, T. E., and Welbourne, F. (1962). The cytological effects of growth inhibitors on excised roots of *Vicia faba* and *Pisum sativum*. *Proc. S. Dak. Acad. Sci.* **41**, 131–136.

Johnson, G., and Schaal, L. A. (1952). Relation of chlorogenic acid to scab resistance in potatoes. *Science* **115**, 627–629.

Johnson, H. W., and Clark, F. E. (1958). Role of the root nodule in the bacterial-induced chlorosis of soybeans. *Soil Sci. Soc. Amer., Proc.* **22**, 527–528.

Johnson, H. W., Means, U. M., and Clark, F. E. (1959). Responses of seedlings to extracts of soybean nodules bearing selected strains of *Rhizobium japonicum*. *Nature (London)* **183**, 308–309.

Katznelson, H., Rouatt, J. W., and Payne, T. M. B. (1955). The liberation of amino acids and reducing compounds by plant roots. *Plant Soil* **7**, 35–48.

Kaurov, I. A. (1970). Interaction of bird's foot and yellow lupine in pure and mixed cultures. *In* "Physiological-Biochemical Basis of Plant Interactions in Phytocenoses" (A. M. Grodzinsky, ed.), Vol. 1, pp. 66–71. Naukova Dumka, Kiev. (In Russian)

Keever, C. (1950). Causes of succession on old fields of the Piedmont, North Carolina. *Ecol. Monogr.* **20**, 229–250.

Kefeli, V. I., and Turetskaya, R. K. (1967). Comparative effect of natural growth inhibitors, narcotics, and antibiotics on plant growth. *Fiziol. Rast.* **14**, 796–803.

Kingsbury, J. M. (1964). "Poisonous Plants of the United States and Canada." Prentice-Hall, Englewood Cliffs, New Jersey.

Klaus, H. (1939). Das Problem der Bodenmüdikeit unter Berücksichtigung des Obstbaues. *Landwirt. Jahrb.* **89**, 413–459.

Klun, J. A. (1969). Host plant resistance to the European corn borer. *In* "Insect-Plant Interactions" (U.S. Nat. Comm. for IBP, eds.), p. 42. Nat. Acad. Sci., Washington, D.C.

Knudson, L. (1913). Tannic acid fermentation. I. *J. Biol. Chem.* **14**, 159–184.

Koch, L. W. (1955). The peach replant problem in Ontario. I. Symptomatology and distribution. *Can. J. Bot.* **33**, 450–460.

Koeppe, D. E. (1972). Some reactions of isolated corn mitochondria influenced by juglone. *Physiol. Plant.* **27**, 89–94.

Koeppe, D. E., Rohrbaugh, L. M., and Wender, S. H. (1969). The effect of varying U.V. intensities on the concentration of scopolin and caffeoylquinic acids in tobacco and sunflower. *Phytochemistry* **8**, 889–896.

Koeppe, D. E., Rohrbaugh, L. M., Rice, E. L., and Wender, S. H. (1970a). The effect of x-radiation on the concentration of scopolin and caffeoylquinic acids in tobacco. *Radiat. Bot.* **10**, 261–265.

Koeppe, D. E., Rohrbaugh, L. M., Rice, E. L., and Wender, S. H. (1970b). The effect of age and chilling temperatures on the concentration of scopolin and caffeoylquinic acids in tobacco. *Physiol. Plant.* **23**, 258–266.

Koeppe, D. E., Rohrbaugh, L. M., Rice, E. L., and Wender, S. H. (1970c). Tissue age and caffeoylquinic acid concentration in sunflower. *Phytochemistry* **9**, 297–301.

Kofoid, C. A. (1911). Dinoflagellata of the San Diego region. VI. *Univ. Calif., Berkeley, Publ. Zool.* **8**(4).

Kohlmuenzer, S. (1965a). Botanical and chemical studies of the collective species *Galium mollugo* with reference to karyotypes growing in Poland. V. Phytochemical studies, *Diss. Pharm.* **17**, 357, see *Chem. Abstr.* **64**, 10085g (1966).

Kohlmuenzer, S. (1965b). Botanical and chemical studies of the collective species *Galium mollugo* with reference to karyotypes growing in Poland. VI. Effect of extracts and some other chemical components of *Galium mollugo* on the germination of seeds and growth of selected plants. *Diss. Pharm.* **17**, 369, see *Chem. Abstr.* **64**, 10085g (1966).

Koller, D. (1955a). Germination regulating mechanisms in some desert seeds. I. *Bull. Res. Counc. Isr.* **4**, 379–381.

Koller, D. (1955b). Germination regulating mechanisms in some desert seeds. II. *Zygophyllum dumosum* Boiss. *Bull. Res. Counc. Isr.* **4**, 381–387.

Konishi, K. (1931). Effect of soil bacteria on the growth of the root nodule bacteria. *Mem. Coll. Agr., Kyoto Imp. Univ.* **16**, 1–17.

Koths, J. S., and Litsky, W. (1962). Concerning the antibiotic activity of a commercial bacterial culture for the control of poultry pathogens in yard soils. *Poultry Sci.* **41**, 1014–1016.

Kozel, P. C., and Tukey, H. B., Jr. (1968). Loss of gibberellins by leaching from stems and foliage of *Chrysanthemum morifolium* 'Princess Anne.' *Amer. J. Bot,* **55**, 1184–1189.

Krylov, Y. V. (1970). Influence of potatoes on an apple tree and its photosynthesis. *In* "Physiological-Biochemical Basis of Plant Interactions in Phytocenoses" (A. M. Grodzinsky, ed.), Vol. 1, pp. 128–134. Naukova Dumka, Kiev. (In Russian)

Kúc, J. (1957). A biochemical study of the resistance of potato tuber tissue to attack by various fungi. *Phytopathology* **47**, 676–680.

Kúc, J., Henze, R. E., Ulstrup, A. J., and Quackenbush, F. W. (1956). Chlorogenic and caffeic acids as fungistatic agents produced by potatoes in response to inoculation with *Helminthosporium carbonum. J. Amer. Chem. Soc.* **78**, 3123–3125.

Kuhn, R., Jerchel, D., Moewus, F., and Moeller, E. F. (1943). Über die chemische Natur der Blastokoline und ihre Einwirkung auf keimende Samen, Pollenkörner, Hefen, Bakterien, Epithelgewebe und Fibroblasten. *Naturwissenschaften* **31**, 468.

Lahiri, A. N., and Kharabanda, B. C. (1962-1963). Germination studies on arid zone plants. 2. Germination inhibitors in the spikelet glumes of *Lasiurus sindicus, Cenchrus ciliaris,* and *Cenchrus setigerus. Ann. Arid Zone, Jodhpur* **1**, 114–126.

Lane, F. E. (1965). Dormancy and germination in fruits of the sunflower, Ph.D. Dissertation, University of Oklahoma, Norman.

Lastuvka, Z. (1970). Allelopathy and the processes of ion absorption and accumulation. *In* "Physiological-Biochemical Basis of Plant Interactions in Phytocenoses" (A. M. Grodzinsky, ed.), Vol. 1, pp. 37–40. Naukova Dumka, Kiev. (In Russian)

Lastuvka, Z., and Minarz, I. (1970). Mutual effect of maize and pea in water cultures with additional nutrition. *In* "Physiological-Biochemical Basis of Plant Interactions in Phytocenoses" (A. M. Grodzinsky, ed.), Vol. 1, pp. 55–59. Naukova Dumka, Kiev. (In Russian)

Lazauskas, P., and Balinevichiute, Z. (1972). Influence of the excretions from *Vicia villosa* Roth seeds on germination and primary growth of some crops and weeds. *In* "Physiological-Biochemical Basis of Plant Interactions in Phytocenoses" (A. M. Grodzinsky, ed.), Vol. 3, pp. 76–79. Naukova Dumka, Kiev. (In Russian)

Leather, J. W. (1911). Records of drainage in India. *Mem. Dep. Agr., India, Chem.* **2**, 63–140.

Lee, I. K., and Monsi, M. (1963). Ecological studies on *Pinus densiflora* forest. 1. Effects of plant substances on the floristic composition of the undergrowth. *Bot. Mag.* **76**, 400–413.

Lee, T. T. (1966). Effects of hydroxybenzoic acids on oxidation of reduced nicotinamide adenine dinucleotide by enzymes from tobacco leaves. *Physiol. Plant.* **19**, 660–671.

Lee, T. T., and Skoog, F. (1965). Effects of hydroxybenzoic acids on indoleacetic acid inactivation by tobacco callus extracts. *Physiol. Plant.* **18**, 577–585.

Leelavathy, K. M. (1969). Effect of rhizosphere fungi on seed germination. *Plant Soil* **30**, 473–476.

Lefevre, M. (1950). Compatibilités et antagonismes entre algues d'eau douce dans les collections d'eau naturelles. *Proc. Int. Ass. Limnol.* **11**, 224–229.

Lefevre, M. (1952). Auto et heteroantagonisme chez les algues d'eau douce. *Ann. Sta. Cent. Hydrobiol. Appl.* **4**, 5–197.

Lefevre, M., Jakob, H., and Nisbet, M. (1948). Action des substances excretées en culture par certaines espéces d'algues sur le métabolisme d'autres espéces d'algues. *Proc. Int. Ass. Limnol.* **10**, 259–264.

Lehman, R. H., and Rice, E. L. (1972). Effect of deficiencies of nitrogen, potassium and sulfur on chlorogenic acids and scopolin in sunflower. *Amer. Midl. Natur.* **87**, 71–80.

Leopold, A. C. (1955). "Auxins and Plant Growth," Univ. of California Press, Berkeley.

LeTourneau, D., Failes, G. D., and Heggeness, H. G. (1956). The effect of aqueous extracts of plant tissue on germination of seeds and growth of seedlings. *Weeds* **4**, 363–368.

Levitan, H., and Barker, J. L. (1972). Salicylate: A structure-activity study of its effects on membrane permeability. *Science* **176**, 1423–1425.

Lieth, H. (1960). Patterns of change within grassland communities. *In* "The Biology of Weeds" (J. L. Harper, ed.), pp. 27–39. Blackwell, Oxford.

Likens, G. E., Bormann, F. H., and Johnson, N. M. (1969). Nitrification: Importance to nutrient losses from a cutover forested ecosystem. *Science* **163**, 1205–1206.

Lingappa, B. T., Prasad, M., and Lingappa, Y. (1969). Phenethyl alcohol and tryptophol: Autoantibiotics produced by the fungus *Candida albicans*. *Science* **163**, 192–194.

Livingston, B. E. (1905). Physiological properties of bog water. *Bot. Gaz. (Chicago)* **39**, 348–355.

Loche, J., and Chouteau, J. (1963). Incidences des carences en Ca, Mg, or P sur l'accumulation des polyphenol dans la feuille de tabac. *C. R. Hebd. Seances Acad. Agr. Fr.* **49**, 1017–1026.

Lockwood, J. L. (1959). *Streptomyces* spp. as a cause of natural fungitoxicity in soil. *Phytopathology* **49**, 327–334.

Lodhi, M. A. K., and Rice, E. L. (1971). Allelopathic effects of *Celtis laevigata*. *Bull. Torrey Bot. Club* **98**, 83–89.

Loehwing, W. F. (1937). Root interactions in plants. *Bot. Rev.* **3**, 195–239.

Löfgren, N., Lüning, B., and Hedström, H. (1954). The isolation of nebularine and the determination of its structure. *Acta Chem. Scand.* **8**, 670–680.

Logan, R. H., Hoveland, C. S., and Donnelly, E. D. (1968). A germination inhibitor in the seedcoat of sericea (*Lespedeza cuneata* (Dumont) G. Don). *Agron. J.* **61**, 265–266.

Lott, H. V. (1960). Über den Einfluss der kurzwelligen Strahlung auf die Biosyntheses der pflanzlichen Polyphenole. *Planta* **55**, 480–495.

Lucas, C. E. (1947). The ecological effects of external metabolities. *Biol. Rev.* **22**, 270–295.

Lucas, E. H., and Lewis, R. W. (1944). Antibacterial substances in organs of higher plants. *Science* **100**, 597–599.

Lucas, E. H., Lickfeldt, A., Gottshall, R. Y., and Jennings, J. C. (1951). The occurrence of antibacterial substances in seed plants with special reference to *Mycobacterium tuberculosis*. *Bull. Torrey Bot. Club* **78**, 310–321.

Lucas, E. H., Frisbey, A., Gottshall, R. Y., and Jennings, J. C. (1955). The occurrence of antibacterial substances in seed plants with special reference to *Mycobacterium tuberculosis* (Fifth Report). *Mich. Quart. Bull.* **37**, 425–436.

Ludwig, R. A. (1957). Toxin production by *Helminthosporium sativum* P. K. & B. and its significance in disease development. *Can. J. Bot.* **35**, 291–303.

Lukefahr, M. J., Shaver, T. N., and Guerra, A. A. (1969). Development of cotton plants resistant to *Heliothis* spp. and other cotton insects. *In* "Insect-Plant Interactions" (U.S. Nat. Comm. for IBP, eds.), pp. 43–44. Nat. Acad. Sci., Washington, D.C.

Lundegardh, H., and Stenlid, G. (1944). On the exudation of nucleotides and flavanone from living roots. *Ark. Bot.*, **31A**, 1–27.

Lykhvar, D. F., and Nazarova, N. S. (1970). On importance of legume varieties in mixed cultures with maize. *In* "Physiological-Biochemical Basis of Plant Interactions in Phytocenoses" (A. M. Grodzinsky, ed.), Vol. 1, pp. 83–88. Naukova Dumka, Kiev. (In Russian)

Lyon, T. L., and Wilson, J. K. (1921). Liberation of organic matter by roots of growing plants, *Cornell Univ. Agr. Exp. Sta., Mem.* **40**.

Lyon, T. L., Bizzell, J. A., and Wilson, B. D. (1923). Depressive influence of certain higher plants on the accumulation of nitrates in the soil. *J. Amer. Soc. Agron.* **15**, 457–467.

McCalla, T. M., and Duley, F. L. (1948). Stubble mulch studies: Effect of sweetclover extract on corn germination. *Science* **108**, 163.

McCalla, T. M., and Duley, F. L. (1949). Stubble mulch studies. III. Influence of soil microorganisms and crop residues on the germination, growth and direction of root growth of corn seedlings. *Soil Sci. Soc. Amer., Proc.* **14**, 196–199.

McCalla, T. M., and Haskins, F. A. (1964). Phytotoxic substances from soil micro-organisms and crop residues. *Bacteriol. Rev.* **28**, 181–207.

McFee, W. W., and Stone, E. L., Jr. (1968). Ammonium and nitrate as nitrogen sources for *Pinus radiata* and *Picea glauca*. *Soil Sci. Soc. Amer., Proc.* **32**, 879–884.

McKnight, R. S. and Lindegren, C. C. (1936). Bactericidal effects of vapors from crushed garlic on *Mycobacterium Cepae*. *Proc. Soc. Exp. Biol. Med.* **35**, 477–479.

McLachlan, J., and Craigie, J. S. (1964). Algal inhibition by yellow ultraviolet-absorbing substances from *Fucus vesiculosus*. *Can. J. Bot.* **42**, 287–292.

McNaughton, S. J. (1968). Autotoxic feedback in relation to germination and seedling growth in *Typha latifolia*. *Ecology* **49**, 367–369.

McPherson, J. K., and Muller, C. H. (1969). Allelopathic effects of *Adenostoma fasciculatum*, "chamise," in the California chaparral. *Ecol. Monogr.* **39**, 177–198.

Magnus, W. (1920). Hemmungsstoffe und falsche Keimung. *Ber. Deut. Bot. Ges.* **38**, 19–26.

Mallik, M. A. B. (1966). The influence of crop on soil fungistasis. *Pak. J. Sci. Ind. Res.* **9**, 285–286.

Manasse, R. J., and Corpe, W. A. (1965). Bacterial inhibition by two plant extracts. *Bull. Torrey Bot. Club* **92**, 364–371.

Markova, S. A. (1972). Experimental investigations of the influence of oats on growth and development of *Erysimum cheiranthoides* L. *In* "Physiological-Biochemical

Basis of Plant Interactions in Phytocenoses" (A. M. Grodzinsky, ed.), Vol. 3, pp. 66–68. Naukova Dumka, Kiev. (In Russian)

Martin, J. P. (1948). Fungus flora of some California soils in relation to slow decline of citrus trees. *Soil Sci. Soc. Amer., Proc.* 12, 209–214.

Martin, J. P. (1950a). Effects of soil fungi on germination of sweet orange seeds and development of the young seedlings. *Soil Sci. Soc. Amer., Proc.* 14, 184–188.

Martin, J. P. (1950b). Effects of fumigation and other soil treatments in the greenhouse on the fungus population of old citrus soil. *Soil Sci.* 69, 107–122.

Martin, J. P., and Ervin, J. O. (1958). Greenhouse studies on the influence of other crops and of organic materials on growth of orange seedlings in citrus soils. *Soil Sci.* 85, 141–147.

Martin, J. P., Aldrich, D. G., Murphy, W. S., and Bradford, G. R. (1953). Effects of soil fumigation on growth and chemical composition of citrus plants. *Soil Sci.* 75, 137–151.

Martin, J. P., Klotz, L. J., DeWolfe, T. A., and Ervin, J. O. (1956). Influence of some common soil fungi on growth of citrus seedlings. *Soil Sci.* 81, 259–267.

Martin, P. (1957). Die Abgabe von organischen Verbindungen insbesondere von Scopoletin, aus den Keimwurzeln des Hafers. *Z. Bot.* 45, 475–506.

Martin, P., and Rademacher, B. (1960a). Studies on the mutual influences of weeds and crops. *In* "The Biology of Weeds" (J. L. Harper, ed.), pp. 143–152. Blackwell, Oxford.

Martin, P., and Rademacher, B. (1960b). Experimentelle Untersuchungen zur Frage der Nachwirkung von Rapsiwurzelrückständen. *Z. Acker Pflanzenbau* 111, 105–115.

Massart, L. (1957). Inhibiteur de la germination dans des glomérules de la betterave a serce et dans d' autres fruits' secs et grains. *Biokhimiga* 22, 417–420.

Massey, A. B. (1925). Antagonism of the walnuts (*Juglans nigra* L. and *J. cinerea* L.) in certain plant associations. *Phytopathology* 15, 773–784.

Mathes, M. C. (1967). The secretion of antimicrobial materials by various isolated plant tissues. *Lloydia* 30, 177–181.

Meiklejohn, J. (1962). Microbiology of the nitrogen cycle in some Ghana soils. *Emp. J. Exp. Agr.* 30, 115–126.

Meiklejohn, J. (1968). Numbers of nitrifying bacteria in some Rhodesian soils under natural grass and improved pasture. *J. Appl. Ecol.* 5, 291–300.

Mergen, F. (1959). A toxic principle in the leaves of *Ailanthus*. *Bot. Gaz.* (*Chicago*) 121, 32–36.

Millard, W. A., and Taylor, G. B. (1927). Antagonism of microorganisms as the controlling factor in the inhibition of scab by green manuring. *Ann. Appl. Biol.* 14, 202–216.

Miller, H. E., Mabry, T. J., Turner, B. L., and Payne, W. W. (1968). Infraspecific variation of sesquiterpene lactones in *Ambrosia psilostachya* (Compositae). *Amer. J. Bot.* 55, 316–324.

Mills, W. R. (1953). Nitrate accumulation in Uganda soils. *East Afr. Agr. J.* 19, 53–54.

Minamikawa, T., Akazawa, T., and Uritani, I. (1963). Analytical study of umbelliferone and scopoletin synthesis in sweet potato roots infected by *Ceratocystis fimbriata*. *Plant Physiol.* 38, 493–497.

Minamikawa, T., Jayasankar, N. P., Bohm, B. A., Taylor, I. E. P., and Towers, G. H. N. (1970). An inducible hydrolase from *Aspergillus niger*, acting on carbon-carbon bonds, for phlorrhizin and other C-acylated phenols. *Biochem. J.* 116, 889–897.

Mirchink, T. G. (1972). Significance of fungal toxins in relations between soil and plants. *In* "Physiological-Biochemical Basis of Plant Interactions in Phytocenoses" (A. M. Grodzinsky, ed.), Vol. 3, pp. 108–111. Naukova Dumka, Kiev. (In Russian)

Mitin, V. V. (1970). On study of chemical nature of growth inhibitors in the dead leaves of hornbean and beech. *In* "Physiological-Biochemical Basis of Plant Interactions in Phytocenoses" (A. M. Grodzinsky, ed.), Vol. 1, pp. 177–181. Naukova Dumka, Kiev. (In Russian)

Mitin, V. V. (1971). The water-soluble inhibitors of seed germination from beech (*Fagus silvatica* L.) autumn leaves. *In* "Physiological-Biochemical Basis of Plant Interactions in Phytocenoses" (A. M. Grodzinsky, ed.), Vol. 2, pp. 22–25. Naukova Dumka, Kiev. (In Russian)

Miyamoto, T., Tolbert, N. E., and Everson, E. H. (1961). Germination inhibitors related to dormancy in wheat seeds. *Plant Physiol.* **36,** 739–746.

Molisch, H. (1937). "Der Einfluss einer Pflanze auf die andere-Allelopathie." Fischer, Jena.

Moore, C. W. E., and Keraitis, K. (1971). Effect of nitrogen source on growth of eucalypts in sand culture. *Aust. J. Bot.* **19,** 125–141.

Moore, D. R. E., and Waid, J. S. (1971). The influence of washings of living roots on nitrification. *Soil Biol.&Biochem.* **3,** 69–83.

Morgan, G. T., and Collins, W. B. (1964). The effect of organic treatments and crop rotation on soil populations of *Pratylenchus penetrans* in strawberry culture. *Can. J. Plant Sci.* **44,** 272–275.

Morgan, P. W., and Powell, R. D. (1970). Involvement of ethylene in responses of etiolated bean hypocotyl hook to coumarin. *Plant Physiol.* **45,** 553–557.

Mosheov, G. (1937). The influence of the water extract of wheat seeds upon their germination and growth. *Bull., Heb. Univ.* **1,** 1–16.

Mountain, W. B., and Boyce, H. R. (1958). The peach replant problem in Ontario. VI. The relation of *Pratylenchus penetrans* to the growth of young peach trees. *Can. J. Bot.* **36,** 135–151.

Mountain, W. B., and Patrick, Z. A. (1959). The peach replant problem in Ontario. VII. The pathogenicity of *Pratylenchus penetrans* (Cobb, 1917) Filip and Stek, 1941. *Can. J. Bot.* **37,** 459–470.

Mulder, E. G. (1954). Molybdenum in relation to growth of higher plants and micro-organisms. *Plant Soil* **5,** 368–415.

Muller, C. H. (1965). Inhibitory terpenes volatilized from *Salvia* shrubs. *Bull. Torrey Bot. Club* **92,** 38–45.

Muller, C. H. (1966). The role of chemical inhibition (allelopathy) in vegetational composition. *Bull. Torrey Bot. Club* **93,** 332–351.

Muller, C. H. (1969). Allelopathy as a factor in ecological process. *Vegetatio, Haag* **18,** 348–357.

Muller, C. H. (1970). Phytotoxins as plant habitat variables. *Recent Advan. Phytochem.* **3,** 106–121.

Muller, C. H., and del Moral, R. (1966). Soil toxicity induced by terpenes from *Salvia leucophylla. Bull. Torrey Bot. Club* **93,** 130–137.

Muller, C. H., Muller, W. H., and Haines, B. L. (1964). Volatile growth inhibitors produced by shrubs. *Science* **143,** 471–473.

Muller, C. H., Hanawalt, R. B., and McPherson, J. K. (1968). Allelopathic control of herb growth in the fire cycle of California chaparral. *Bull. Torrey Bot. Club* **95,** 225–231.

Muller, W. H. (1965). Volatile materials produced by *Salvia leucophylla:* Effects on seedling growth and soil bacteria. *Bot. Gaz (Chicago)* **126,** 195–200.

Muller, W. H., and Muller, C. H. (1964). Volatile growth inhibitors produced by *Salvia* species. *Bull. Torrey Bot. Club* **91**, 327–330.

Muller, W. H., Lorber, P., Haley, B., and Johnson, K. (1969). Volatile growth inhibitors produced by *Salvia leucophylla*: Effect on oxygen uptake by mitochondrial suspensions. *Bull. Torrey Bot. Club* **96**, 89–96.

Munro, P. E. (1966a). Inhibition of nitrite oxidizers by roots of grass. *J. Appl. Ecol.* **3**, 227–229.

Munro, P. E. (1966b). Inhibition of nitrifiers by grass roots. *J. Appl. Ecol.* **3**, 231–238.

Nagy, J. G., Vidacs, G., and Ward, G. M. (1964). Separation of the essential oils of *Artemisia* spp. by gas chromatography and the effects of the oils on bacteria. *J. Colo.-Wyo. Acad. Sci.* **5**, 41–42.

Nakanishi, K. (1969). Ecdysones and ecdysone analogues. *In* "Insect-Plant Interactions" (U.S. Nat. Comm. for IBP, eds.), pp. 6–9. Nat. Acad. Sci., Washington, D.C.

Neal, J. L., Jr. (1969). Inhibition of nitrifying bacteria by grass and forb root extracts. *Can. J. Bot.* **15**, 633–635.

Neal, J. L., Jr., Bollen, W. B., and Zak, B. (1964). Rhizosphere microflora associated with mycorrhizae of douglas fir. *Can. J. Microbiol.* **10**, 259–265.

Neill, R. L., and Rice, E. L. (1971). Possible role of *Ambrosia psilostachya* on patterning and succession in old-fields. *Amer. Midl. Natur.* **86**, 344–357.

Neish, A. C. (1964). Major pathways of biosynthesis of phenols. *In* "Biochemistry of Phenolic Compounds" (J. B. Harborne, ed.), pp. 295–359. Academic Press, New York.

Neustruyeva, S. N., and Dobretsova, T. N. (1972). Influence of some summer crops on white goosefoot. *In* "Physiological-Biochemical Basis of Plant Interactions in Phytocenoses" (A. M. Grodzinsky, ed.), Vol. 3, pp. 68–73. Naukova Dumka, Kiev. (In Russian)

Nickell, L. G. (1960). Antimicrobial activity of vascular plants. *Econ. Bot.* **13**, 281–318.

Nielsen, K. F., and Cunningham, R. K. (1964). The effects of soil temperature and form and level of nitrogen on growth and chemical composition of Italian rye-grass. *Soil Sci. Soc. Amer., Proc.* **28**, 213–218.

Nielsen, K. F., Cuddy, T., and Woods, W. (1960). The influence of the extract of some crops and soil residues on germination and growth. *Can. J. Plant Sci.* **40**, 188–197.

Nierenstein, M. (1934). "The Natural Organic Tannins." Churchill, London.

Norstadt, F. A., and McCalla, T. M. (1963). Phytotoxic substance from a species of *Penicillium. Science* **140**, 410–411.

Nowinski, M. (1961). Review of studies on allelopathy. *Postepy Nauk Roln.* **8**, 39–57.

Nye, R. H., and Greenland, D. J. (1960). "The Soil under Shifting Cultivation," Tech. Commun. No. 51. Commonwealth Bureau of Soils, Harpenden.

Oertli, J. J. (1963). Effect of the form of nitrogen and pH on growth of blueberry plants. *Agron. J.* **55**, 305–307.

Oleksevich, V. M. (1970). On the allelopathic activity of trees and shrubs used for landscape gardening. *In* "Physiological-Biochemical Basis of Plant Interactions in Phytocenoses" (A. M. Grodzinsky, ed.), Vol. 1, pp. 186-190. Naukova Dumka, Kiev. (In Russian)

Olmsted, C. E., III, and Rice, E. L. (1970). Relative effects of known plant inhibitors on species from first two stages of old-field succession. *Southwest. Natur.* **15**, 165–173.

Olsen, R. A., Odham, G., and Linderberge, G. (1971). Aromatic substances in leaves of *Populus tremula* as inhibitors of mycorrhizal fungi. *Physiol. Plant.* **25**, 122–129.

Oppenheimer, H. (1922). Keimungshemmende Substanzen in der Frucht von-*Solanum lycopersicum* und in anderen pflanzen. *Sitzungsber. Akad. Wiss., Wien. Kl., Abt. 1* **131**, 59–65.

Osborn, E. M. (1943). On the occurrence of antibacterial substances in green plants. *Brit. J. Exp. Pathol.* **24**, 227–231.

Owens, L. D. (1969). Toxins in plant disease: Structure and mode of action. *Science* **165**, 18–25. (Copyright 1969 by Amer. Ass. Advan. Sci.)

Owens, L. D., Lieberman, M., and Kunishi, A. (1971). Inhibition of ethylene production by rhizobitoxine. *Plant Physiol.* **48**, 1–4.

Owens, L. D., Thompson, J. F., Pitcher, R. G., and Williams, T. (1972). Structure of rhizobitoxine, an antimetabolic enol-ether amino-acid from *Rhizobium japonicum*. *J. Chem. Soc., Chem. Commun.* p. 714.

Parenti, R. L., and Rice, E. L. (1969). Inhibitional effects of *Digitaria sanguinalis* and possible role in old-field succession. *Bull. Torrey Bot. Club* **96**, 70–78.

Parks, J. M., and Rice, E. L. (1969). Effects of certain plants of old-field succession on the growth of blue-green algae. *Bull. Torrey Bot. Club* **96**, 345–360.

Parpiev, Y. P. (1971). Influence of excretions of seeds and fall of some tree shrubby species of middle Asia deserts on seed germination of subcrown plants. *In* "Physiological-Biochemical Basis of Plant Interactions in Phytocenoses" (A. M. Grodzinsky, ed.), Vol. 2, pp. 46–51. Naukova Dumka, Kiev. (In Russian)

Patrick, Z. A. (1955). The peach replant problem in Ontario. II. Toxic substances from microbial decomposition products of peach root residues. *Can. J. Bot.* **33**, 461–486.

Patrick, Z. A. (1971). Phytotoxic substances associated with the decomposition in soil of plant residues. *Soil Sci.* **111**, 13–18.

Patrick, Z. A., and Koch, L. W. (1958). Inhibition of respiration, germination and growth by substances arising during the decomposition of certain plant residues in the soil. *Can. J. Bot.* **36**, 621–647.

Patrick, Z. A., and Koch, L. W. (1963). The adverse influence of phytotoxic substances from decomposing plant residues on resistance of tobacco to black root rot. *Can. J. Bot.* **41**, 747–758.

Patrick, Z. A., Toussoun, T. A., and Snyder, W. C. (1963). Phytotoxic substances in arable soils associated with decomposition of plant residues. *Phytopathology* **53**, 152–161.

Patrick, Z. A., Toussoun, T. A., and Koch, L. W. (1964). Effect of crop residue decomposition products on plant roots. *Annu. Rev. Phytopathol.* **2**, 267–292.

Pecket, R. C. (1960). Phenolic constituents of leaves and flowers in the genus *Lathyrus*. *In* "Phenolics in Plants in Health and Disease" (J. B. Pridham, ed.), pp. 119-126. Pergamon, Oxford.

Petrii, E., and Chrastil, J. (1955). The exosmosis of flavanone from root explantations of *Arachis hypogaea* L. *Folia Biol. (Prague)* 310-312.

Pharis, R. P., Barnes, R. L., and Naylor, A. W. (1964). Effects of nitrogen level, calcium level, and nitrogen source upon growth and composition of *Pinus taeda* L. *Physiol. Plant.* **17**, 560–572.

Pickering, S. V. (1917). The effect of one plant on another. *Ann. Bot. (London)* **31**, 181–187.

Pickering, S. V. (1919). The action of one crop on another. *J. Roy. Hort. Soc.* **43**, 372–380.

Podtelok, M. P. (1972). Effect of physiologically active substances of maple, oak and ash roots and their role in seedling growth. *In* "Physiological-Biochemical Basis of Plant Interactions in Phytocenoses" (A. M. Grodzinsky, ed.), Vol. 3, pp. 104–106. Naukova Dumka, Kiev. (In Russian)

Pratt, R. (1940). Influence of the size of the inoculum on the growth of *Chlorella vulgaris* in freshly prepared culture medium. *Amer. J. Bot.* **27**, 52–56.

Pratt, R. (1942). Studies on *Chlorella vulgaris*. V. Some properties of the growth inhibitor formed by *Chlorella* cells. *Amer. J. Bot.* **29**, 142–148.

Pratt, R. (1944). Studies on *Chlorella vulgaris*. IX. Influence on the growth of *Chlorella* of continuous removal of chlorellin from the solution. *Amer. J. Bot.* **31**, 418–421.

Pratt, R. (1948). Studies on *Chlorella vulgaris*. XI. Relation between surface tension and accumulation of chlorellin. *Amer. J. Bot.* **35**, 634–637.

Pratt, R., and Fong, J. (1940). Studies on *Chlorella vulgaris*. II. Further evidence that *Chlorella* cells form a growth-inhibiting substance. *Amer. J. Bot.* **27**, 431–436.

Prescott, G. W. (1948). Objectionable algae, with reference to the killing of fish and other animals. *Hydrobiologia* **1**, 1–13.

Proctor, V. W. (1957). Studies of algae antibiosis using *Haematococcus* and *Chlamydomonas*. *Limnol. Oceanogr.* **2**, 125–139.

Proebsting, E. L. (1950). A case history of a "peach replant" situation. *Proc. Amer. Soc. Hort. Sci.* **56**, 46–48.

Proebsting, E. L., and Gilmore, A. E. (1941). The relation of peach root toxicity to the re-establishing of peach orchards. *Proc. Amer. Soc. Hort. Sci.* **38**, 21–26.

Pronin, V. A., and Yakovlev. A. A. (1970). Influence of nutrition conditions and rhizospheric microorganisms on the interrelations of maize and fodder beans in mixed culture. *In* "Physiological-Biochemical Basis of Plant Interactions in Phytocenoses" (A. M. Grodzinsky, ed.), Vol. 1, pp. 93–101. Naukova Dumka, Kiev. (In Russian)

Prutenskaya, N. I. (1972). Presence of inhibitors and stimulators of *Sinapis arvensis* L. in germinating seeds of cultivated plants. *In* "Physiological-Biochemical Basis of Plant Interactions in Phytocenoses" (A. M. Grodzinsky, ed.), Vol. 3, pp. 73–75. Naukova Dumka, Kiev. (In Russian)

Prutenskaya, N. I., Yurchak, L. D., and Soroka, M. A. (1970). Physiologically active substances of microorganisms and decomposing plant residue. *In* "Physiological-Biochemical Basis of Plant Interactions in Phytocenoses" (A. M. Grodzinsky, ed.), Vol. 1, pp. 218–222. Naukova Dumka, Kiev. (In Russian)

Randon, Y. (1966). Action inhibitrice de l'extrait du lichen *Rocelle fucoides* (Dicks) Vain sur la germination. *Bull. Soc. Bot. Fr.* **113**, 1–2.

Rasmussen, J. A., and Rice, E. L. (1971). Allelopathic effects of *Sporobolus pyramidatus* on vegetational patterning. *Amer. Midl. Natur.* **86**, 309–326.

Reid, A., (1964). Further studies on growth inhibitors produced by shrubs. *J. Colo.-Wyo. Acad. Sci.* **5**, 42.

Rice, E. L. (1964). Inhibition of nitrogen-fixing and nitrifying bacteria by seed plants. I. *Ecology* **45**, 824–837.

Rice, E. L. (1965a). Inhibition of nitrogen-flxing and nitrifying bacteria by seed plants. II. Characterization and identification of inhibitors. *Physiol. Plant.* **18**, 255–268.

Rice, E. L. (1965b). Inhibition of nitrogen-fixing and nitrifying bacteria by seed plants. III. Comparison of three species of *Euphorbia*. *Proc. Okla. Acad. Sci.* **45**, 43–44.

Rice, E. L. (1965c). Inhibition of nitrogen-fixing and nitrifying bacteria by seed plants. IV. The inhibitors produced by *Ambrosia elatior* L. and *Ambrosia psilostachya* DC. *Southwest. Natur.* 248–255.

Rice, E. L. (1968). Inhibition of nodulation of inoculated legumes by pioneer plant species from abandoned fields. *Bull. Torrey Bot. Club* **95**, 346–358.

Rice, E. L. (1969). Inhibition of nitrogen-fixing and nitrifying bacteria by seed plants. VI. Inhibitors from *Euphorbia supina* Raf. *Physiol. Plant.* **22**, 1175–1183.

Rice, E. L. (1971a). Inhibition of nodulation of inoculated legumes by leaf leachates from pioneer plant species from abandoned fields. *Amer. J. Bot.* **58**, 368–371.

Rice, E. L. (1971b). Some possible roles of inhibitors in old-field succession. *In* "Biochemical interactions among Plants" (U.S. Nat. Comm. for IBP, eds.), pp. 128–132. Nat. Acad. Sci., Washington, D.C.

Rice, E. L. (1972). Allelopathic effects of *Andropogon virginicus* and its persistence in old fields. *Amer. J. Bot.* **59**, 752–755.

Rice, E. L., and Pancholy, S. K. (1972). Inhibition of nitrification by climax vegetation. *Amer. J. Bot.* **59**, 1033–1040.

Rice, E. L., and Pancholy, S. K. (1973). Inhibition of nitrification by climax ecosystems. II. Additional evidence and possible role of tannins. *Amer. J. Bot.* **60**, 691–702.

Rice, E. L., and Parenti, R. L. (1967). Inhibition of nitrogen-fixing bacteria by seed plants. V. Inhibitors produced by *Bromus japonicus* Thunb. *Southwest. Natur.* **12**, 97–103.

Rice, E. L., and Penfound, W. T. (1955). An evaluation of the variable-radius and paired-tree methods in the blackjack-post oak forest. *Ecology* **36**, 315–320.

Rice, E. L., Penfound, W. T., and Rohrbaugh, L. M. (1960). Seed dispersal and mineral nutrition in succession in abandoned fields in central Oklahoma. *Ecology* **41**, 224–228.

Rice, T. R. (1954). Biotic influences affecting population growth of planktonic algae. *U.S., Fish Wildl. Serv., Fish. Bull.* **54**, 227–245.

Richardson, H. L. (1935). The nitrogen cycle in grassland soils. *Trans. Int. Cong. Soil Sci., 3rd, 1935* Vol. 1, pp. 219–221.

Richardson, H. L. (1938). Nitrification in grassland soils. *J. Agr. Sci.* **28**, 73–121.

Riddiford, L. M. (1969). Oak leaves and the mating and ovipositional behavior of the polyphemus moth. *In* "Insect-Plant Interactions" (U.S. Nat. Comm. for IBP, eds.), p. 60. Nat. Acad. Sci., Washington, D.C.

Riddiford, L. M., and Williams, C. M. (1967). Volatile principle in oak leaves: Role in sex life of the *Polyphemus* moth. *Science* **155**, 589–590.

Riov, J., Monselise, S. P., and Kahan, R. S. (1969). Ethylene-controlled induction of phenylalanine ammonia-lyase in citrus fruit peel. *Plant Physiol.* **44**, 631–635.

Robinson, R. K. (1972). The production by roots of *Calluna vulgaris* of a factor inhibitory to growth of some mycorrhizal fungi. *J. Ecol.* **60**, 219–224.

Robinson, T. (1963). "The Organic Constituents of Higher Plants." Burgess, Minneapolis, Minnesota.

Rodhe, W. (1948). Environmental requirements of fresh-water plankton algae. *Symb. Bot. Upsal.* **10**, 1–149.

Rovira, A. D. (1956). Plant root excretions in relation to the rhizosphere effect. I. The nature of root exudate from oats and peas. *Plant Soil* **7**, 178–194.

Rovira, A. D. (1965). Plant root exudates and their influence upon soil microorganisms. *In* "Ecology of Soil-Borne Plant Pathogens" (K. F. Baker and W. C. Snyder, eds.), pp. 170-184. Univ. of California Press, Berkeley.

Rovira, A. D. (1969). Plant root exudates. *Bot. Rev.* **35**, 35–59.

Rovira, A. D. (1971). Plant root exudates. *In* "Biochemical Interactions among Plants" (U.S. Nat. Comm. for IBP, eds.), pp. 19–24. Nat. Acad. Sci., Washington, D.C.

Rudinsky, J. A. (1966). Host selection and invasion by the Douglas-fir beetle, *Dendroctonus pseudotsugae* Hopkins, in coastal Douglas-fir forest. *Can. Entomol.* **98**, 98–111.

Rudinsky, J. A. (1969). Studies on timber beetles. *In* "Insect-Plant Interactions" (U.S. Nat. Comm. for IBP, eds.), pp. 64–65. Nat. Acad. Sci., Washington, D.C.

Russell, E. J. (1914). The nature and amount of the fluctuations in nitrate contents of arable soils.*J. Agr. Sci.* **6**, 50–53.

Russell, E. J. and Russell, E. W. (1961). "Soil Conditions and Plant Growth," 9th ed. Wiley, New York.

Sampson, A. W. (1944). Plant succession on burned chaparral lands in northern California. *Univ. Calif., Davis, Agr. Exp. Sta., Bull.* **685**.

Samtsevich, S. A. (1968). Gel-like excretions of plant roots and their influence upon soil and rhizosphere microflora. *In* "Methods of Productivity Studies in Root Systems and Rhizosphere Organisms" (Sov. Nat. Comm. for IBP, eds.), pp. 200–204. Nauka, Leningrad.

Sandfaer, J. (1968). Induced sterility as a factor in the competition between barley varieties.*Nature (London)* **218**, 241–243.

Santos, S. P., Lat, B. S., and Palo, M. A. (1964). The antibiotic activities of some Philippine lichens.*Philipp. J. Sci.* **93**, 325–336.

Saunders, G. W. (1957). Interrelations of dissolved organic matter and phytoplankton. *Bot. Rev.* **23**, 389–409.

Savage, D. A., and Runyon, H. E. (1937). Natural revegetation of abandoned farm land in the central and southern Great Plains. *In* "Report of Section 1 (Grassland Ecology) of International Grassland Congress," pp. 178–182. Int. Grassland Congr. Aberystwyth.

Schaal, L. A., and Johnson, G. (1955). The inhibitory effect of phenolic compounds on the growth of *Streptomyces scabies* as related to the mechanism of scab resistance. *Phytopathology* **45**, 626–628.

Schlatterer, E. F., and Tisdale, E. W. (1969). Effects of litter of *Artemisia, Chrysothamnus*, and *Tortula* on germination.*Ecology* **50**, 869–873.

Schneiderhan, F. J. (1927). The black walnut (*Juglans nigra* L.) as a cause of the death of apple trees.*Phytopathology* **17**, 529–540.

Schreiner, O., and Lathrop, E. C. (1911). Examination of soils for organic constituents. *U.S., Bur. Soils, Bull.* **80**.

Schreiner, O., and Reed, H. S. (1907a). Certain organic constituents of soil in relation to soil fertility.*U.S., Bur. Soils, Bull.* **47**.

Schreiner, O., and Reed, H. S. (1907b). The production of deleterious excretions by roots. *Bull. Torrey Bot. Club* **34**, 279–303.

Schreiner, O., and Reed, H. S. (1908). The toxic action of certain organic plant constituents. *Bot. Gaz. (Chicago)* **45**, 73–102.

Schreiner, O., and Shorey, E. D. (1909). The isolation of harmful organic substances from soils. *U.S., Bur. Soils, Bull.* **53**.

Schreiner, O., and Sullivan, M. X. (1909). Soil fatigue caused by organic compounds. *J. Biol. Chem.* **6**, 39–50.

Schwimmer, S. (1958). Influence of polyphenols and potato components on potato phosphorylase.*J. Biol. Chem.* **232**, 715–721.

Schwinghamer, E. A. (1964). Association between antibiotic resistance and ineffectiveness in mutant strains of *Rhizobium* spp. *Can. J. Microbiol.* **10**, 221–233.

Schwinghamer, E. A. (1967). Effectiveness of *Rhizobium* as modified by mutation for resistance to antibiotics.*Antonie van Leeuwenoek; J. Microbiol. Serol.* **33**, 121–136.

Scott, F. M., Schroeder, M. R., and Turrell, F. M. (1948). Development, cell shape, suberization of internal surface, and abscission in the leaf of the Valencia orange, *Citrus sinensis. Bot. Gaz. (Chicago)* **109**, 381–411.

Scott, R. M. (1952). Algal toxins.*Pub. Works, March*, 54–55, 65–66.

Seegal, B. C., and Holden, M. (1945). The antibiotic activity of extracts of Ranunculaceae. *Science* **101**, 413–414.

Selleck, G. W. (1972). The antibiotic effects of plants in laboratory and field. *Weed Sci.* **20**, 189–194.

Sevilla-Santos, P., Encinas, C. J., and Leus-Palo, S. (1964). The antibacterial activities of aqueous extracts from Philippine Basidiomycetes. *Phillipp. J. Sci.* **93**, 479–498.

Shen, T. C. (1969). The induction of nitrate reductase and the preferential assimilation of ammonium in germinating rice seedlings. *Plant Physiol.* **44**, 1650–1655.

Shields, L. M., and Durrell, L. W. (1964). Algae in relation to soil fertility. *Bot. Rev.* **30**, 92–128.

Shilo, M., and Aschner, M. (1953). Factors governing the toxicity of cultures containing the phytoflagellate *Prymnesium parvum. J. Gen. Microbiol.* **8**, 333–343.

Shimshi, D. (1963a). Effect of chemical closure of stomata on transpiration in varied soil and atmospheric environments. *Plant Physiol.* **38**, 709–712.

Shimshi, D. (1963b). Effect of soil moisture and phenylmercuric acetate upon stomatal aperture, transpiration, and photosynthesis. *Plant Physiol.* **38**, 713–721.

Shtina, E. A. (1960). The interrelationship of soil algae and agricultural plants in different environmental conditions. *Dokl. Vysshei Shkolg. Biol. Nauk* **1**, 75–79; See *Biol. Abstr.* **42**, 269 (No. 3275) (1963).

Sidhu, K. S., and Pfander, W. H. (1968). Metabolic inhibitor(s) in orchard grass (*Dactylis glomerata* L.). *J. Dairy Sci.* **51**, 1042–1045.

Sieburth, J. M. (1959). Antibacterial activity of Antarctic marine phytoplankton. *Limnol. Oceanogr.* **4**, 419–424.

Sigmund, W. (1924). Über die Einwirking von Stoffwechselendprodukten auf die Pflanzen. III. Einwirking N-freier pflanzlicher Stoffweckselendprodukte aud die Keimung von Samen (Aetherische Oele, Terpene u.a.). *Biochem. Z.* **146**, 380–419.

Sikka, H. C., Shimabukuro, R. H., and Zweig, G. (1972). Studies on effect of certain quinones I. Electron transport, photophosphorylation and CO_2 fixation in isolated chloroplasts. *Plant Physiol.* **49**, 381–384.

Silverstein, R. M. (1969). Terpenes and insect behavior. *In* "Insect-Plant Interactions" (U.S. Nat. Comm. for IBP, eds.), pp. 73–75. Nat. Acad. Sci., Washington, D.C.

Silverstein, R. M., Rodin, J. P., and Wood, D. L. (1966). The principal sex attractants in the frass produced by *Ips confusus. Science* **154**, 509–510.

Smale, B. C., Wilson, R. A., and Keil, H. L. (1964). A survey of green plants for antimicrobial substances. *Phytopathology* **54**, 748.

Smart, W. W. G., Jr., Bell, T. A., Stanley, N. W., and Cope, W. A. (1961). Inhibition of rumen cellulase by extract of sericea forage. *J. Dairy Sci.* **44**, 1945–1946.

Smith, W., Bormann, F. H., and Likens, G. E. (1968). Response of chemoautotrophic nitrifiers to forest cutting. *Soil Sci.* **106**, 471–473.

Society of American Bacteriologists. (1957). "Manual of Microbiological Methods." McGraw-Hill, New York.

Somers, T. C., and Harrison, A. F. (1967). Wood tannins-isolation and significance in host resistance to *Verticillium* wilt disease. *Aust. J. Biol. Sci.* **20**, 475–479.

Sondheimer, E. (1962). The chlorogenic acids and related compounds. *In* "Plant Phenolics and their Industrial Significance" (V. C. Runeckles, ed.), pp. 15–37. Imperial Tobacco Company of Canada, Montreal.

Sondheimer, E., and Griffin, D. H. (1960). Activation and inhibition of indoleacetic acid oxidase activity from peas. *Science* **131**, 672.

Starkey, R. L. (1929). Some influences of the development of higher plants upon the microorganisms in the soil. II. Influence of the stage of plant growth upon abundance of organisms. *Soil Sci.* **27**, 355–378.

Stenlid, G. (1968). On the physiological effects of phloridzin, phloretin and some related substances upon higher plants. *Physiol. Plant.* **21**, 882–894.

Stewart, J. R., and Brown, R. M., Jr. (1969). *Cytophaga* that kills or lyses algae. *Science* **164**, 1523–1524.

Stewart, W. D. (1966). "Nitrogen Fixation in Plants." Oxford Univ. Press, London and New York.

Stickney, J. S., and Hoy, P. R. (1881). Toxic action of black walnut. *Trans. Wis. State Hort. Soc.* **11**, 166–167.

Stillwell, M. A. (1966). A growth inhibitor produced by *Cryptosporiopsis* sp., an imperfect fungus isolated from yellow birch, *Betula alleghaniensis*. *Can. J. Bot.* **44**, 259–267.

Stiven, G. (1952). Production of antibiotic substances by the roots of a grass (*Trachypogon plumosus*) (H.B.K. Nees) and of *Pentanisia variabilis* (E. Mey.) Harv. (Rubiaceae). *Nature (London)* **170**, 712–713.

Swain, T. (1965). The tannins. *In* "Plant Biochemistry" (J. Bonner and J. E. Varner, eds.), 2nd ed., pp. 552–580. Academic Press, New York.

Swan, H. S. D. (1960). "The Mineral Nutrition of Canadian Pulpwood Species. I. The Influence of Nitrogen, Phosphorus, Potassium, and Magnesium Deficiencies on the Growth and Development of White Spruce, Black Spruce, Jack Pine, and Western Hemlock Seedlings Grown in a Controlled Environment," Tech. Rep. No. 168. Pulp and Paper Research Institute of Canada, Montreal.

Sweeney, J. R. (1956). Responses of vegetation to fire, a study of the herbaceous vegetation following chaparral fires. *Univ. Calif., Berkeley, Publ. Bot.* **28**, 143–250.

Szczepańska, W. (1971). Allelopathy among the aquatic plants. *Pol. Arch. Hydrobiol.* **18**, 17–30.

Szczepański, A. (1971). Allelopathy and other factors controlling the macrophytes production. *Hydrobiologia* **12**, 193–197.

Tam, R. K., and Clark, H. E. (1943). Effects of chloropicrin and other soil disinfectants on the nitrogen nutrition of the pineapple plant. *Soil Sci.* **56**, 245–261.

Taylor, A. O. (1965). Some effects of photoperiod on the biosynthesis of phenylpropane derivatives in *Xanthium*. *Plant Physiol.* **40**, 273–280.

Theron, J. J. (1951). The influence of plants on the mineralization of nitrogen and the maintenance of organic matter in soil. *J. Agr. Sci.* **41**, 289–296.

Thorne, D. W., and Brown, P. E. (1937). The growth and respiration of some soil bacteria in juices of leguminous and non-leguminous plants. *J. Bacteriol.* **34**, 567–580.

Thorsteinson, A. J. (1969). Olfactory influences of plants on behavior and physiology of phytophagous insects. *In* "Insect-Plant Interactions" (U.S. Nat. Comm. for IBP, eds.), pp. 82–83. Nat. Acad. Sci., Washington, D.C.

Tillberg, J-E. (1970). Effects of abscisic acid, salicylic acid and trans-cinnamic acid on phosphate uptake, ATP-level and oxygen evolution in *Scenedesmus*. *Physiol. Plant.* **23**, 647–653.

Tinnin, R., and Muller, C. H. (1971). The allelopathic potential of *Avena fatua*: Influence on herb distribution. *Bull. Torrey Bot. Club.* **98**, 243–250.

Todd, G. W., Getahun, A., and Cress, D. C. (1971). Resistance in barley to the greenbug, *Schizaphis graminum*. I. Toxicity of phenolic and flavonoid compounds and related substances. *Ann. Entomol. Soc. Amer.* **64**, 718–722.

Tomanek, G. W., Albertson, F. W., and Riegel, A. (1955). Natural revegetation on a field abandoned for thirty-three years in central Kansas. *Ecology* **36**, 407–412.

Tomaszewski, M., and Thimann, K. V. (1966). Interactions of phenolic acids, metallic ions and chelating agents on auxin-induced growth. *Plant Physiol.* **41**, 1443–1454.

Toussoun, T. A., and Patrick, Z. A. (1963). Effect of phytotoxic substances from decomposing plant residues on root rot of bean. *Phytopathology* **53**, 265–270.

Towers, G. H. N. (1964). Metabolism of phenolics in higher plants and microorganisms. *In* "Biochemistry of Phenolic Compounds" (J. B. Harborne, ed.), pp. 249–294. Academic Press, New York.

Tso, T. C., Socokin, T. P., Engelhaupt, M. E., Anderson, R. A., Bortner, C. E., Chaplin, J. F., Miles, J. D., Nichols, B. C., Shaw, L. and Street, O. E. (1967). Nitrogenous and phenolic compounds of *Nicotiana* plants. I. Field and greenhouse grown plants. *Tob. Sci.* **11**, 133–136.

Tso, T. C., Kasperbauer, M. J., and Sorokin, T. P. (1970). Effect of photoperiod and end-of-day light quality on alkaloids and phenolic compounds of tobacco. *Plant Physiol.* **45**, 330–333.

Tukey, H. B., Jr. (1966). Leaching of metabolites from above-ground plant parts and its implications. *Bull. Torrey Bot. Club* **93**, 385–401.

Tukey, H. B., Jr. (1969). Implications of allelopathy in agricultural plant science. *Bot. Rev.* **35**, 1–16.

Tukey, H. B., Jr. (1971). Leaching of substances from plants. *In* "Biochemical Interactions among Plants" (U.S. Nat. Comm. for IBP, eds.), pp. 25–32. Nat. Acad. Sci., Washington, D.C.

Turner, N. C. (1972). Stomatal behavior of *Avena sativa* treated with two phytotoxins, victorin and fusicoccin. *Amer. J. Bot.* **59**, 133–136.

U.S. Department of Agriculture. (1960). "Soil Classification, a Comprehensive System. Seventh Approximation." US Govt. Printing Office, Washington, D.C.

Vacca, D. D., and Walsh, R. A. (1954). The antibacterial extract obtained from *Ascophyllum nodosum. J. Amer. Pharm. Ass., Sci. Ed.* **43**, 24–26.

Van der Merwe, K. J., Van Jaarsveld, P. P., and Hattingh, M. J. (1967). The isolation of 2,4-diacetyl-phloroglucinol from a *Pseudomonas* sp. *S. Afr. Med. J.* **41**, 1110.

Van Sumere, C. F., and Massart, L. (1959). Natural substances in relation to germination. *In* "Biochemistry of Antibiotics" (K. H. Spitzy and R. Brunner, eds.), Vol. 5, pp. 20–32. Pergamon, Oxford.

Van Sumere, C. F., Cottenie, J., De Greef, J., and Kint, J. (1971). Biochemical studies in relation to the possible germination regulatory role of naturally occurring coumarin and phenolics. *Recent Adv. Phytochem.* **4**, 165–221.

Varga, M., and Köves, E. (1959). Phenolic acids as growth and germination inhibitors in dry fruits. *Nature (London)* **183**, 401.

Vieitez, E., and Ballester, A. (1972). Compuestos fenólicos y cumáricos en *Erica cinerea* L. *An. Inst. Bot. A. J. Cavanilles* **29**, 129–142.

Vikherkova, M. (1970). Influence of active substances from rhizome of wheatgrass on growth and water balance of flax. *In* "Physiological-Biochemical Basis of Plant Interactions in Phytocenoses" (A. M. Grodzinsky, ed.), Vol. 1, pp. 135–140. Naukova Dumka, Kiev. (In Russian)

Vincent, J. G., and Vincent, H. W. (1944). Filter paper disc modification of the Oxford cup penicillin determination. *Proc. Soc. Exp. Biol. Med.* **55**, 162–164.

Viro, P. J. (1963). Factorial experiments on forest humus decomposition. *Soil Sci.* **95**, 24–30.

Virtanen, A. I., Erkama, J., and Linkola, H. (1947). On the relation between nitrogen fixation and leghaemoglobin content of leguminous root nodules. II. *Acta Chem. Scand.* **1**, 861–870.

Visona, L., and Pesce, E. (1963). Action de quelques antibiotiques sur la symbiose du tréfle rouge *(Trifolium pratense* L.). *Ann. Inst. Pasteur Paris* **105**, 368–382.

Visona, L., and Tardieux, P. (1964). Antagonistes des *Rhizobium* dans la rhizosphére du tréfle et de la luzerne. *Ann. Inst. Pasteur, Paris Sup. to No. 3*, 297–302.

von Liebig, J. (1843). "Die Chemie in ihrer Anwendung auf Agriculture und Physio-logie." Vieweg, Braunschweig.

Wahlroos, O., and Virtanen, A. I. (1959). The precursors of G-methoxybenzoxazolinone in maize and wheat plants, their isolation and some of their properties. *Acta Chem. Scand.* **13**, 1906–1908.

Waks, C. (1936). The influence of extract from *Robinia pseudoacacia* on the growth of barley. *Publ. Fac. Sci. Univ. Charles, Prague* **150**, 84–85.

Waksman, S. A. (1937). Soil deterioration and soil conservation from the viewpoint of soil microbiology. *J. Amer. Soc. Agron.* **29**, 113–122.

Waksman, S. A. (1947). "Microbial Antagonisms and Antibiotic Substances." Commonwealth Fund, New York.

Waller, C. W., Patrick, J. B., Fulmor, W., and Meyer, W. E. (1957). The structure of nucleocidin. I. *J. Amer. Chem. Soc.* **79**, 1011–1012.

Walton, L., Herbold, M., and Lindegren, C. C. (1936). Bactericidal effects of vapors from crushed garlic. *Food Res.* **1**, 163–169.

Wang, T. S. C., Yang, T., and Chuang, T. (1967). Soil phenolic acids as plant growth inhibitors. *Soil Sci.* **103**, 239–246.

Ward, G. M., and Durkee, A. B. (1956). The peach replant problem in Ontario. III. Amygdalin content of peach tree tissues. *Can. J. Bot.* **34**, 419–422.

Warren, M. (1965). A study of soil-nutritional and other factors operating in secondary succession in highveld grassland in the neighborhood of Johannesburg. Ph.D. Dissertation, University of Witwatersrand, Johannesburg.

Watanabe, R., McIlrath, W. J., Skok, J., Chorney, W., and Wender, S. H. (1961). Accumulation of scopoletin glucoside in boron-deficient tobacco leaves. *Arch. Biochem. Biophys.* **94**, 241–243.

Way, J. T. (1847). On the fairy-rings of pastures, as illustrating the use of inorganic manures. *J. Roy. Agr. Soc. Engl.* **7**, 549–552.

Weetman, G. F. (1961). "The Nitrogen Cycle in Temperate Forest Stands (Literature Review)," Res. Note No. 21. Pulp and Paper Research Institute of Canada, Montreal.

Weissman, G. S. (1972). Influence of ammonium and nitrate nutrition on enzymatic activity in soybean and sunflower. *Plant Physiol.* **49**, 138–141.

Welbank, P. J. (1960). Toxin production from *Agropyron repens. In* "The Biology of Weeds" (J. L. Harper, ed.), pp. 158–164. Blackwell, Oxford.

Welch, R. M., and Epstein, E. (1969). The plasmalemma: Seat of the type 2 mechanisms of ion absorption. *Plant Physiol.* **44**, 301–304.

Went, F. W. (1942). The dependence of certain annual plants on shrubs in southern California deserts. *Bull. Torrey Bot. Club* **69**, 100–114.

Went, F. W. (1948). Ecology of desert plants. I. Observations on the germination in the Joshua Tree National Monument, California. *Ecology* **29**, 242–253.

Went, F. W., and Westergaard, M. (1949). Ecology of desert plants. III. Development of plants in the Death Valley National Monument, California. *Ecology* **30**, 26–38.

White, G. A., and Starratt, A. N. (1967). The production of a phytotoxic substance by *Alternaria zinniae. Can. J. Bot.* **45**, 2087–2090.

Whitehead, D. C. (1964). Identification of p-hydroxybenzoic, vanillic, p-coumaric and ferulic acids in soils. *Nature (London)* **202**, 417.

Whittaker, R. H. (1971). The chemistry of communities. *In* "Biochemical Interactions among Plants" (U.S. Nat. Comm. for IBP, eds.), pp. 10–18. Nat. Acad. Sci., Washington, D.C.

Whittaker, R. H., and Feeny, P. P. (1971). Allelochemics: Chemical interactions between species. *Science* **171**, 757–770.

Williams, A. H. (1960). The distribution of phenolic compounds in apple and pear trees. *In* "Phenolics in Plants in Health and Disease" (J. B. Pridham, ed.), pp. 3–7. Pergamon, Oxford.

Williams, A. H. (1963). Enzyme inhibition by phenolic compounds. *In* "Enzyme Chemistry of Phenolic Compounds" (J. B. Pridham, ed.), pp. 87–96. Macmillan, New York.

Wilson, R. E., and Rice, E. L. (1968). Allelopathy as expressed by *Helianthus annuus* and its role in old-field succession. *Bull. Torrey Bot. Club* **95**, 432–448.

Winkler, B. C. (1967). Quantitative analysis of coumarins by thin layer chromatography, related chromatographic studies, and the partial identification of a scopoletin glycoside present in tobacco tissue culture. Ph.D. Dissertation, University of Oklahoma, Norman.

Winter, A. G. (1961). New physiological and biological aspects in the interrelationships between higher plants. *Symp. Soc. Exp. Biol.* **15**, 229–244.

Woods, F. W. (1960). Biological antagonisms due to phytotoxic root exudates. *Bot. Rev.* **26**, 546–569.

Wright, J. M. (1956). The production of antibiotics in soil. IV. Production of antibiotics in coats of seeds sown in soil. *Ann. Appl. Biol.* **44**, 561–566.

Wurzburger, J., and Leshem, Y. (1969). Physiological action of the germination inhibitor in the husk of *Aegilops kotschyi* Boiss. *New Phytol.* **68**, 337–341.

Zelitch, I. (1967). Control of leaf stomata—Their role in transpiration and photosynthesis. *Amer. Sci.* **55**, 472–486.

Zucker, M. (1963). The influence of light on synthesis of protein and of chlorogenic acid in potato tuber tissue. *Plant Physiol.* **38**, 575–580.

Zucker, M. (1969). Induction of phenylalanine ammonia-lyase in *Xanthium* leaf discs. Photosynthetic requirement and effect of daylength. *Plant Physiol.* **44**, 912–922.

Zucker, M., Nitsch, C., and Nitsch, J. P. (1965). The induction of flowering in *Nicotiana*. II. Photoperiodic alteration of the chlorogenic acid concentration. *Amer. J. Bot.* **52**, 271–277.

Zweig, G., Carroll, J., Tamas, I., and Sikka, H. C. (1972). Studies on effects of certain quinones. II. Photosynthetic incorporation of $^{14}CO_2$ by *Chlorella. Plant Physiol.* **49**, 385–387.

Index

A

Abies amabilis, 172
Abies concolor, 172
Abies grandis, 172
Abies procera, 172
Abutilon theophrasti, 263
  inhibition by seeds, 208
Acer circinatum, 172
Acer species, inhibition by, 219
Acetaldehyde, 189
Acetone, 189
Acorus calamus, inhibition by, 149
Actinomycetes, production of toxins, 194
Adenostoma fasciculatum
  clearing effects on herbs, 115, 116
  effects of leaf leachates, 119
  heat effects on toxicity of soil under, 118, 119
  inhibition by, 114-120
Aegilops kotschyi, 274
Aesculus hippocastanum, 257
Agropyrene, 269
Agropyron repens, 269, 275, 284
Alcohols, 247
Aldehydes, 247
Alfalfa, inhibition by, 185-188
  effects on germination, 185-187
    on root growth, 185, 187
    on shoot growth, 185, 187
Algae, *see* specific types
Alkaloids, 264
Allelochemics, 312-316
  algae vs animals, 315, 316

ecdysones, 313, 314
gall-forming insects, 313
microbial production of toxins, 315
pheromones, 313, 314
phytophagous insect feeding, 313
plants vs animals, 314-316
  vs insects, 313, 314
resistance of plants to animal grazing, 315
  to insect predation, 313
Allelopathic agents, *see* Inhibitors
Allelopathy
  definition, 1, 2
  fire cycle, 104-106
    role of, in California grasslands, 104-125
  grafting and budding, 219, 220
  higher plants vs higher plants, 3-11
    vs microorganisms, 11-15
  historical account of, 3-22
  impact on agriculture, 184-217
    on forestry, 234-236
    on horticulture, 218-234
  infection promotion, 212, 213
  infection resistance, 213-216
  inhibition of seed germination of crop plants, 210, 211
  interactions with other types of chemical interactions, 312-316
  microorganisms vs higher plants, 15-18
    vs microorganisms, 18-22
  nitrogen fixation vs, 210
  origin of term, 1, 2
  prevention of seed decay, 174-183

Allelopathy (*continued*)
   related phenomena, 216, 217
   role in old-field succession, 35-76
      in patterning of vegetation, 126-173
      in phytoplankton succession, 23-34
   slowing of old-field succession, 52-74
Allicin, as toxin, 12
Allium sativum, 265
   toxin in, 12
Amanita, 315
Amaranthus retroflexus, inhibition by
      seeds, 208
Ambrosia artemisiifolia, inhibition by
      seeds, 208
Ambrosia psilostachya, *see* Ragweed,
      western
Amino acids, 262-264
   inhibition by, 209
Amygdalin, as source of toxins, 222-228
   amounts in organs of peach, 227
   benzaldehyde from, 222-226
   cyanide from, 222-226
   decomposition of, 222-226
      by microorganisms, 227
   emulsin effects, 222
   respiration effects, 224
   of breakdown products, 224, 225
Anabaena, 316
   inhibition of, by phenolic acids, 72
Anacystis nidulans, 32
Andropogon scoparius, as inhibitor of
      Anabaena, 72, 73
Andropogon virginicus, *see* Broomsedge
Antibiotics, 2
Aphanizomenon, 316
Apple, inhibition by, 229-231
   by fruits, 220
   patulin production in soil, 231
   Penicillium species vs patulin, 231
   phlorizin as toxin, 230, 231
      breakdown products of, 230, 231
   replant problems, 229-231
   root residue effects, 229-231
Arbutus menziesii, 172
Arctostaphylos, allelopathic effects,
      120-124
   clearing effects on herbs, 121-122
   decaying material, 123
   leachates of tops, 122
Aristida oligantha, as inhibitor of *Ana-
      baena*, 73
Artemisia absinthium, 6, 7, 251, 260

Artemisia californica, inhibition by,
      106-113
Artemisia tridentata, inhibition by, 217
Avena fatua, inhibition by, 145-148
   cleared plots, 147, 148
   toxins in dry straw of, 148
Avena sativa, *see* Oats

B

Bacteria
   control of poultry pathogens, 217
   nitrogen-fixing, inhibition of
      methods of testing, 55
      of nodulation, 57, 58
      successional species inhibitory to, 56,
         57
   in soil, inhibition by, 194
Barbarea vulgaris, inhibition by seeds,
      208
Barberry, inhibition by, 219
Barley
   inhibition by, 186
      by seeds, 209
   residues, 203
   resistance to greenbug, 217
Beet, 189
   inhibition by seeds, 209
Benzaldehyde
   respiration effects, 226
   as toxin, 222-226
Benzoic acid, 256, 257
Birdsfoot trefoil, interaction with yellow
      lupine, 188
Black walnut, 3-6, 272
   inhibition by, 218
   toxin in, 6
Blue-green algae, inhibition of, 69-74
   toxic to animals, 316
Brassica juncea, inhibition by seeds, 208
Brassica nigra, 267
   inhibition by, 131-133
      effects of decaying leaves and stems,
         133
      of leachate, 133
      volatile toxins from, 132
Brefeldin A, *see* Nectrolide
Broadbean residues, 203
Broccoli residues, 203
Brome grass, 191
Bromus inermis, *see* Smooth brome

Broomsedge, inhibition by
  of *Azotobacter,* 75
  of higher plants, 75
  of nodulation, 75
  of *Rhizobium,* 75

C

Caffeic acid, 214, 215
Calligonum species, 173
Camelina alyssum vs flax, 205
Carrot, 189
Catalase, effect of inhibitors on, 291
Cattail, *see Typha latifolia*
Cell division, effect of inhibitors on,
  271-272
Cellulase, effect of inhibitors on, 291
Celtis laevigata, see Hackberry
Cercidium floridum, 293
Chamise, *see Adenostoma fasciculatum*
Chenopodium album, 70
  inhibition by seeds, 208
  as inhibitor of *Anabaena,* 72, 73
Chlamydomonas reinhardi, 32
Chlorella, inhibitor from, 29
Chlorella vulgaris, 24-31
  autotoxin from, 24-26
Chlorellin, as inhibitor, 29
Chlorogenic acid, 214, 215, 300, 301,
  304-308
Chrysanthemum morifolium, inhibition
  by, 189, 190
Cinnamic acid, 256, 257
  as toxin, 8
Citrinin, 236
Citrus
  decline, 231-234
  soil microflora, 232-234
Coelosphaerium, 316
Colletotrichum circinans, inhibition of,
  214
  by catechol, 214
  by protocatechuic acid, 214
Competition, 1, 2
Convallaria majalis, 253
Cordycepin, 269
Corn, 191, 291
  inhibition by, 185-188
    effects on root growth, 185, 187
    on shoot growth, 185,187

germination effects, 185-187
residues, 196, 197
Corn stalk mulch, stimulation of fungal
  growth, 193
p-Coumaric acid, 186, 194
Coumarins, 257, 258
  production increased by viruses, 215
Crabgrass, inhibition by, 48, 49, 206
  effects of root exudates, 48, 49
  by seeds, 208
Crop plants, inhibition by, 184-210
  extracts of, 184-188
  exudates and volatile inhibitors, 188,
    189
  leachates of, 189, 190
  by other crop plants, 184-204
  by weeds, 205, 206
Crop residues, inhibition by, 190-204
  effects of roots, 203, 204
  field studies, 202-204
  respiratory effects, 197-202
Crop seeds, inhibition of weeds, 209
Cryptosporiopsis, inhibitor of *Fomes fomentarius,* 21
Cucumber, 189
Cyanide, as toxin, 222-226
  respiration effects, 226
Cyanohydrins, 265

D

Dactylis glomerata, see Orchard grass
Datura stramonium, inhibition by seeds,
  208
Daylength, 299, 300
Dendroctonus pseudotsugae, 314
Dhurrin, 265
Digitalis purpurea, 253, 315
Digitaria sanguinalis, see Crabgrass
3,4-Dihydroxyflavone, 186
Douglas fir beetle, *see Dendroctonus
  pseudotsugae*

E

Ecdysones, 313, 314
Echinochloa crusgalli, inhibition by
  seeds, 208
Encelia farinosa, 7
Enzymes, effect of inhibitors on, 290, 291

Eragrostis cilianensis, inhibition by seeds, 208
Erigeron canadensis, 9
  as inhibitor of *Anabaena,* 72, 73
Essential oils, 217
Ethanol, 189
Ethylene, 269, 293
Eucalyptus camaldulensis, inhibition by, 155-160
  competition studies, 157, 158
  effects of litter, 159, 160
    of soil, 160
  volatile inhibitors, 158
  water-soluble toxins, 159
  zonation around, 155, 156
Eucalyptus globulus, inhibition by, 154, 155
  effect of fog drip, 155
Euphorbia species, 260-261
Euphorbia supina, inhibition by, 50, 51
  effect of decaying material, 50, 51
    of root exudate, 50

F

Fatty acids, 249
Ferulic acid, 186, 194
Fir, inhibition by, 219
Flavonoids, 217, 258-260, 283, 300
Fodder beans, interaction with corn, 188
Foxtail, giant, inhibition by, 206-208
Fraxinus excelsior, inhibition by, 219
Fungi, toxin production, 236
  in soil, 194

G

Galium mollugo, 260
Glyceria aquatica, inhibition by, 149
Gonyaulax catenella, 315
Gonyaulax tamerensis, 315
Guayule, 7, 8
  toxin in, 8
Gymnodinium brevis, 315, 316

H

Hackberry, inhibition by, 167-171
  competition studies, 168

effects of decaying leaves, 168, 169
  of leaf leachate, 169
  of patterning, 167, 168
  of soil, 169, 170
  toxins produced, 171
Haematococcus pluvialis, 32
Hairy vetch, inhibition by, 209
Haloxylon aphyllum, 173
Heleocharis palustris, inhibition by, 149
Helianthus annuus, see Sunflower
Helianthus rigidus, see Sunflower, prairie
Helminthosporium carbonum, 263
  inhibition of, 214
    by caffeic acid, 214
    by chlorogenic acid, 214
Helminthosporium victoriae, 263
Hemoglobin, synthesis of, 59
  effects of leachates of successional species, 65
    of tannic acid on, 68
  inhibition of, 210, 289
Hordeum vulgare, see Barley
Horse chestnut, inhibition by, 219
Hydroquinone as toxin, 124
p-Hydroxybenzoic acid, 186, 194, 230
p-Hydroxyhydrocinnamic acid, 230

I

Infection in plants, 212-216
Inhibitors, *see also* specific types
  alkaloids, 264
  amino acids and polypeptides, 262-264
  biosynthetic pathways, 246
  chemical nature of, 245-270
  cinnamic acid and derivatives, 256, 257
  classification of, 246
  coumarins, 257, 258
  cyanohydrins, 265
  effect on catalase and peroxidase, 291
    on cell division, 271, 272
    on cellulase, 291
    on hemoglobin synthesis, 289
    on hormone-induced growth, 273, 274
    on lipid synthesis, 285-288
    on membrane permeability, 289, 290
    on mineral uptake, 274-278
    on phosphorylases, 292
    on protein synthesis, 285-288
    on proteolytic enzymes, 290, 291

on respiration, 281-283
on synthesis of organic acids, 285-288
flavonoids, 258-260
in higher plants, 237-239
   exudation from roots, 242, 243
   leaching of, 241, 242
   methods of egress, 238-244
   organs containing, 237-239
   release by plant decay, 243, 244
   source
      fruits, 239
      leaves, 238
      roots, 238, 239
      seeds, 239
      stems, 237, 238
   volatilization of, 239, 240
long-chain fatty acids, 249
mechanisms of actions, 171-194, 292-294
miscellaneous, 270
production of, 295-311
   age of plant organs, 310, 311
   effects of allelopathic agents, 308, 309
      of daylength, 299, 300
      genetic, 311
      of ionizing radiation, 296
      of light intensity, 299
      of mineral deficiency, 300-305
         boron, 300
         calcium, 300
         magnesium, 301
         nitrogen, 301-303
         phosphorus, 303
         potassium, 304
         sulfur, 305
      of red and far-red light, 297, 298
      synergistic, 306, 307
      of temperature, 307, 308
      of ultraviolet radiation, 296, 297
      of water stress, 305-307
purines and nucleosides, 267-269
quinones, 249, 250
retardation of photosynthesis, 279-281
simple organic acids, alcohols, aldehydes and ketones, 247
simple phenols, benzoic acid and derivatives, 256, 257
simple unsaturated lactones, 247
stimulation of ethylene synthesis, 293
stomatal opening vs, 283-285
sulfides and mustard oil glycosides, 265-267

tannins
   condensed, 262
   hydrolyzable, 260, 261
   terpenoids and steroids, 250-253
   water-repellant soils, 293, 294
Insects, 313, 314, *see also* specific genera
Ipomeamarone, 215
Ips confusus, 314
Isochlorogenic acid, 215, 300, 306
   production increased by viruses, 215

J

Jack pine, inhibition of, 235, 236
   by *Prunus*, 235
   by *Salix pellita*, 235
   by *Solidago*, 235
Johnson grass, 70, 265
   inhibition by, 37-41
      decaying tops and rhizomes, 38
      root and rhizome exudates, 39
   inhibitors produced, 41
      of *Anabaena*, 73
Juglans nigra, *see* Black walnut
Juglone (5-hydroxy-α-naphthaquinone), 6
Juniperus species, inhibition by, 151, 152

K

Kaempferol, 215
   production increased by viruses, 215
Ketones, 247
Kolines, 2

L

Lactones, 175, 247
Larix decidua, 172
Larrea divaricata, 293
Legumes, *see also* specific types
   inhibition of nodulation, 210
      decaying materials of forbs, 62-64
         of grasses, 62, 64
      exudates of successional species, 60
      by gallic acid, 66, 67
      leachates of successional species, 65
      by tannic acid, 66, 67
Lepidium virginicum, inhibition by, 206
Lilac, inhibition by, 219

Lipids, effect of inhibitors on, 285-288
Lupinus albus, 291
Lyngbya, inhibition of, by phenolic acids, 72

M

Malcomia maritima, inhibition by, 219
Manzanita, *see Arctostaphylos*
Marasmins, 2, 263
Marine algae, antibacterial and antifungal compounds produced by, 19
Medicago sativa, see Alfalfa
Melilotus alba, see Sweet clover
Membranes, effect of inhibitors on, 289, 290
Methanol, 189
3-Methyl-6-methoxy-8-hydroxy-3,4-dihydroxyisocoumarin, 215
Microbial inhibitors
    direct production by seed plants, 174-182
    higher plants, 216
    phenolic inhibitors in seeds and fruits, 175-182
    production in seed coats by microorganisms, 182, 183
    species with seeds containing, 179-182
    unsaturated lactones in seeds, 175
Microcystis, 316
Minerals
    deficiency, 300-305
    uptake, 274-278
Mockorange, inhibition by, 219
Mustard, *see Brassica nigra*
Mustard oil glycosides, 265-267

N

Nebularine, 269
Nectrolide (Brefeldin A), 17
Nitrification, inhibition of, 77-103
    ammonium nitrogen in soil, 90
    analysis of ammonium nitrogen, 89
        of nitrate, 89
        of nitrifiers, 89
    general evidence for, 77-87
    nitrate in soil, 91
    Nitrobacter in soil, 93
    Nitrosomonas in soil, 92

specific evidence for, 88-103
    theoretical basis for, 87, 88
Nitrobacter in soil, 93
Nitrogen fixation, 236
    extracts of forest species, 236
    inhibition of, 210, 236
        of hemoglobin synthesis in nodules, 59
        of successional species vs blue-green algae, 69-74
        of sunflower vs blue-green algae, 70
Nitrogen-fixing bacteria, *see* Bacteria
Nitrosomonas in soil, 92
Nitzschia frustulum, 26-31
Nodularia, 316
Nodulation of legumes, *see* Legumes
Nucleocidin, 269
Nucleosides, 267-269

O

Oat straw, 191
Oat straw mulch, stimulation of fungal growth, 193
Oats
    inhibition by, 185-188
        effects on root growth, 185, 187
            on shoot growth, 185, 187
        germination effects, 185-187
    residues, 196
Oenothera biennis, inhibition by, 206
Old-field succession, 35-76
    inhibitors identified, 51, 52
        effects on species from first two stages, 51
    nitrogen and phosphorus in relation to, 54, 55
    rapid disappearance of pioneer weed stage, 36-52
Orchard grass, inhibition by, rumen effects, 217
Orchinol, 215
Organic acids, 247
    effect of inhibitors on, 285-288

P

Parthenium argentatum, see Guayule
Patterning of vegetation
    concepts, 126-128

herbaceous species and, 128-150
woody species and, 150-173
Patulin, 193, 236
Peach, inhibition by, 220-228
amygdalin in bark, 222-228
replant problem, 220-228
nematodes vs, 228
root extracts, 222
roots as inhibitors, 221
Pear, inhibition by fruits, 220
Penicillic acid, 236
Penicillium urticae, inhibition by, 193
Peroxidase, effect of inhibitors on, 291
Phaseollin, 215
Phenolic compounds, 217
Phenolic inhibitors
inhibition of *Ceratocystis fimbriata,*
214
of *Gloeosporium kawakamii,* 214
of *Helminthosporium,* 214
of *Podosphaera leucotricha,* 214
of rust fungi, 214, 215
of *Venturia inaequalis,* 214
phytoalexins, 215, 216
role in hypersensitivity, 215
Phenols, 256, 257
Pheromones, 313, 314
Phleum pratense, see Timothy
Phloretin, 231
Phlorizin, 17, 230
Phloroglucinol, 230
Phosphorylases, effect of inhibitors on,
292
Photosynthesis, effect of inhibitors on,
279-281
Phytoalexins, 215, *see also* specific substances
Phytoflagellate, 316
Phytoncide, 2
Phytotoxins in soil, under crop plants,
194-196
Picea engelmannii, 172
Picea excelsa, 172
Pinus banksiana, see Jack pine
Pinus densiflora, inhibition by, 152-154
effects of dew-drip, 152
of soil, 153
Pinus edulis, inhibition by, 151, 152
Pinus resinosa, 247
Pinus silvestris, 172
Pinus strobus, 172

Pisatin, 215
Platanus occidentalis, see Sycamore
Polygonum pennsylvanicum, inhibition
by seeds, 208
Polypeptides, 262-264
Polyphemus moth, *trans*-2-hexenal, 314
Populus pruinosa, 173
Portulaca oleracea, inhibition by seeds,
208
Potato, inhibition by, 219
Potato vines, inhibition by, 185-188
effect on root growth, 185, 187
on shoot growth, 185, 187
germination effects, 185-187
Pratylenchus penetrans, 217
control by crop residues, 217
Propionic aldehyde, 189
Prosopis juliflora, 293
Proteins, effect of inhibitors on, 285-88
Protocatechuic acid, 214
Prymnesium parvum, 316
Pseudohylesinus nebulosus, 314
Pseudomonas tumefaciens, 221
Purines, 267-269

Q

Quercetin, 215
production increased by viruses, 215
Quercus robur, inhibition by, 219
Quinones, 249, 250

R

Radiation, 296-300
Radish, 189
Ragweed, western, 70, 311
inhibition by, 49, 50, 140-145
effect of decaying leaves, 50, 142-144
of leaf leachate, 50
of root exudate, 50, 144
of soil, 49, 50, 141, 142
patterns in field, 140, 141
as inhibitor of *Anabaena,* 72, 73
Ranunculus, 315
Rape roots, inhibition by, 197
Respiration, effect of inhibitors on,
281-283

Rhizobitoxine, 17
Rhizobium, inhibition of, 210
Rhizobium phaseoli, tannic acid-resistant
    strains of, 67
    inhibition of nodulation, 68
Rhizosolenia shrubsolei, toxin produced
    by, 315
Rhododendron albiflorum, 172
Rhus glabra, 70
    as inhibitor of *Anabaena,* 72, 73
Rhus radicans, 315
Rose, inhibition by, 219
Rubrotoxin, 236
Rye
    inhibition by, 186
    residues, 197, 203
        toxins produced by, 204

S

Salix rubra, 273
Salsola richteri, 173
Salvia apiana, inhibition by, 109, 110
    terpenes of, 110
Salvia leucophylla, inhibition by, 106-113
    terpenes of, 110
Salvia mellifera, inhibition by, 110
    terpenes of, 110
Scab resistance, 212
Schoenoplectus lacustris, inhibition by,
    149
Scolytus unispinosus, 314
Scopoletin, 186, 214, 215, 307, 308
    production increased by viruses, 215
Scopolin, 214, 301, 304, 305, 308
Secale, see Rye
Seed decay, inhibitors of
    postharvest, 212
    preharvest, 212
Seed germination, inhibition of, prehar-
    vest, 211
Sericea, inhibition by, leaf extract vs cellu-
    lase, 217
Setaria faberii, see Foxtail, giant
Setaria lutescens, inhibition by seeds, 208
Smooth brome, 7
Soil
    fungistasis of, 22
    water-repellant, 293, 294

Sorbus aucuparia, 247
Sorghum
    dhurrin in, 265
    residues, 196
Sorghum halepense, see Johnson grass
Sorghum stalks, 191
Soybean, 191
Sporobolus pyramidatus, inhibition by,
    133-140
    effect of decaying tops, 137
    of leachate, 137
    of root exudate, 137, 138
    of soil, 135, 136
    rate of spread in field, 138
Steroids, 250-253
Sudan grass residues, 203
Sulfides, 265-267
Sunflower, 70
    age of plant organs, 310
    inhibition by, 41-48
        effects of decaying leaves, 44
        of leaf leachate, 46
        of root exudate, 44
    patterning by, 129-131
    by soil, 42
    as inhibitor of *Anabaena,* 72, 73
    water stress, 306
    zones of reduced growth in field, 41
Sunflower, prairie
    autotoxic effects of, 9
    inhibition by, 128, 129
Sweet clover, inhibition by, 190-193
Sweet potato, 189
Sycamore, inhibition by, 160-167
    bare areas under, 161
    competition studies, 162, 163
    effects of decaying leaves, 163, 164
        of leaf leachates, 164, 165
        of soil, 165-166
    species outside canopy, 161
    toxins produced, 166
Syringic acid, 194

T

Tamarix hispida, 173
Tannic acid
    effect on hemoglobin synthesis, 68
    in soil under *Rhus copallina,* 67, 74

Tannins
  condensed, 262
  Erysiphe polygoni inhibition, 213
  hydrolyzable, 260, 261
  in sorghum grain and forage, effect on
      digestibility, 217
  Verticillium albo-atrum inhibition, 213
Taxus brevifola, 172
Temperature, 307, 308
Terpenes,
  inhibition by
    adsorption by soil, 111, 112
    of *Ceratocystis*, 215
    of *Fomes annonus*, 215
    uptake by paraffin, 110
  production of, by other plants, 113
Terpenoids, 250-253
Thalassiosira nordenskioldii, toxin pro-
      duced by, 315
Thamnosma montana, 258
Thuja occidentalis, 172
Thuja plicata, 172
Timothy
  inhibition by, 185-188
    effects on root growth, 185, 187
      on shoot growth, 185, 187
    germination effects, 185-187
  residues, 197
Tobacco residues, 197
Tomato, 189
Toxins, *see* Inhibitors, specific substances
Trifolirhizin, 215
Triticum, see Wheat
Trypodendron lineatum, 314
Typha angustifolia, inhibition by, 149
Typha latifolia, inhibition by, 148-149

U

Umbelliferone, 214

V

Vanillic acid, 186, 194
Vegetation, patterning of, *see* Patterning
Vetch residues, 203
Viburnum, inhibition by, 219
Vicia villosa, see Hairy vetch

W

Water stress, 305-307
Weeds, inhibition by
  crop plants inhibited by, 205-208
  seeds, 208, 209
Wheat
  inhibition by, 186
  residues, 196, 203
Wheat straw, inhibition by, 190-193
  effects of different varieties, 196
Wheat straw mulch, stimulation of fungal
  growth, 193

X

Xanthium pennsylvanicum, 300

Z

Zea mays, see Corn
Zinniol, 17